PRIMARY CARE: EVALUATION AND MANAGEMENT OF OBESITY

PRIMARY CARE: EVALUATION AND MANAGEMENT OF OBESITY

EDITORS

Robert F. Kushner, MD, MS
Professor, Medicine, Endocrinology Division
Professor, Medical Education
Northwestern University Feinberg School of Medicine

Daniel H. Bessesen, MD
Professor of Medicine
University of Colorado School of Medicine

Adam H. Gilden, MD, MSCE, FACP
Kaiser Permanente Colorado, Internal Medicine & Weight Management
Associate Professor, University of Colorado School of Medicine

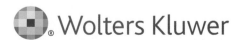

Philadelphia • Baltimore • New York • London
Buenos Aires • Hong Kong • Sydney • Tokyo

Acquisitions Editor: Colleen Dietzler
Development Editor: Thomas Celona
Editorial Coordinators: Blair Jackson, Christopher Rodgers
Editorial Assistant: Victoria Giansante
Marketing Manager: Kirsten Watrud
Production Project Manager: Bridgett Dougherty
Design Coordinator: Stephen Druding
Art Director, Illustration: Jennifer Clements
Illustrator: SPi
Senior Manufacturing Coordinator: Beth Welsh
Prepress Vendor: TNQ Technologies

Copyright © 2022 Wolters Kluwer.

9 8 7 6 5 4 3 2 1

Printed in China

Library of Congress Cataloging-in-Publication Data

ISBN-13: 978-1-975145-75-0

Cataloging-in-Publication data available on request from the Publisher.

shop.lww.com

CONTRIBUTORS

Vance L. Albaugh, MD, PhD
Assistant Professor of Metabolic Surgery
Pennington Biomedical Research Center at Louisiana
    State University
Bariatric & Metabolic Institute
Baton Rouge, Louisiana

Melanie K. Bean, PhD, LCP
Associate Professor
Co-Director, Healthy Lifestyles Center
Department of Pediatrics
Children's Hospital of Richmond at Virginia
    Commonwealth University
Richmond, VA

Peter N. Benotti, MD
Senior Clinical Investigator
Geisinger Obesity Institute
Geisinger Medical Center
Danville, PA

Daniel H. Bessesen, MD
Professor of Medicine
University of Colorado School of Medicine,
Aurora, CO

Jessica Briscoe, MD
Gastroenterology Fellow
Department of Medicine
Section of Gastroenterology and Hepatology
Lewis Katz School of Medicine at Temple University
Philadelphia, PA

Victoria A. Catenacci, MD
Associate Professor
Anschutz Health and Wellness Center
Division of Endocrinology, Metabolism, and Diabetes
University of Colorado Anschutz Medical Campus
Aurora, CO

Ariana M. Chao, PhD, CRNP
Assistant Professor
Department of Biobehavioral Health Sciences
University of Pennsylvania School of Nursing
Philadelphia, PA

Maria L. Collazo-Clavell, MD
Professor of Medicine
Division of Endocrinology, Diabetes, Metabolism &
    Nutrition
Mayo Clinic
Rochester, MN

Seth A. Creasy, PhD
Assistant Professor
Department of Medicine
University of Colorado Anschutz Medical Campus
Aurora, CO

Wayne J. English, MD
Associate Professor
Surgery
Vanderbilt University Medical Center
Nashville, TN

W. Timothy Garvey, MD
Charles E. Butterworth, Jr. Professor
Department of Nutrition Sciences
University of Alabama at Birmingham
Birmingham, AL

Adam H. Gilden, MD, MSCE, FACP
Kaiser Permanente Colorado, Internal Medicine &
    Weight Management
Associate Professor, University of Colorado School of
    Medicine,
Aurora, CO

Sharon J. Herring, MD, MPH
Associate Professor
Department of Medicine
Temple University
Philadelphia, PA
Staff Physician
Department of Medicine
Temple University Health System
Philadelphia, PA

Deborah Bade Horn, DO, MPH
Assistant Professor, Medical Director
Center for Obesity Medicine and Metabolic
    Performance
Department of Surgery
UT McGovern Medical School
Houston, TX

Keerthana Kesavarapu, DO
Fellow
Department of Gastroenterology and Hepatology
Temple University
Philadelphia, PA

Rekha Kumar, MD, MS
Assistant Professor of Medicine
Endocrinology, Diabetes, and Metabolism
Weill Cornell Medical College
New York, NY

Robert F. Kushner, MD, MS
Professor, Medicine, Endocrinology Division
Professor, Medical Education
Northwestern University Feinberg School of Medicine
Evanston, IL

Ethan A. Lazarus, MD
Senior Clinical Instructor
Aurora, Colorado
Family Medicine
University of Colorado Health Sciences Center
Clinical Nutrition Center
Physician/Owner
Greenwood Village, CO

Shannon Marie McShea, MSPAS, PA-C
Physician Assistant
Nutrition and Weight Management
Geisinger Medical Center
Danville, PA

Danielle Marie Ostendorf, PhD
Postdoctoral Fellow
Department of Medicine, Division of Endocrinology,
    Metabolism, and Diabetes
University of Colorado Anschutz Medical Campus
Anschutz Health and Wellness Center
Aurora, CO

Kerry M. Quigley, BA
Centre for Weight and Eating Disorders
Department of Psychiatry
University of Pennsylvania
Philadelphia, PA

Donna H. Ryan, MD
Professor Emerita
Pennington Biomedical Research Center
BatonRouge, LA

David R. Saxon, MD
Assistant Professor
Division of Endocrinology, Metabolism, and Diabetes
Department of Medicine
University of Colorado School of Medicine
Aurora, CO
Endocrinologist
Medicine
University of Colorado Hospital and Rocky Mountain
    VA Medical Center
Hospital or Institution
Aurora, CO

Christopher D. Still, DO
Professor of Medicine
Department of Medical Sciences
Geisinger Commonwealth School of Medicine
Scranton, PA
Medical Director
Department of Nutrition and Weight Management
Geisinger Health System
Danville, PA

Thomas A. Wadden, PhD
Albert J. Stunkard Professor of Psychology in
    Psychiatry
Perelman School of Medicine at the University of
    Pennsylvania
Philadelphia, Pennsylvania

Edmond Pryce Wickham III, MD, MPH
Associate Professor
Departments of Internal Medicine and Pediatrics
Virginia Commonwealth University
Richmond, VA

Fahad Zubair, MD
Medical Director, Obesity Medicine
Allegheny Health Network
Pittsburgh, PA

PREFACE

We are facing a challenging dilemma in health care. The rising tide of obesity is driving an unprecedented increase in prevalence of noncommunicable diseases (NCD), which are the leading cause for increased disability-adjusted life years in the United States and around the world. Type 2 diabetes, cardiovascular disease, nonalcoholic fatty liver disease, and some forms of cancer, among other NCDs, represent a significant health and economic threat for the nation. Currently, over 40% of American adults and 20% of adolescents are affected by obesity, with a disproportionately higher prevalence among minority race/ethnicity groups and those of lower socioeconomic strata. Epidemiological studies suggest that the prevalence and burden of obesity will continue to worsen over the coming decades.

Despite this health crisis, physician surveys repeatedly report insufficient training and self-efficacy of the knowledge, skills, attitudes, and behaviors needed to adequately manage patients with obesity. At the time of this writing, we are also in the midst of the global COVID-19 viral pandemic, a communicable disease that places people with obesity at a higher risk for hospitalization, need for mechanical ventilatory support, and death. Thus, more than ever we need to ensure that healthcare professionals acquire the competence to assess and treat patients with obesity to reduce overall risk from NCDs and infectious diseases alike and improve quality of life. In short, there is a demand for a comprehensive and practical text that meet these needs.

Written with the primary healthcare professional in mind, *Primary Care: Evaluation and Management of Obesity* presents step-by-step, practical, and evidence-based information for the assessment and treatment of patients who present with overweight or obesity. Each chapter is authored by established clinical experts in the field who use their knowledge, experience, and educational acumen to shape the chapter's content. Different from other textbooks on the subject, the editors painstakingly used an educational design for all chapters to include uniform special features that enhance learning. Each chapter begins with a case study to illustrate the clinical context for the information covered. Additional special features include a succinct paragraph that frames the clinical significance, bulleted clinical highlights and guidance on when to refer, practical resources, and a series of case studies with discussion to cover key concepts and nuances of patient care. Each chapter includes instructive tables and ends with selected references and two case-based multiple-choice questions with an annotated discussion.

Primary Care: Evaluation and Management of Obesity begins with an introductory chapter that familiarizes readers with recognizing obesity as a disease, an important consideration for clinicians, patients, healthcare systems and payers, and the public. The essential topics of epidemiology; the biology of body weight and appetite regulation; the genetic, behavioral, and environmental determinants of weight gain; the physiological adaptive response from weight loss; and the pathophysiology that underlies the burden of obesity are succinctly covered to provide a foundation of knowledge for the modern care of patients with obesity.

The next three chapters address the clinical assessment process for obesity, an essential first step prior to initiating treatment. Key elements of how to structure the clinical encounter, make the diagnosis, take an informed and comprehensive weight history, conduct an obesity-focused physical examination, and use appropriate communication techniques are covered in Chapter 2. Chapter 3 "fine tunes" the assessment process by discussing strategies for identifying high-risk patients using staging systems, a new model in obesity medicine. The concept of adiposity-based chronic disease (ABCD) is addressed, along with the multiple determinants of weight gain and obesity. Two novel staging system approaches—the cardiometabolic disease staging and the Edmonton obesity staging system—are introduced, along with practical applications. In Chapter 4, we turn our attention to the assessment, treatment, and monitoring of the most common obesity-related comorbidities. Since most patients with obesity have associated chronic diseases, it is important for the healthcare professional to comanage these conditions. Succinct reviews of selected conditions, including hypertension, cardiovascular disease, type 2 diabetes, polycystic ovarian syndrome, infertility and hypogonadism, sleep apnea, and nonalcoholic fatty liver disease, among others, are included.

In Chapters 5 to 10, we turn our attention to the management of patients with obesity, beginning with lifestyle counseling. The cornerstone of treatment—diet, physical activity, and behavioral therapy—are covered in Chapters 5 to 7. The rationale, scientific principles, supporting clinical studies, evidence-based counseling tips, and resources for each lifestyle component of treatment are discussed. The aim of these chapters is to enable healthcare professionals to provide credible, effective, and efficient lifestyle counseling to their patients. Chapter 8 on pharmacotherapy reviews the rationale, mechanisms of action, indications, side effects, and use of currently available antiobesity medications. Although woefully underutilized, medications for obesity are an effective adjunctive tool and should be part of the treatment toolkit in primary care. Chapters 9 and 10 review bariatric surgery and management of the post–bariatric surgery patient. Bariatric surgery is the most effective and durable treatment approach for patients with severe obesity and should be offered when appropriate. Accordingly, healthcare professionals need to be knowledgeable about the surgical procedures offered and the process for selecting potential candidates. Furthermore, as bariatric surgery patients will be followed by their primary care clinician in the long term, it is important to know how to monitor and medically manage these patients for nutritional and metabolic complications that can arise following surgery.

Chapter 11 is devoted to the comprehensive assessment and management of the pediatric patient. Whether a healthcare professional cares only for adults or for the entire family, it is imperative to be informed about the impact of excess weight on growth and development, the methods used for diagnosis, and the strategies employed for treatment.

Chapters 12 and 13 conclude by providing an overview of practice management, team care, referrals, and practice resources that are pertinent to the effective and efficient care of patients with obesity. Specific topics include a detailed description of the roles, credentials, and structure of team members; models and ethics of care; team communication; office equipment; protocols and policies; the role of advocacy; and the importance of eliminating weight bias.

We have purposefully used the term healthcare professional throughout the book to describe the target audience of physicians, nurse practitioners, and physician assistants who practice outpatient primary care. However, other health professionals who care for patient with obesity, including registered dietitian nutritionists, nurses, health psychologists, and exercise specialists, would also benefit from the practical information provided.

As editors of *Primary Care: Evaluation and Management of Obesity*, we strove to write an informative, practical, and appealing textbook that would benefit healthcare professionals and the patients they serve. We hope we have accomplished this goal.

Robert F. Kushner
Daniel H. Bessesen
Adam H. Gilden

ACKNOWLEDGMENTS

We wish to thank our families and colleagues for their support and encouragement, and our patients from whom we learn far more than we could ever teach.

ABBREVIATIONS

AACE	American Association of Clinical Endocrinologists	CBT	Cognitive behavioral therapy
AAP	American Academy of Pediatrics	CCK	Cholecystokinin
AASLD	American Association for the Study of Liver Diseases	CDC	Centers for Disease Control and Prevention
ABCD	Adiposity-based chronic disease	CDR	Commission on Dietetic Registration
ACC	American College of Cardiology	CHF	Congestive heart failure
ACS	American College of Surgeons	CKD	Chronic kidney disease
ADA	American Diabetes Association	CMDS	Cardiometabolic Disease Staging
ADHD	Attention-deficit hyperactivity disorder	CMS	Center for Medicare and Medicaid Services
AE	Adverse effects	CPAP	Continuous positive airway pressure
AGB	Adjustable gastric banding	CPT	Current procedural technology
AgRP	Agouti-related peptide	CRP	C-reactive protein
AHA	American Heart Association	CT	Computed tomography
AHI	Apnea-hypopnea index	CVD	Cardiovascular disease
ALT	Alanine aminotransferase	CXR	Chest X-ray
AMA	American Medical Association	DASH	Dietary Approaches to Stop Hypertension
AOM	Antiobesity medications	DCR	Daily calorie restriction
APP	Advanced Practice Practitioner	DPP-4	Dipeptidyl peptidase 4
ART	Assisted reproductive technology	DPP	Diabetes Prevention Program
ASCVD	Atherosclerotic cardiovascular disease	DSE	Diabetes support and education
ASMBS	American Society of Metabolic and Bariatric Surgery	DSM	Diagnostic and Statistical Manual
AST	Aspartate aminotransferase	DXA	Dual-energy X-ray absorptiometry
BBS	Bardet-Biedl syndrome	EASO	European Association for the Study of Obesity
BED	Binge eating disorder	ECG	Electrocardiogram
BiPAP	Bilevel (with an enhanced ventilatory component) positive airway pressure	EHR	Electronic health record
BP	Blood pressure	EIM	Exercise is Medicine
BPD	Biliopancreatic diversion	eNOS	Endothelial nitric oxide synthase
BMI	Body mass index	ESS	Epworth Sleepiness Scale
BMR	Basal metabolic rate	FDA	US Food and Drug Administration
BPA	Bisphenol A	FFA	Free fatty acids
BPD/DS	Biliopancreatic diversion with duodenal switch	FPG	Fasting plasma glucose
		FSH	Follicle-stimulating hormone
BRFSS	Behavioral Risk Factor Surveillance System	FTO	Fat mass and obesity-associated protein
		GDM	Gestational diabetes mellitus
CAC	Coronary artery calcium	GERD	Gastroesophageal reflux disease
CAD	Coronary artery disease	GI	Gastrointestinal
CART	Cocaine amphetamine-related transcript	GLP-1	Glucagon-like peptide-1
		HBA1c	Hemoglobin A1c

HCP	Healthcare professional
HDL-c	High-density lipoprotein cholesterol
hGH	Human growth hormone
HPI	History of present illness
HSAT	Home sleep apnea testing
HTN	Hypertension
IBT	Intensive behavioral treatment
ICD	International Classification of Diseases
IEP	Individualized education program
IFG	Impaired fasting glucose
IGT	Impaired glucose tolerance
ILI	Intensive lifestyle intervention
JNC	Joint National Committee
LDL-c	Low-density lipoprotein cholesterol
LFTs	Liver function tests
LH	Lateral hypothalamus; luteinizing hormone
Look AHEAD	Action for Health in Diabetes
MAOIs	Monoamine oxidase inhibitors
MBS	Metabolic and bariatric surgery
MBSAQIP	Metabolic and Bariatric Surgery Accreditation and Quality Improvement Program
MC4R	Melanocortin 4 receptor
MDD	Major depressive disorder
METS	Metabolic equivalents
MetS	Metabolic syndrome
MHO	Metabolically healthy obesity
MVPA	Moderate to vigorous physical activity
NAFLD	Nonalcoholic fatty liver disease
NASH	Nonalcoholic steatohepatitis
NEAT	Nonexercise activity thermogenesis
NFS	NAFLD fibrosis score
NHANES	National Health and Nutrition Examination Survey
NP	Nurse practitioner
NSAIDs	Nonsteroidal anti-inflammatory drugs
NPY	Neuropeptide Y
OA	Osteoarthritis
OCP	Oral contraceptive pill
OGTT	Oral glucose tolerance test
OHS	Obesity hypoventilation syndrome
OPQRST	Mnemonic for taking a weight history
OSA	Obstructive sleep apnea
OTC	Over the counter
PA	Physical activity; physician assistant
PAEE	Physical activity energy expenditure
PAG	Physical Activity Guidelines
PAP	Positive airway pressure
PBH	Postbypass hypoglycemia
PCOS	Polycystic ovarian syndrome
PFCs	Perfluorinated chemicals
PHQ9	Patient Health Questionnaire 9
POMC	Proopiomelanocortin
PPI	Proton pump inhibitor
PSG	Polysomnography
PTH	Parathyroid hormone
PVD	Peripheral artery disease
PWS	Prader-Willi syndrome
PYY	Peptide YY
RDN	Registered dietitian nutritionist
ROS	Review of systems
RPE	Rating of Perceived Exertion
RYGB	Roux-en-Y gastric bypass
SSB	Sugar-sweetened beverages
SCFE	Slipped capital femoral epiphysis
SGLT-2	Sodium-glucose transport protein 2
SMR	Sexual Maturity Rating
SSRIs	Selective Serotonin Reuptake Inhibitor
T2D	Type 2 Diabetes
TDEE	Total daily energy expenditure
TEF	Thermic effect of feeding
TRE	Time-restricted eating
TZD	Thiazolidinedione
USDA	US Department of Agriculture
US FDA	US Food and Drug Administration
USPSTF	US Preventive Services Task Force
VLCD	Very-low-calorie diet
VLCKD	Very-low-carbohydrate ketogenic diet
VSG	Vertical sleeve gastrectomy
WHO	World Health Organization
WLM	Weight loss maintainers
WOMAC	Western Ontario and McMasters Universities Osteoarthritis Index

CONTENTS

OBESITY AS A DISEASE

David R. Saxon, Daniel H. Bessesen

CASE STUDY

A 45-year-old man with obesity (body mass index [BMI] 39 kg/m²) and prediabetes is frustrated with his weight and comes to clinic asking for help. He noticed a progressive weight gain of nearly 50 lb over the last 11 years. He had not been paying much attention to his diet or physical activity until he was diagnosed with prediabetes 6 months ago with an HbA_{1c} of 6.0%. Since then, he reports following a strict diet of 1,200 kcal/day and running on a treadmill 4 days/week for 30 minutes each session. While he initially lost 15 lb (5% of his starting weight), his weight has stabilized over the past 3 months despite adhering to his diet and exercise routine. Both his mother and father have obesity and type 2 diabetes. His best friend from work weighs about the same that he does now and yet "can eat whatever he wants and he never exercises." He is frustrated and comes in today to see if he has a metabolic problem. He wants to know why it is so difficult for him to lose weight. On examination, his blood pressure is 132/86, heart rate 88, and BMI 39 kg/m². The remainder of the examination is unremarkable.

CLINICAL SIGNIFICANCE

Obesity is often viewed differently than diabetes or hypertension by patients, the general public, and even healthcare professionals (HCPs). The unstated belief that the problem is simply a result of poor lifestyle choices can lead to weight bias and suboptimal care. A greater understanding of the physiology behind weight regulation and the adaptive responses to weight loss that promote weight regain can help patients and HCPs have a more realistic view of the complexity of the problem and the challenges of treatment. While labeling obesity as a disease is useful, there are also limitations to this designation including controversies about "metabolically healthy obesity" and the "obesity paradox." However, seeing the problem of obesity as a biological problem that can be addressed with a range of treatments from lifestyle to medications and surgery will be more productive and effective for HCPs and patients alike.

EPIDEMIOLOGY

Obesity is defined as a BMI ≥30 kg/m² and class 3 obesity as a BMI ≥40 kg/m². There are two data sets that provide information on the prevalence of obesity in the United States. The National Health and Nutrition Examination Survey (NHANES) directly measures height and weight annually in a nationally representative sample of 5,000 people of all ages. Because the heights and weights are directly measured, this is the most reliable data set for determining obesity prevalence; however the limited sample size cannot provide data at a state level. The most recent data from NHANES demonstrate that the prevalence of obesity among US adults aged 20 years and older increased from 26.4% in 2006 to 42.4% in 2018. The second data set is the Behavioral Risk Factor Surveillance System (BRFSS), which annually surveys a nationally representative sample of >400,000 adults by phone to get self-reported height and weight among other health data. Because people tend to overreport height and underreport weight, the data from this survey likely underestimates actual prevalence rates. However, a recent analysis used a statistical approach to correct the BRFSS data for the limitations of self-reported height and weight. The results of this analysis predict that by 2030, 48.9% of adults in the United States will have obesity and that 24.2% of adults will have severe obesity (Figure 1.1). This analysis further predicted that severe obesity will

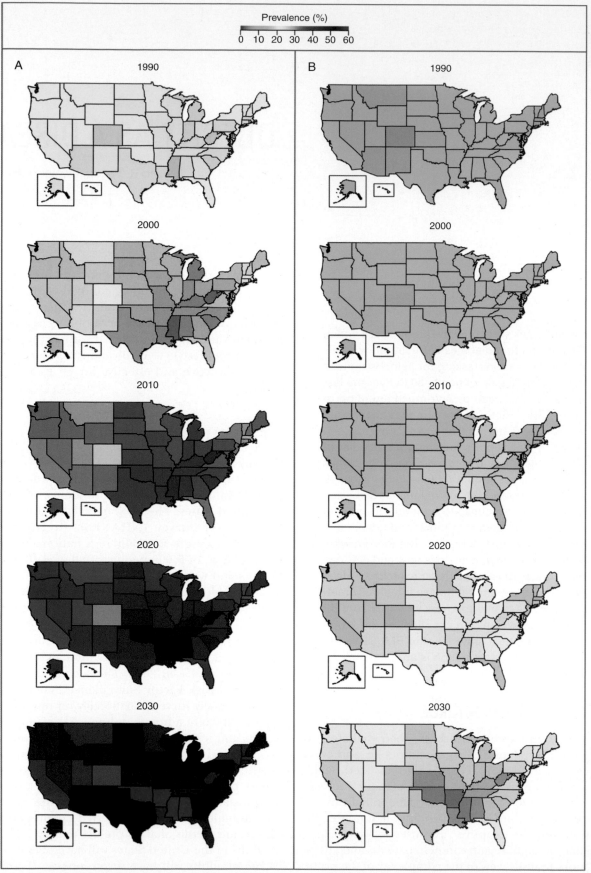

FIGURE 1.1 The estimated prevalence of obesity (BMI > 30 to 35 kg/m²) (A) or severe obesity (BMI > 35 kg/m²) (B) in each state from 1990 to 2030. BMI, body mass index. (Reprinted from Ward ZJ, Bleich SN, Cradock AL, et al. Projected U.S. state-level prevalence of adult obesity and severe obesity. *N Engl J Med.* 2019;381:2440-2450.)

become the most common BMI category (among four: normal weight, overweight, obesity, severe obesity) affecting women (27.6%), non-Hispanic black adults (31.7%), and low-income adults (31.7%) and thereby demonstrating the important effects of race/ethnicity and income on obesity prevalence. Obesity is common and growing in prevalence making it an important issue to address in primary care.

VALUE OF LABELING OBESITY A DISEASE

In 2013, the American Medical Association voted to recognize obesity as a disease that requires prevention and treatment. A large number of professional societies and organizations including the World Health Organization, National Institutes of Health, American College of Physicians, American Academy of Family Physicians, American Heart Association, and American Diabetes Association (ADA) among many others have agreed that obesity is a disease. The purpose of recognizing obesity as a disease was, in part, to shift the stigma that obesity is simply due to personal failings or lack of responsibility, to the modern concept that obesity results from a complex interaction of multiple factors including genetics, biology, behavior, and environment. In doing so, the medical community hoped that a greater investment would be made in understanding the causes of obesity, which would eventually lead to improved prevention and treatment options. Recognition that obesity is a disease has implications for patients, clinicians, and healthcare systems.[1]

For Patients

From a patient perspective, the value of recognizing obesity as a disease is that it may better allow patients to accept the disorder, seek treatment, and have treatment covered by insurance. One major barrier to obesity treatment has been that some HCPs either stigmatize patients with obesity (both implicitly and explicitly) or fail to offer obesity treatment within routine practice environments. Categorizing obesity as a disease opens up the opportunity for it to be treated in the same manner as other common metabolic diseases like diabetes, hypertension, and hyperlipidemia. Lack of consistent insurance coverage for treatment of obesity is an additional barrier from the patient perspective.

For Healthcare Professionals

From a provider perspective, the recognition of obesity as a disease opens the door to treating the condition within the context of routine clinical practice. For many HCPs, this is appealing since many of the conditions they spend time treating are a direct consequence of increased body weight. Although training in weight management and nutrition have historically been lacking for physicians, obesity competencies have been developed for undergraduate and graduate medical education,[2] and there has been an exponential growth in the number of physicians seeking certification in obesity medicine (ABOM.org) by attaining additional continuing medical education (CME) credits in obesity-related educational content.[3] With obesity recognized as a disease, clinicians are more readily able to have meaningful conversations with patients about their weight and about newer treatment approaches like antiobesity medications and bariatric surgery. Accordingly, recent treatment guidelines from the ADA have begun to shift toward a more obesity-focused approach.[4] This includes prioritization of diabetes medications such as glucagon-like peptide 1 (GLP-1) agonists and sodium-glucose cotransporter-2 (SGLT-2) inhibitors that promote weight loss as well as recommendations for frequent discussions about lifestyle management and bariatric surgery (if indicated) during visits that are focused on diabetes management.

For the Healthcare System

Lastly, from a healthcare system perspective, the value of identifying obesity as a disease is that it promotes increased reimbursement for weight management care. Increased coverage of obesity care is beneficial in that it potentially allows systems to mobilize and centralize resources around population health and clinical obesity-focused care. Since comprehensive weight management requires a multidisciplinary team approach, reimbursement for weight management commensurate with that received for the treatment of other chronic health conditions allows systems to focus on identifying resources to build teams and clinics that can address weight management. Currently, the US healthcare system does not consistently reimburse for the treatment of obesity, creating additional hurdles for HCPs and patients.

LIMITATIONS TO LABELING OBESITY AS A DISEASE

Stigma

Some patients may find the designation of their weight as a "disease" stigmatizing. While many patients want to discuss weight management with their HCPs, they often do not appreciate a clinician "blaming everything on my weight." For many, being labeled as "a person with obesity" is taken as a criticism.[5] Therefore, clinicians should be sensitive to ask permission to discuss weight with patients and in general avoid the use of the term obesity in favor of a more neutral term like "weight." Also, caution should be taken in labeling 40% of the US population with a chronic disease. Not all individuals with a BMI ≥ 30 kg/m² would consider themselves to have a chronic disease if they are in good overall health.

Metabolically Healthy Obesity

Labeling something as a disease suggests that those with the condition will invariably suffer adverse consequences. While many people with obesity do develop comorbid conditions, a substantial minority of people with obesity have normal blood glucose, normal blood pressure, no evidence of cardiovascular disease, and no other problems attributable to their weight. A number of studies have shown that these so-called metabolically healthy obese (MHO) individuals have a lower risk of mortality than normal weight individuals who are metabolically unhealthy.[6] However, long-term follow-up of MHO individuals shows that they do develop more metabolic illness than those of normal weight who were metabolically healthy.[7] It may be that these MHO individuals have higher levels of cardiorespiratory fitness that mediates reduced risk for health problems.[8] These data highlight that the health risks of obesity are variable and that BMI alone is not an adequate predictor of who will develop complications and, as a result, who is most likely to benefit from weight loss treatment. The issue of risk assessment and stratification is addressed in more detail in Chapter 3.

The Obesity Paradox

A large number of studies have been conducted to identify the relationship between BMI and adverse health consequences. These studies have consistently shown that obesity is associated with an increased risk for developing hypertension, coronary heart disease, heart failure, and atrial fibrillation among other weight-related illnesses. However, when studies examining the relationship between BMI and mortality in individuals with established heart disease, investigators were surprised to find the opposite relationship: individuals with established heart failure, coronary artery disease, acute myocardial infarction, and those with atrial fibrillation with obesity had lower mortality than those of normal weight.[9,10] This protective effect of obesity, though counterintuitive, has been seen in numerous studies and confirmed in meta-analyses. In addition to these cardiovascular diseases, evidence of an obesity paradox has been found in end-stage renal disease, diabetes, renal cell carcinoma, and even ICU-related mortality. How can obesity be a disease if having the condition lowers the risk of mortality in those with associated medical illness? This area has been the subject of much ongoing controversy, but emerging data suggest that the obesity paradox may be more relevant in individuals with low levels of cardiorespiratory fitness.[10]

Aging and Sarcopenia

There is a curvilinear relationship between BMI and mortality. Specifically, mortality is increased in those with both low and high BMIs compared with those in the middle range of BMIs. This curvilinear relationship changes as people age with low BMIs becoming associated with greater risk and high BMI levels having a smaller relative increase in mortality in people older than 65 years.[11] This may in part be a reflection of the fact that body composition plays an important role in determining health. Individuals with reduced lean mass or sarcopenia (which lowers BMI), especially in older individuals, have an increased mortality while those with increased fat mass and reduced lean mass have the highest mortality.[12] Since weight loss often leads to a loss in both fat and lean mass and the risks of being overweight or obese are less in older individuals, the benefits of weight loss are less clear in older people.

COMMON MISCONCEPTIONS ABOUT OBESITY AND ITS TREATMENT

Changing the view of obesity from a problem of lifestyle choices to that of a chronic, often progressive metabolic disease leads to changes in the way we talk about treatment. Many patients initially are looking to make short-term drastic dietary changes to lose weight without understanding that changes need to be long-term and sustainable. It is important for clinicians to emphasize this point up front when discussing treatment. Many people also think that exercise alone is an effective method to lose weight. While increased levels of physical activity are undoubtedly good for health, consideration of the number of calories that can be burned with 30 to 60 minutes of moderate intensity exercise for someone who is not physically fit will make it clear how difficult it is to create an energy deficit through exercise alone. This issue is discussed in detail in Chapter 6. Importantly, most people seeking treatment are unaware that weight is regulated, that there is a biological tendency for progressive weight gain through adult life, and that if a person loses weight, the body responds with adaptive responses that promote weight regain. They assume that if caloric restriction is sustained, weight will continue to fall. The idea of a "weight plateau" as a new steady state is a concept that most patients have not considered. A fuller understanding of the nature of weight regulation can lead to an acknowledgment that treatment needs to be ongoing and a consideration for more aggressive therapies such as a structured approach to diet, prescription of anti-obesity medications, or surgery as potentially reasonable treatment options.

BODY WEIGHT AS A REGULATED PARAMETER

One might initially think that a person could choose what they weigh by making voluntary decisions about food intake and physical activity. On closer consideration, and with some simple math, it is clear that each of us eats somewhere between 15,000 and 25,000 lb of food over the course of our adult life during which our weight changes on average only 1 to 2 lb/year. When examined over long periods of time, the maintenance of energy balance is remarkably accurate despite dramatic variations in day-to-day levels of energy intake and expenditure. It is clear that maintaining long-term energy balance, weight, fat mass, or some related parameter is the focus of a highly complex regulatory system.[13] However, it is not clear exactly what parameter is being regulated. The observed biology suggests the regulation is not around a "set point" but rather around a "trajectory" of gradual weight gain over the life span with a modest decline in weight in the later years of life. The rate of weight gain tends to be higher in individuals with a greater genetic propensity for obesity and lower in those with constitutional thinness. It also varies depending on qualities of the environment including access to highly palatable food and opportunities for physical activity.

Body weight is largely determined by the energy balance equation, where the currency of energy-in and energy-out is in the form of calories. If there is an imbalance between energy intake and energy expenditure, weight will change. Either the person will lose weight (energy contained in fat stores is consumed) or will gain weight (energy contained in fat stores will increase). How do the body and brain govern and respond to changes in energy balance? An understanding of this regulation requires a more detailed consideration of the components of energy expenditure and the regulation of energy balance by the brain.

Energy Expenditure (the Burning of Calories)

Total daily energy expenditure (TDEE) is the number of calories that the body burns per day and is an important number because it is equal to the number of calories per day that a person must consume to maintain weight. To lose weight, a person must consume fewer calories than TDEE. The components of TDEE are depicted in Figure 1.2. Basal metabolic rate (BMR) is the energy needed to support basic body functions such as maintaining heart and kidney function, body

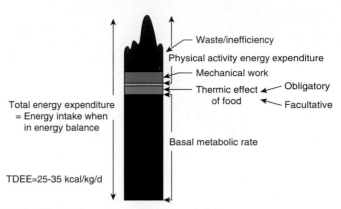

Components of energy expenditure

Waste/inefficiency
Physical activity energy expenditure
Mechanical work
Thermic effect of food — Obligatory
— Facultative
Basal metabolic rate

Total energy expenditure = Energy intake when in energy balance

TDEE=25-35 kcal/kg/d

FIGURE 1.2 Components of total daily energy expenditure (TDEE). Height of the bar represents an estimate of what fraction of TDEE is made up by each component.

temperature, basal brain functioning, and ion gradients in cells. BMR accounts for about 65% to 75% of TDEE. BMR can be estimated with formulae such as the Mifflin-St Jeor equation, which takes into account sex, age, height, and weight (https://www.calculator.net/bmr-calculator.html). The thermic effect of feeding (TEF) is the energy requirements of food digestion and metabolism and accounts for about 8% of TDEE. The third and most variable component of TDEE is physical activity energy expenditure (PAEE). This can be energy expended in planned exercise or in so-called non-exercise activity thermogenesis—the calories burned by daily body movements. Because skeletal muscle and vital organs are the biggest energy consumers in the body, TDEE is linearly related to lean body mass (Figure 1.3), although there is some interindividual variability in this relationship. Women have lower energy requirements than men and TDEE declines for everyone as we age by roughly 5 cal/year. While this may seem like a small number, over 40 to 50 years, it amounts to a reduction in TDEE of several hundred calories. TDEE can be estimated by multiplying the calculated BMR by an activity factor of 1.2 to 1.5 based on the amount of PAEE a person does.

The linear nature of the relationship between energy expenditure and lean body mass means that people with obesity consume more energy than thin people. Many people who struggle with their weight report eating very little and not losing weight. A classic study by Lichtman measured energy expenditure and energy intake in a group of these people.[14] They found no evidence of "metabolic efficiency" as a cause of obesity. Rather they found strong evidence of underreporting of food intake in all of the subjects studied, as well as overreporting of physical activity levels. What is a clinician to do with this information? It may be that when people with obesity report low levels of energy intake, they are either

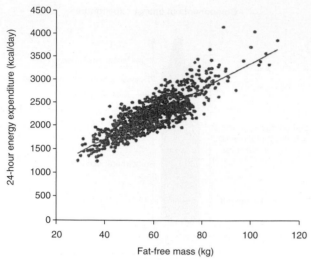

FIGURE 1.3 **Relationship between total daily energy expenditure (TDEE) and lean body mass.** Each point on this figure comes from the measurement of 24-hour energy expenditure by indirect calorimetry in one person. The figure demonstrates both the linear relationship of TDEE with lean body mass and the interindividual variability in this relationship. (Reprinted from Weyer C, Snitker S, Rising R, Bogardus C, Ravussin E. Determinants of energy expenditure and fuel utilization in man: effects of body composition, age, sex, ethnicity and glucose tolerance in 916 subjects. *Int J Obes Relat Metab Disord.* 1999;23(7):715-722.)

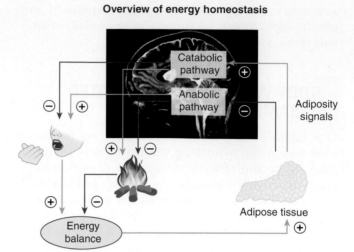

FIGURE 1.4 **Overview of the homeostatic regulation of energy balance by the brain.** The hypothalamus of the brain contains parallel neural pathways that either promote food intake and reduce energy expenditure (anabolic pathways) or the opposite (catabolic pathways). These pathways receive information about fat stores via the adiposity signals insulin and leptin.

not correctly perceiving how much they eat or they are relating "response bias" (they may feel pressure to give answers that are socially acceptable or desirable). It is also possible that energy density plays a role in the underreporting of calorie intake. Specifically, patients with obesity are not eating large volumes of food, but the foods they are eating are high in energy density (more fried foods and processed/snack foods, fewer vegetables). It is generally not useful to try to convince a person that they are actually eating more than they think they are or that they are being untruthful. Rather it is typically more helpful to discuss how difficult it is to know what we are eating unless we consciously monitor food intake with a diet record. Rather than challenging the person's perception of their food intake, the HCP can focus on the value of the person's current effort to lose weight, discuss available treatment options, and emphasize that a new course of action will be needed if the person is going to lose weight.

Appetite Regulation

The other side of the energy balance equation is food intake. A great deal of progress has been made over the last 20 years on the role various brain regions play in regulating energy balance.[15] The hypothalamus has been a

particular focus of study since the discovery of leptin in 1994. The arcuate nucleus of the hypothalamus plays a central role in sensing energy balance through a number of hormones including insulin, leptin, and ghrelin. This brain region functions as a classical feedback system sensing energy balance and in the presence of positive energy balance, activating neural systems that decrease food intake and increase energy expenditure (catabolic pathways). The opposite occurs in the presence of negative energy balance, where activation of neural pathways leads to increased food intake and reduced energy expenditure (anabolic pathways, Figure 1.4). In the presence of sustained positive energy balance, fat mass expands and leptin, which is secreted from adipose tissue in proportion to adipose tissue mass, increases along with increased circulating levels of insulin. These two hormones act on two populations of neurons in the arcuate nucleus of the hypothalamus to regulate energy balance. A number of neurotransmitters have been identified in the hypothalamus that are involved in the catabolic and anabolic pathways. Specifically, neuropeptide Y and agouti-related peptide increase food intake and decrease energy expenditure (Figure 1.5). Conversely, proopiomelanocortin (POMC) and cocaine- and amphetamine-related transcript decrease food intake and increase energy expenditure. When weight is lost, leptin and insulin levels fall, and the activities in these pathways change in a manner that promotes food intake and reduces energy expenditure.

While it was anticipated that the discovery of leptin would lead to new treatments that worked on these hypothalamic neuronal systems, this hope was not

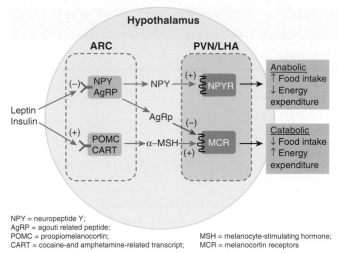

NPY = neuropeptide Y;
AgRP = agouti related peptide;
POMC = proopiomelanocortin;
CART = cocaine-and amphetamine-related transcript;
MSH = melanocyte-stimulating hormone;
MCR = melanocortin receptors

FIGURE 1.5 Hypothalamic regulation of energy balance.
The central pathways for regulating energy balance
are in the arcuate nucleus of the hypothalamus where
two sets of neurons, one containing the neuropeptides
neuropeptide Y/agouti-related peptide (NPY/AgRP)
and another containing proopiomelanocortin/cocaine-
and amphetamine-related transcript (POMC/CART),
form the core circuitry of the parallel anabolic and
catabolic pathways. These cells have receptors for and
respond to the adiposity signals leptin and insulin. NPY
released from arcuate neurons bind to NPY receptors
on downstream neurons in the paraventricular nucleus
and lateral hypothalamic area (PVN/LHA). Alpha-
melanocyte-stimulating hormone (melanocortin or
α-MSH) signals through melanocortin receptors (MCRs)
in PVN/LHA neurons.

realized. This is because typical human obesity is not
due to leptin deficiency but rather leptin resistance.
In typical human obesity, the cellular signaling mechanisms that mediate leptin's actions to reduce appetite and increase energy expenditure do not function
normally. A number of other hormones have also
been discovered that are secreted by the gastrointestinal (GI) tract and interact with these hypothalamic
nuclei and other brain regions to regulate food intake.
These include the "hunger hormone" ghrelin, which is
secreted by the stomach and works on the same arcuate nuclei neurons that insulin and leptin do but in an
opposite manner stimulating food intake. The GI hormones cholecystokinin, peptide YY (PYY), and GLP-1
are satiety hormones that reduce food intake. The
vagus nerve also plays an important role in providing
input from the GI tract to the central nervous system
about taste, gastric distention, and nutrient availability.
Changes in GI hormones following bariatric surgery
are thought to be involved in the effectiveness of this
weight loss treatment.

Other areas of the brain like the ventral striatum
mediate the rewarding qualities of food intake. When a
person loses weight, food becomes a stronger and more

attractive stimulus for the brain.[16] The prefrontal cortex
plays an important role in exerting control over impulses
to pursue short-term rewarding stimuli. This is a key process in how an individual can sustain a calorie-restricted
diet in the face of biological forces that promote weight
regain. Finally, the cerebral cortex is involved in complex decision-making and interpretation of complex
data. Food intake and physical activity have powerful
social meaning, and social factors play an important
role in ultimately determining these lifestyle behaviors.
Social, emotional, and psychological factors clearly play
an important role in determining food intake acting
through a number of brain regions. All of these systems
work in concert to ultimately control when and what
we eat rather than how and why we eat. For example,
hypothalamic systems sense energy balance and affect
the brain regions that regulate attractiveness and plea-
sure associated with food. Social factors are interpreted
by the cerebral cortex and work through the prefrontal
cortex to limit food intake in the face of adverse health
consequences or social stigma. Areas of the brain that
are involved in food intake are listed in Table 1.1.

Effects of Weight Loss on Appetite and Energy Expenditure

If weight is regulated, it is not surprising that weight
loss induces adaptive responses that work to promote
weight regain. These include an increase in appetite
and desire for food, reduction in energy expenditure,
and changes in metabolism favoring nutrient storage
(Table 1.2). Following weight loss, leptin, insulin, and
PYY levels fall and ghrelin levels rise.[17] These changes
in appetite-related hormones would be predicted to
promote increased food intake. Experimental studies
have demonstrated that these hormonal changes and
associated increase in appetite persist for at least a year
following weight loss. TDEE falls with weight loss in

TABLE 1.1 Brain Regions That Regulate Food Intake

BRAIN REGION	FUNCTIONS
Hypothalamus	Maintaining energy homeostasis
Ventral striatum	Rewarding aspects of food intake
Frontal and prefrontal cortex	Impulsivity, executive function
Brainstem, vagus nerve	Communication with gastrointestinal tract
Cortex	Social meaning of food

TABLE 1.2 Adaptive Responses to Weight Loss That Promote Weight Regain

DOMAIN	PARAMETER	RESPONSE TO WEIGHT LOSS
Appetite	Subjective experience Hormones and neurotransmitters Rewarding properties of food	Hunger increases Satiety falls Leptin falls Ghrelin rises Neuropeptide Y rises Increased brain activity in areas relating to reward and attention
Energy expenditure	Total energy expenditure Resting energy expenditure Physical activity	Falls due to a decrease in each component: resting energy expenditure, physical activity, and thermic effect of food Decreased lean mass Decreased thyroid hormone Decreased catecholamine levels Decreased workload due to decreased weight Increased efficiency at same workload Possibly a decrease in spontaneous physical activity
Metabolism	Insulin sensitivity Fat metabolism Adipose tissue	Increased insulin sensitivity increases favors fat storage Decreased lipolysis (fat release) Increased adipose tissue lipoprotein lipase (triglyceride storage in fat) Reduced fat oxidation Increased number of new adipocytes

part because lean body mass falls. However, the decline in TDEE is greater than what would be predicted by weight loss alone, suggesting an increase in energy efficiency. PAEE falls in part due to the decrease in weight, resulting in less mechanical work for the same degree of exercise (an individual who weighs 200 lb expends less energy walking a mile than a person who weighs 300 lb simply because they weigh less). However, here again the reduction in exercise associated PAEE decreases more than would be predicted by weight loss alone.[18] This suggests that mechanical efficiency may also increase with weight loss. These changes in energy expenditure are associated with and may be caused by reductions in leptin, thyroid hormone, and catecholamines. These changes in energy expenditure also appear to persist for at least a year after weight loss, possibly indefinitely and are clinically meaningful. For example, a 200 lb woman losing 20 to 30 lb experiences a 350 kcal/day reduction in TDEE as a result of weight loss. This fall in TDEE is the explanation for the plateau that patients experience as they lose weight. The body enters a new steady state where fewer calories are required to maintain the new reduced weight. If the person increases food intake without increasing physical activity at this point, they will regain weight. With so many physiologic changes occurring, it is not surprising that it is so difficult for most people to maintain a reduced weight state with lifestyle measures alone.

Fortunately, humans possess a remarkable ability to learn new behaviors and weight loss and weight maintenance can be achieved by adopting certain lifestyle changes. The National Weight Control Registry is a group of people who have used lifestyle alone to maintain a weight loss of at least 30 lb for at least a year, although the actual average weight loss of this group was 70 lb that was maintained for an average of 5.7 years. These individuals demonstrate that weight loss maintenance is possible. They have succeeded using a variety of strategies including self-monitoring of weight and food intake and maintaining high levels of physical activity (generally 60-70 minutes/day).[19,20] These individuals use cognitive strategies and learned behaviors to counteract the biological forces that promote weight regain.

FACTORS INVOLVED WITH THE DEVELOPMENT OF OBESITY

What is responsible for the dramatic increase in the prevalence of obesity over the last 60 years? Despite a large number of studies, no clear answer has emerged, and taken together, the evidence suggests multiple factors are likely involved. Some possible contributors include changes in diet and physical activity.

Diet

Studies point to a number of dietary factors that are consistently associated with weight gain and the development of obesity. These include increased intake of dietary fat, high fructose corn syrup, and saturated fat along with reduced intake of whole grains, fiber, fruits, legumes, and vegetables. Moderate-quality data support the idea that increased intake of high glycemic index foods and highly processed foods (defined as foods undergoing multiple physical, biological, and/or chemical processes that are associated with industrial as opposed to culinary food production and typically containing food additives) are detrimental as well. Increases in the intake of specific foods have been associated with either weight gain (potato chips, French fries, processed meats, red meat, sweets/desserts) or protection against weight gain (yogurt, fruit, whole grains, nuts, vegetables).[21] The US Department of Agriculture (USDA) follows food consumption from food production data. These data show that overall food consumption increased between 1970 and 2014, although these data have limitations because of difficulties estimating food waste. These data from the USDA suggest that Americans are eating more fat, sugar, proteins, and grains than guidelines would recommend and less fruit, vegetables, and dairy than recommended.

Physical Activity

Reduced levels of physical activity also appear to have played an important role in the increased prevalence of obesity. The Amish who have a traditional lifestyle and a low prevalence of obesity take 14,000 to 16,000 steps per day compared with the average American who takes 5,000 to 6,000. This amounts to an energetic difference of 400 to 600 kcal/day. The workforce in the United States has gradually transitioned from one where almost 50% of workers were moderately active on the job in 1960 to one where >70% of workers are either sedentary or only have a light workload on the job in 2010. The effect of these changes in the work environment is estimated to be responsible for an average decline in work-related energy expenditure of 140 kcal/day in men and 120 kcal/day in women, an amount that mathematically could be a strong driver of the increased prevalence of obesity.[22] One study compared physical activity and food intake in Pima Indians living a traditional agrarian lifestyle in Northern Mexico who had a low prevalence of obesity to genetically related Pima people living in Arizona where almost 80% had obesity. The main difference between the two groups was not more food intake in the Pima people living in Arizona but much higher levels of physical activity in the Pima people living in Mexico.[23] These results emphasize that reduced levels of physical activity likely play an important role in the increased rates of obesity seen over the last 20 years.

Genetics

Studies of weight in twin pairs raised together or apart suggest that the genetic contribution to BMI is 40% to 70%.[24] In the era of "personalized medicine," there is a hope that prevention and treatment efforts could potentially be tailored to the individual by identifying those with genes that predict risk and targeting therapy to pathogenic processes identified by genetic screening. Genome-wide association studies have identified about 100 genetic loci that are associated with obesity. Unfortunately, all of these genes together only account for 3% to 5% of the individual variation in weight. As a result, genetic screening is not useful diagnostically or therapeutically in common forms of obesity at this time. The most common weight-related genetic abnormality associated with increased weight is a polymorphism in the "fat mass and obesity-associated protein" or FTO gene. The gene product appears to affect appetite responses and the development of "beige fat," a type of fat tissue that burns fat, generates heat, and is thought to protect against weight gain.[25] However, the effect is small, with those possessing the at-risk allele weighing on average only a few pounds more than those with the low-risk allele.

Rare mutations in a number of genes have been associated with severe obesity that develops in early childhood. The most common of these are Prader-Willi syndrome and melanocortin 4 receptor deficiency. Other monogenic forms of obesity resulting in early-onset severe obesity include leptin deficiency, leptin receptor deficiency, and POMC deficiency.[26] These unusual forms of obesity typically present with other signs and symptoms that may include reproductive dysfunction, intellectual disability, altered pigmentation, unique facial features, and others. Genetic panels are now available to screen for these rare gene mutations in the clinical setting of early-onset severe obesity. The topic of monogenic obesity is also discussed in Chapter 3.

Other Causes

The modern world is quite different than the environment we evolved in. Increases in the prevalence of obesity have been correlated with a wide variety of factors that have also changed over the last 60 years, including changes in the built environment favoring reduced physical activity, socioeconomic changes, changes in food availability and marketing, increased levels of stress, changes in the gut microbiome including the effects of exposure to antibiotics in people or commercial livestock, increasing exposure to a variety of endocrine-disrupting chemicals such as bisphenol A and perfluorinated chemicals, lower rates of smoking (smokers weigh less than nonsmokers), increasing use of psychotropic medications, changes in social norms and social networks, and increasing average home temperature to name just a few potential factors.[15] Correlations, however, do not necessarily indicate causation; therefore, mechanistic studies and controlled clinical trials are required to unravel whether these associations are valid.

Shortened sleep time and so-called circadian misalignment have been proposed as potential causative factors in the recent increase in obesity prevalence.[27] Average sleep duration has declined in the United States over the last 60 years, and the number of people performing night shift work has increased. Epidemiological studies show a strong, clear, and consistent association between shortened sleep time, night shift work, and the development of obesity, insulin resistance, and type 2 diabetes. Experimental studies demonstrate that individuals who have shortened sleep time or a night shift schedule may spend more time in sedentary activities and less time in moderate and vigorous physical activity as compared with people on a normal sleep schedule. These changes lead to a reduction in TDEE. Studies have also shown that measured food intake increases with sleep restriction, in particular intake of high-fat foods. Levels of satiety hormones are reduced, and levels of ghrelin are higher following sleep restriction.[28]

Another area that has received a good deal of attention as a potential cause of the obesity epidemic is the role of fetal and early childhood factors.[29] Epidemiological studies show strong associations between both maternal undernutrition and maternal obesity on the risk of obesity in offspring. Increased nutrient delivery to the fetus appears to promote increased adiposity at birth in the infant and may favor development of neural systems controlling food intake in a manner that promotes weight gain. Since more women of reproductive age have obesity now, compared to 60 years ago, it is likely that some of the increase in childhood obesity is due to maternal obesity and gestational diabetes.

Secondary Causes

While many patients come to the doctor asking if they have a hormone problem causing weight gain, it is rare that a specific endocrine cause can be found and it is typically not productive to embark on an extensive workup for medical causes of obesity in the usual patient. Hypothyroidism is a common endocrine disorder and it is reasonable to check thyroid-stimulating hormone at an initial visit if one has not been done in the last year. However, hypothyroidism typically causes modest weight gain and T4 replacement therapy usually does not lead to dramatic weight loss. Weight gain and central adiposity are common components of pathological hypercortisolism or Cushing syndrome. However, there are usually other features including proximal muscle weakness, easy bruisability, and wide purple striae. Hypertension, hirsutism, irregular menses, glucose intolerance, and osteoporosis are other features that increase the concern for hypercortisolism. The evaluation of patients for secondary causes of obesity is discussed in Chapter 3.

WEIGHT AND HEALTH

Weight-Related Illnesses

Obesity is defined as a degree of excess weight that is associated with an increased risk of comorbid illness and/or increased mortality.[30] Obesity is associated with a wide range of illnesses involving virtually every organ of the body (Figure 1.6). An example of the relationship between BMI and the risk of developing type 2 diabetes is depicted in Figure 1.7. Because the risk of illness begins to increase above a BMI of 25 kg/m^2 and increases markedly above a BMI of 30 kg/m^2 in Caucasian adults, these were chosen as the cut points between healthy weight, overweight, and obesity. Because visceral obesity is a risk factor for metabolic complications of obesity and because waist circumference is a measurement that provides information about visceral fat, BMI and waist circumference can be used together to make an initial assessment of weight-related health risks (Figure 1.8). The relationship between BMI

Medical complications of obesity

Pulmonary disease
Abnormal function
Obstructive sleep apnea
Hypoventilation syndrome

Nonalcoholic fatty liver disease
Steatosis
Steatohepatitis
Cirrhosis

Gall bladder disease

Gynecologic abnormalities
Abnormal menses
Infertility
Polycystic ovarian syndrome

Osteoarthritis

Skin

Gout

Idiopathic intracranial hypertension
Stroke
Cataracts

Coronary heart disease
Diabetes
Dyslipidemia
Hypertension
Severe pancreatitis

Cancer
Breast, uterus, cervix, colon, esophagus, pancreas, kidney, prostate

Phlebitis
Venous stasis

FIGURE 1.6 Medical complications of obesity.

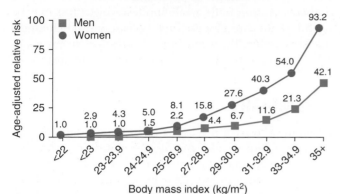

Relationship between BMI and risk of type 2 diabetes mellitus

FIGURE 1.7 Relationship between body mass index (BMI) and risk of type 2 diabetes mellitus. The age-adjusted increase in the relative risk for developing type 2 diabetes is depicted as a function of increasing BMI in men and women. (Adapted from Chan JM, Rimm EB, Colditz GA, Stampfer MJ, Willett WC. Obesity, fat distribution, and weight gain as risk factors for clinical diabetes in men. *Diabetes Care*. 1994;17(9):961-969 and Colditz GA, Willett WC, Rotnitzky A, Manson JE. Weight gain as a risk factor for clinical diabetes mellitus in women. *Ann Intern Med*. 1995;122(7):481-486.)

and mortality is curvilinear with increased mortality at very low BMIs and definitely increased mortality above 35 kg/m². The BMI associated with the lowest mortality has been the subject of some controversy recently. The bulk of the evidence suggests that the BMI associated

Assessing obesity: BMI, waist circumference, and disease risk

Category	BMI	Disease risk relative to normal weight and waist circumference	
		Men ≤40 in Women ≤35 in	Men >40 in Women >35 in
Underweight	<18.5	—	—
Normal	18.5-24.9	—	—
Overweight	25.0-29.9	Increased	High
Obesity	30.0-34.9	High	Very high
	35.0-39.9	Very high	Very high
Extreme obesity	≥40	Extremely high	Extremely high

FIGURE 1.8 Using body mass index (BMI) and waist circumference to diagnose obesity. (Adapted from Jensen MD, Ryan DH, Apovian CM, et al; American College of Cardiology/American Heart Association Task Force on Practice Guidelines; Obesity Society. 2013 AHA/ACC/TOS guideline for the management of overweight and obesity in adults: a report of the American College of Cardiology/American Heart Association Task Force on Practice Guidelines and the Obesity Society. *Circulation*. 2014;129(25 suppl 2):S102-S138.)

with the lowest mortality is somewhere between 25 and 30 kg/m², but this depends on characteristics of the population studied.[31]

How Does Obesity Cause Illness?

Obesity is associated with a wide range of comorbid conditions.[30] Some of these are due simply to excess weight and the accumulation of fat tissue in specific regions. Osteoarthritis is due to increased mechanical stress on joints that is potentially exacerbated by the systemic inflammation that accompanies obesity. Although existing joint damage does not improve with weight loss, functional capacity can improve. Urinary incontinence and gastroesophageal reflux are exacerbated by the increase in intra-abdominal pressure that accompanies the accumulation of visceral fat. Obstructive sleep apnea is due in part to reductions in airway dimensions that result from fat accumulation in the retropharynx. Increased fat mass can alter the metabolism of estrogen and testosterone, resulting in changes in reproductive function. Increased lipid in the liver and skeletal muscle can lead to insulin resistance predisposing to type 2 diabetes. The resulting hyperinsulinemia can predispose to a variety of cancers. Changes in physical appearance that accompany excess adiposity are noticed by others and can result in social stigmatization and weight bias. This social stigma and weight bias can lead to anxiety, social isolation, and depression. These issues are discussed in greater depth in Chapters 4 and 5.

Health Benefits of Weight Loss

It would naturally follow that if obesity is a disease, then treating the "disease" should result in better health. Among the multiple comorbidities associated with obesity, the most extensively studied has been diabetes. There is strong evidence of the benefits of weight loss on glucose metabolism. The Diabetes Prevention Program study and other similar studies such as the Finnish Diabetes Prevention Study and the Da Qing Diabetes Prevention Study demonstrated that a modest weight loss could prevent or delay the development of type 2 diabetes in individuals with prediabetes or women with a history of gestational diabetes.[32] A number of recent studies of weight loss from bariatric surgery have shown dramatic improvements in glucose levels and even remission in people with type 2 diabetes. The Look AHEAD trial of a lifestyle behavioral weight loss program in people with type 2 diabetes showed that weight loss improved glucose control, blood pressure, lipid levels, and sleep apnea. Randomized trials of medical therapy or bariatric surgery show that the greater weight loss provided by bariatric surgery provides more extensive benefits for most weight-related comorbidities.[33,34] Recent detailed mechanistic studies such as those done by Klein and colleagues confirm that a 5% weight loss has measurable benefits on glucose metabolism with greater benefits being provided with greater weight loss.[35] Thirty-year follow-up of the Da Qing study participants provided evidence that weight loss provided by a lifestyle program could reduce long-term mortality.[36] Epidemiological studies and nonrandomized prospective, controlled trials of individuals undergoing bariatric surgery provide evidence that weight loss reduces long-term mortality as a result of both a reduction in cardiovascular disease death and lower rates of cancer especially in women. These results support the idea that obesity is causative in the development of diabetes, cardiovascular disease, and cancer. The details of how to treat obesity are extensively discussed in Chapters 5-9 of this book.

Limitations of Existing Evidence

Evidence of the health benefits of weight loss, however, is not entirely positive. Epidemiological studies of individuals who lose weight have shown that repeated episodes of weight loss followed by weight regain, so-called weight cycling or yo-yo dieting, are associated with increased mortality. Since most people who lose weight regain the lost weight, these data raise concerns about the advisability of advocating weight loss. The studies demonstrating this relationship, however, have a number of methodological concerns. For example, subjects in some of these studies were of normal weight to start with and details of how and why these individuals lost and regained the weight are not known, allowing the possibility that some intervening illness may have been the cause of both the weight loss and increased mortality. Taken together, there is currently no definitive evidence that weight cycling has harmful effects.

The Look AHEAD trial was a randomized controlled trial of over 5,000 subjects that was designed to test the hypothesis that weight loss provided by a lifestyle program reduced mortality in people with type 2 diabetes. The subjects in the study did lose weight and as noted above experienced a range of health benefits. However, the study did not show any reduction in mortality. The study was negative largely because the observed rate of cardiovascular events was markedly lower than what had been projected making the study underpowered to show a benefit. Importantly, as a requirement of the protocol, the individuals who participated in this study were adherent with care, often were on statins and angiotensin-converting enzyme (ACE) inhibitors, and were able to engage in regular physical activity. A later subgroup analysis demonstrated that those subjects who lost >10% of their baseline weight had a significant 21% lower risk of cardiovascular disease compared with those who maintained a stable weight or gained weight.[37] The take-home message from this study may be that moderate weight loss is not a powerful intervention to prevent cardiovascular disease as compared to medications like statins, ACE inhibitors, and glucose lowering medications in people with established type 2 diabetes. Additionally, while modest weight loss may be useful in altering glucose metabolism and biochemical markers of health, it may take weight loss in excess of 10% to have a significant impact on mortality rates.

SUMMARY

Labeling obesity a disease is an acknowledgment that there is a biological basis for the condition and that weight is a regulated parameter much like blood pressure or blood glucose. Obesity is a disorder of body weight regulation. As is true with hypertension and diabetes, lifestyle choices are involved in the development of these metabolic disorders, but no one chooses to have diabetes, hypertension, or obesity. We do not look at patients as being "at fault" for developing hypertension or diabetes, and we should extend the same thinking to those who struggle with their weight. Not all individuals with an elevated blood pressure or blood glucose will suffer complications, nor do they all need treatment, and the same is true for patients with obesity. Lifestyle treatments alone are important in hypertension and diabetes but have limited effectiveness because of the powerful biological processes that underlie these conditions. These principles apply to the evaluation and treatment of obesity as well. Clinicians are used to discussing the risks and benefits of a variety of strategies to address hypertension and diabetes. HCPs can apply these same skills to the care of their patients with obesity. They can acknowledge the variety of causes, the variability in the risks for complications, and the risks and benefits of treatment. They can use authoritative guidelines along with good clinical judgment and communication skills to tailor the diagnostic and therapeutic approach to that person in a way that will be helpful to them.

CASE STUDY

Discussion

The patient presented is frustrated that he is not losing as much weight as he thinks he should based on his perception of how restricted his diet is and how much he is exercising. He has had some success having changed his lifestyle habits and achieving a 5% weight loss. This weight loss would result in a reduction of his TDEE to a level that would be lower than his friend who is of similar weight but has not lost weight. This is because of a reduction in BMR, TEF, and energy expended in physical activity that is greater than what would be predicted based on the change in weight alone. This is part of the explanation for why he senses that he needs to eat less than his friend to maintain weight. However, because TDEE is related to lean body mass, he still requires much more than 1,200 kcal/day to maintain his new weight. His difficulty is also due to increased hunger signals that occur as a result of successful weight loss. Studies of individuals like this show that they routinely underreport calorie intake and overreport physical activity. The HCP could calculate energy needs and provide a calorie prescription based on this calculation, but this is not usually helpful as he already thinks he is eating a 1,200 kcal/day diet which would be predicted to produce continued weight loss. While the HCP in this situation feels pressure to explain the situation or do further testing, the best approach is to acknowledge how challenging weight loss is because of the biological nature of weight regulation, provide positive reinforcement for the work he has already done, and offer help if he wants to make further changes. Specific treatment options will be discussed in later chapters, but a sample conversation is offered here that demonstrates motivational interviewing support for the patient and opens the door to discussing further treatment options.

Sample Conversation About Body Weight Regulation

Pt: I just don't get it; I am eating almost nothing and cannot lose any weight. I am just ready to give up.

HCP: That sounds incredibly frustrating. It sounds like you are working as hard as you can to watch your diet and eat less and yet are not seeing the results you were expecting.

Pt: That is right. I must have some kind of problem with my metabolism or with my thyroid.

HCP: Perhaps you are hoping that I can help make a diagnosis about why you are having trouble losing weight by doing a blood test?

Pt: All I know is there has to be something wrong because I am doing everything right and yet my weight is just not budging. It doesn't make any sense.

HCP: Your frustration is understandable. Believe me, my whole goal here is to help you to the best of my ability in your desire to lose weight. If I could do a test that would explain why you are experiencing this situation I would do it. Unfortunately, our understanding of the biology of how weight is regulated is not as good as you or I would like. What we do know is that weight is regulated much like blood pressure or blood glucose. No one chooses to have high blood pressure or diabetes and no one chooses to have excess weight. Some of us come from a genetic background where our bodies just want to weigh more.

Pt: Yeah, my father was obese and developed diabetes. I don't want that to happen to me.

HCP: Sounds like you are worried that your weight gain may lead to diabetes and you are trying to do everything you can to prevent that.

Pt: Yeah, but it is just not working.

HCP: What the research tells us is that most people tend to gradually gain weight over their entire adult life. A person can restrict calories and exercise more and that will lead to weight loss. However, the body will push back against those efforts because it wants to keep on the trajectory of gradual weight gain. The efforts needed to restrict food intake and increase physical activity need to be sustained or the lost weight will come back. A lot of my patients think of weight like they might think about a bladder infection: treat it for a while then it goes away. Weight problems are more like hypertension or diabetes, they need long term treatments.

Pt: But I am eating only 1,200 cal/day, I should be losing weight! I used to eat fast food five times a week and drink three cans of beer every day. I don't do any of that anymore.

HCP: Sounds like you are working hard on your diet. Congratulations. What do you think you would weigh today if you were eating like you used to?

Pt: (laughing) Sky's the limit!

HCP: So the truth is you are actually having a good deal of success because you would be weighing much more if you hadn't made the changes you have made already. It seems you are not giving yourself the credit you deserve for the efforts you have already made. This is probably because you haven't reached your goal weight. I have found with many of my patients that focusing too much on a weight goal can be frustrating and may lead to a person throwing in the towel and giving up on what they were already doing that was actually providing benefits. Sounds like you would like to lose more weight and would like to talk about other options?

Pt: I need to do something because I can't live like this.

HCP: I am here to help you in this process. It is important to think about what you can control and what you can't. You did not choose to have a weight problem and it is not your fault. Having said that you do have choices. You can try changing your diet and exercise habits more than you have so far to create more of an energy deficit to lose more weight, you could try using a weight loss medication or even consider surgery to lose weight. Whatever you do will only work as long as you do it and unfortunately your body will push back against your weight loss efforts because it has its own ideas of what it wants to weigh, but I think it is terrific that you are interested in exploring these choices to improve your health and I am here to help you in any way I can. What would be most helpful to talk about, your diet, exercise routine, medications or surgery?

CLINICAL HIGHLIGHTS

- Body weight is the product of a complex regulatory system that works to balance energy intake with energy expenditure over time.
- Obesity is a disease of body weight regulation where over time energy intake exceeds expenditure resulting in the accumulation of excess adipose tissue, which then leads to a range of health problems.
- Labeling obesity as a disease acknowledges the biological basis of the condition, reduces guilt and stigma, and can open the door to more effective communication about the disorder and more effective treatment.
- A number of factors are involved in the increased prevalence of obesity including changes in usual dietary patterns, reductions in habitual physical activity, and changes in sleep patterns. Genetic factors and the fetal environment also play important roles.
- While the health risks of obesity are not the same for everyone, in general, increased adiposity is associated with an increased risk for a wide range of other health conditions, and weight loss ameliorates many of these comorbidities.
- Because body weight is regulated, when people lose weight, a range of adaptive responses are recruited including reductions in energy expenditure, increases in appetite, and changes in metabolism that promote weight regain.
- Because adaptive responses to weight loss are biological and therefore persist over time, any weight loss treatment will only work as long as the person adheres to the treatment.

QUIZ QUESTIONS

1. MJ is a 60-year-old man who comes to see you for weight gain. He has had slow steady progressive weight gain for the last 40 years. He is an engineer and says he is eating exactly the same as he did 40 years ago and his exercise habits (walking 2 miles 5 days a week) have not changed either over this time period. He says that he must have a metabolic problem underlying his weight gain.

   Which of the following is the most likely cause of his progressive weight gain?

   A. He actually has been eating more and more calories per day over the years and he is underreporting his food intake.

   B. His basal metabolic rate (BMR) has gradually declined as he aged, which results in a positive energy balance because he is still taking in the same number of calories each day.

   C. His exercise habits have actually declined over the years, and he is underreporting his physical activity.

   D. He has become more insulin resistant as he has aged and this is the underlying cause of his weight gain.

   Answer: B. *Weight gain occurs when energy intake exceeds energy expenditure. For this person to gain weight, he must have been consuming more calories than he was burning over time (energy intake > total daily energy expenditure [TDEE]). While it is possible that he is underreporting food intake and/or overreporting physical activity, neither of these is necessary to explain his progressive weight gain. The Mifflin-St Jeor equation can be used to estimate BMR, which typically makes up 75% of TDEE. The formula takes into account the effects of sex, age, height, and weight. This is because BMR is lower for women than for men of a similar size, higher for larger individuals, and declines as we age. This is why women need to eat less than men of a similar body size to maintain weight and smaller people need to eat fewer calories each day compared with larger people to maintain energy balance and maintain weight. The factor that accounts for age in this formula is −5 × age. This means that between the ages of 20 and 60 years, BMR falls by 5 × 40 = 200 calories. That means all things being equal, a person would need to gradually decrease their food intake by 200 cal/day between the ages of 20 and 60 years to maintain energy balance. While it is likely that energy expended in physical activity declines with age due to changes in habits, and also likely that food intake may increase, the question emphasizes the impact aging alone has on energy balance. While weight gain is associated with insulin resistance, insulin resistance alone does not cause weight gain. Weight gain requires that energy intake > TDEE.*

2. DJ is a 47-year-old woman who is being seen for routine health maintenance. She feels that her health is good and she has no complaints. She reports eating a Mediterranean style diet and exercises at a moderate intensity for 40 minutes 5 days a week. She also does bouts of muscle strengthening activities 3 days a week. She has no family history of diabetes, hypertension, or cardiovascular disease. On examination, her

BMI is 32 kg/m², waist circumference 34 inches, and blood pressure 122/74. Laboratory tests show a fasting glucose of 85 mg/dL, HbA$_{1C}$ of 5.3%, triglycerides 98 mg/dL, HDL cholesterol 52 mg/dL, and LDL cholesterol 93 mg/dL.

Which of the following best describes her future risk for developing metabolic complications of obesity such as type 2 diabetes or cardiovascular disease?

A. Her risk is the same as other people with a BMI of 30 to 35 kg/m² as weight is the primary driver of these comorbidities.

B. Her risk is the same as a normal weight individual with hypertension, hyperlipidemia, and prediabetes.

C. Her risk is the same as a normal weight individual with normal lipids, glucose, and blood pressure, as these markers are the drivers of future comorbidities.

D. Her risk is higher than a normal weight individual with normal metabolic markers but lower than a normal weight individual who has abnormal metabolic markers.

Answer: D. *Obesity is a disorder of body weight regulation that often, but not always, leads to other health problems as either a result of the presence of excess amounts of adipose tissue (osteoarthritis, gastroesophageal reflux, obstructive sleep apnea, for example) or metabolic disorders that stem from excess lipid in a variety of tissues and the resulting insulin resistance and hyperinsulinemia (type 2 diabetes, hyperlipidemia, cardiovascular disease, increased rates of certain cancers, for example). However, not everyone who is categorized as having obesity based on BMI criteria will experience one of these consequences. While these so-called metabolically healthy obese (MHO) individuals who have normal blood pressure, glucose, and lipid levels account for only 20% to 30% of all individuals with obesity, they do not have the same risk for metabolic complications as those who have the more commonly observed elevations in these parameters. Patients like this are encountered in clinical practice and the question is: how concerned should the healthcare professional (HCP) be about the future health of these individuals? A number of studies have examined the natural history of MHO. These studies show that while these individuals are at substantially lower risk for metabolic complications than either healthy weight individuals or people with obesity who have abnormal metabolic markers, they are at greater risk for metabolic complications than healthy weight individuals with normal metabolic markers. Some of the protection from health complications in MHO individuals may relate to their lifestyle habits as demonstrated by DJ. Patients with MHO are still at risk for the mechanical complications of obesity, and this may be a reason to advise treatment. As is true with all patients seen with obesity, the goal for the HCP is to communicate accurately what the future health risks associated with obesity are and to help the person decide on a course of action that aligns with their goals. The issue of risk assessment of the patient with obesity is discussed in greater detail in Chapter 3.*

REFERENCES

1. Upadhyay J, Farr O, Perakakis N, Ghaly W, Mantzoros C. Obesity as a disease. *Med Clin North Am.* 2018;102(1): 13-33.

2. Kushner RF, Horn DB, Butsch WS, et al. Development of obesity competencies for medical education: a report from the Obesity Medicine Education Collaborative. *Obesity (Silver Spring).* 2019;27(7):1063-1067.

3. Kushner RF, Brittan D, Cleek J, et al; ABOM Board of Directors. The American Board of Obesity Medicine: five-year report. *Obesity (Silver Spring).* 2017;25(6): 982-984.

4. American Diabetes Association. 1. Improving care and promoting health in populations: Standards of Medical Care in Diabetes-2020. *Diabetes Care.* 2020;43(suppl 1):S7-s13.

5. Phelan SM, Burgess DJ, Yeazel MW, Hellerstedt WL, Griffin JM, van Ryn M. Impact of weight bias and stigma on quality of care and outcomes for patients with obesity. *Obes Rev.* 2015;16(4):319-326.

6. Kramer CK, Zinman B, Retnakaran R. Are metabolically healthy overweight and obesity benign conditions?: a systematic review and meta-analysis. *Ann Intern Med.* 2013;159(11):758-769.

7. Hansen L, Netterstrøm MK, Johansen NB, et al. Metabolically healthy obesity and ischemic heart disease: a 10-year follow-up of the Inter99 study. *J Clin Endocrinol Metab.* 2017;102(6):1934-1942.

8. Ortega FB, Cadenas-Sanchez C, Migueles JH, et al. Role of physical activity and fitness in the characterization and prognosis of the metabolically healthy obesity phenotype: a systematic review and meta-analysis. *Prog Cardiovasc Dis.* 2018;61(2):190-205.

9. Antonopoulos AS, Oikonomou EK, Antoniades C, Tousoulis D. From the BMI paradox to the obesity paradox: the obesity-mortality association in coronary heart disease. *Obes Rev.* 2016;17(10):989-1000.

10. Lavie CJ, De Schutter A, Parto P, et al. Obesity and prevalence of cardiovascular diseases and prognosis-the obesity paradox updated. *Prog Cardiovasc Dis.* 2016;58(5):537-547.

11. Winter JE, MacInnis RJ, Nowson CA. The influence of age the BMI and all-cause mortality association: a meta-analysis. *J Nutr Health Aging.* 2017;21(10):1254-1258.

12. Atkins JL, Whincup PH, Morris RW, Lennon LT, Papacosta O, Wannamethee SG. Sarcopenic obesity and risk of cardiovascular disease and mortality: a population-based cohort study of older men. *J Am Geriatr Soc.* 2014;62(2):253-260.

13. Bessesen DH. Regulation of body weight: what is the regulated parameter? *Physiol Behav.* 2011;104(4):599-607.

14. Lichtman SW, Pisarska K, Berman ER, et al. Discrepancy between self-reported and actual caloric intake and exercise in obese subjects. *N Engl J Med.* 1992;327(27):1893-1898.

15. Schwartz MW, Seeley RJ, Zeltser LM, et al. Obesity pathogenesis: an endocrine society scientific statement. *Endocr Rev.* 2017;38(4):267-296.

16. Cornier MA, Von Kaenel SS, Bessesen DH, Tregellas JR. Effects of overfeeding on the neuronal response to visual food cues. *Am J Clin Nutr.* 2007;86(4):965-971.

17. Sumithran P, Prendergast LA, Delbridge E, et al. Long-term persistence of hormonal adaptations to weight loss. *N Engl J Med.* 2011;365(17):1597-1604.

18. Leibel RL, Rosenbaum M, Hirsch J. Changes in energy expenditure resulting from altered body weight. *N Engl J Med.* 1995;332(10):621-628.

19. Catenacci VA, Grunwald GK, Ingebrigtsen JP, et al. Physical activity patterns using accelerometry in the National Weight Control Registry. *Obesity (Silver Spring).* 2011;19(6):1163-1170.

20. Catenacci VA, Odgen L, Phelan S, et al. Dietary habits and weight maintenance success in high versus low exercisers in the National Weight Control Registry. *J Phys Act Health.* 2014;11(8):1540-1548.

21. Mozaffarian D, Hao T, Rimm EB, Willett WC, Hu FB. Changes in diet and lifestyle and long-term weight gain in women and men. *N Engl J Med.* 2011;364(25):2392-2404.

22. Church TS, Thomas DM, Tudor-Locke C, et al. Trends over 5 decades in U.S. occupation-related physical activity and their associations with obesity. *PLoS One.* 2011;6(5):e19657.

23. Schulz LO, Bennett PH, Ravussin E, et al. Effects of traditional and western environments on prevalence of type 2 diabetes in Pima Indians in Mexico and the U.S. *Diabetes Care.* 2006;29(8):1866-1871.

24. Farooqi IS, O'Rahilly S. The genetics of obesity in humans. In: Feingold KR, Anawalt B, Boyce A, et al, eds. *Endotext.* MDText.com, Inc.; 2000.

25. Claussnitzer M, Dankel SN, Kim KH, et al. FTO obesity variant circuitry and adipocyte browning in humans. *N Engl J Med.* 2015;373(10):895-907.

26. Farooqi S. Insights from the genetics of severe childhood obesity. *Horm Res.* 2007;68(suppl 5):5-7.

27. McHill AW, Wright KP Jr. Role of sleep and circadian disruption on energy expenditure and in metabolic predisposition to human obesity and metabolic disease. *Obes Rev.* 2017;18(suppl 1):15-24.

28. Spiegel K, Tasali E, Leproult R, Scherberg N, Van Cauter E. Twenty-four-hour profiles of acylated and total ghrelin: relationship with glucose levels and impact of time of day and sleep. *J Clin Endocrinol Metab.* 2011;96(2):486-493.

29. Fernandez-Twinn DS, Hjort L, Novakovic B, Ozanne SE, Saffery R. Intrauterine programming of obesity and type 2 diabetes. *Diabetologia.* 2019;62(10):1789-1801.

30. Bray GA, Heisel WE, Afshin A, et al. The science of obesity management: an endocrine society scientific statement. *Endocr Rev.* 2018;39(2):79-132.

31. Flegal KM, Kit BK, Orpana H, Graubard BI. Association of all-cause mortality with overweight and obesity using standard body mass index categories: a systematic review and meta-analysis. *J Am Med Assoc.* 2013;309(1):71-82.

32. Ackermann RT, O'Brien MJ. Evidence and challenges for translation and population impact of the Diabetes Prevention Program. *Curr Diab Rep.* 2020;20(3):9.

33. Sjöström L. Bariatric surgery and reduction in morbidity and mortality: experiences from the SOS study. *Int J Obes (Lond).* 2008;32(suppl 7):S93-S97.

34. Arterburn DE, Olsen MK, Smith VA, et al. Association between bariatric surgery and long-term survival. *J Am Med Assoc.* 2015;313(1):62-70.

35. Magkos F, Fraterrigo G, Yoshino J, et al. Effects of moderate and subsequent progressive weight loss on metabolic function and adipose tissue biology in humans with obesity. *Cell Metab.* 2016;23(4):591-601.

36. Gong Q, Zhang P, Wang J, et al; Da Qing Diabetes Prevention Study Group. Morbidity and mortality after lifestyle intervention for people with impaired glucose tolerance: 30-year results of the Da Qing Diabetes Prevention Outcome Study. *Lancet Diabetes Endocrinol.* 2019;7(6):452-461.

37. Look AHEAD Research Group; Gregg EW, Jakicic JM, Blackburn G, et al. Association of the magnitude of weight loss and changes in physical fitness with long-term cardiovascular disease outcomes in overweight or obese people with type 2 diabetes: a post-hoc analysis of the Look AHEAD randomised clinical trial. *Lancet Diabetes Endocrinol.* 2016;4(11):913-921.

2

THE OBESITY ENCOUNTER

Robert F. Kushner

CASE STUDY 1

A 42-year-old single man is seen for an initial appointment after relocating to the area for a new job. Medical problems include hypertension, dyslipidemia, gastroesophageal reflux disease (GERD), arthritis of knees, and a weight gain of 20 lb over the past 10 years. He attributes the weight gain to eating out more often, longer commute times in the car, and less physical activity. Medications include metoprolol succinate ER 50 mg q d, omeprazole 20 mg q d, and diclofenac sodium 100 mg ER q d. Family history is notable for hypertension, type 2 diabetes, and obesity. His diet is unplanned and unstructured, consuming the majority of foods at restaurants or ordered from meal delivery services. Physical activity is limited to walking. He drinks about 10 beers a week and does not smoke cigarettes.

On physical examination, height is 70 inches, weight 237 lb, blood pressure 134/88, heart rate 92, body mass index (BMI) 34 kg/m^2, and waist circumference 102 cm. The remainder of examination is notable for acanthosis nigricans around the neck, flesh-colored striae, no goiter, bruising or proximal muscle weakness, normal reflexes, abdominal panniculus, and palpable crepitus of both the knees. Laboratory tests are significant for fasting glucose 110 mg/dL, HbA1c 6.0%, total cholesterol 220 mg/dL, triglycerides 170 mg/dL, low-density lipoprotein (LDL) cholesterol 148 mg/dL, high-density lipoprotein (HDL) cholesterol 38 mg/dL, and thyroid-stimulating hormone (TSH) 2.25 mIU/L.

CLINICAL SIGNIFICANCE

Obesity is one of the most common medical conditions seen in primary care that affects nearly 40% of adults and 18% of children and adolescents.[1] Obesity affects every organ system and is linked to the most prevalent and costly medical problems seen in daily practice. However, despite its high occurrence rate, associated medical problems, and impact on daily functioning and quality of life, patients infrequently present to the healthcare team with "obesity" as their chief concern. For this reason, it commonly falls on the healthcare professional (HCP) to proactively broach the subject of weight management even if the patient does not raise the subject. Depending upon the patient's readiness to address his or her weight, the HCP needs to be able conduct a thorough assessment that includes taking a comprehensive history, performing a physical examination, and ordering pertinent laboratory diagnostic tests. This information is then assimilated to develop a personalized treatment plan. This chapter will focus on the elements of the clinical encounter that encompass a comprehensive obesity-focused assessment.

DIAGNOSIS

Measurement of Body Mass Index

Although the definition of obesity is "an abnormal or excessive fat accumulation that presents a risk to health,"[2] in clinical practice, it is routinely assessed by measuring BMI, an anthropometric calculation of body weight (kg) divided by height squared (m^2). Current assessment and management guidelines recommend measuring the patient's height and weight and calculating BMI at annual visits or more frequently depending upon the patient's risk factors.[3] The US Preventive Services Task Force also recommends screening all adults for obesity.[4] Since BMI is routinely and automatically displayed in the electronic health record, it is readily available as a reference in all patient charts. BMI is useful due to its simplicity and practicality in the office setting, its utility to assess population-based mortality and disease-specific morbidity, and high correlation with excess body fat (adiposity).

Although BMI has been adapted as a universal screener for obesity, there are four major limitations that HCPs need to be aware of when using BMI to diagnose obesity: (1) inaccurate assessment of body fat, (2) inability to measure distribution of body fat, (3) lack of assessment of individuals' health status, and (4) need to interpret according to ethnic and racial differences.

Inaccurate Assessment of Body Fat

BMI does not distinguish between weight associated with muscle and weight associated with fat, the variability of fatness across ethnically and racially diverse populations, and changes in body composition that occur with aging. This is particularly concerning regarding the elderly population who may be misclassified as having a healthy BMI but have a reduced lean body mass. Since aging is often associated with loss of skeletal muscle mass and function (strength or performance) while fat mass is preserved or even increased, the BMI may be in the normal range. This condition has been called sarcopenic obesity, which is a clinical diagnosis (i.e., no specific diagnostic criteria). Nonetheless, despite the low sensitivity to identify body fat, BMI has been shown to be a strong predictor of cardiovascular disease mortality and disease-specific morbidity.[5]

Inability to Distinguish Body Fat Distribution

Measuring fat distribution aids in identifying higher risk individuals because increased abdominal (visceral) fat predicts development of metabolic syndrome, type 2 diabetes, and total and cardiovascular risk mortality better than total body fat.[6] From a practical view, if two presenting patients have the same gender, age, height, and weight (and thus BMI), the patient who has upper body fat "apple-shaped" or android obesity will have a higher risk for metabolic diseases compared with the patient who has lower body fat "pear-shaped" or gynoid obesity (Figure 2.1). The distribution of body fat can be estimated by a variety of techniques; however, for practical purposes, waist circumference is used as a surrogate measurement of visceral fat (measurement of waist circumference is discussed further under physical examination). Although women more commonly seek treatment for obesity, men more commonly have "apple-shaped" obesity and are at higher risk for the metabolic complications of obesity.

Does Not Assess Individual Risk Status

The lack of inclusion of individual and social determinants of health such as genetic, biological, behavioral, social, environmental, racial, or medical factors is not

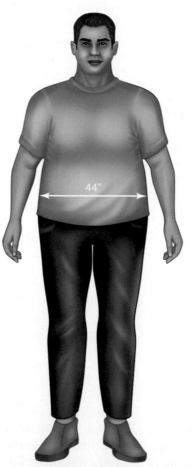

Lower-body obesity   **Upper-body obesity**

FIGURE 2.1 Body fat distribution. The location of body fat as lower (gynoid) or upper (android) fat distribution is independently associated with risk for metabolic syndrome, type 2 diabetes, hypertension, and cardiovascular disease. Body mass index (BMI) does not measure body fat distribution and needs to be assessed in addition to height and weight in individuals with a BMI <35 kg/m². In patients with BMI ≥35 kg/m², nearly all have elevated waist circumference, and thus measurement of waist does not aid in risk assessment.

assessed by the BMI. Treatment decisions should not be based on BMI alone. Rather, the BMI should be interpreted as a screener to identify patients who may be at risk for obesity-related complications. Obesity staging systems that help with risk stratification and facilitate decisions on which patients with obesity warrant more intensive treatment are discussed in Chapter 3.

Need to Interpret According to Ethnic and Racial Differences

Although the BMI calculation is universally used to assess obesity, its interpretation into risk categories or classes varies by race and ethnicity. The BMI cutoff points for overweight and obesity displayed in Table 2.1 were primarily generated from Caucasian populations. However, Asian populations are at higher risk for diabetes, high blood pressure, and high cholesterol at lower BMI thresholds.[7] Using standard BMI definitions for overweight and obesity among Asian Americans may fail to identify people at increased cardiovascular risk. For this reason, the World Health Organization suggests using lower cutoff points of ≥23 kg/m² for overweight and ≥27.5 kg/m² for obesity for this population.[7]

Due to the limitations of using BMI alone, a more appropriate clinical use of this anthropometric measurement is to assist in identifying patients who present with weight-related complications. This is consistent with a complication-centered approach to obesity care as advocated by the American Association of Clinical Endocrinologists.[8]

BROACHING THE TOPIC OF OBESITY

Patients seldom present to healthcare providers with "obesity" as their chief concern. Therefore, it is incumbent upon the healthcare provider to proactively broach the topic if excess weight or obesity is considered a significant contributor to the patients' overall health. However, there are often competing barriers and demands that preclude raising the topic of obesity.

TABLE 2.1 Body Mass Index (BMI) Classification	
Healthy body weight	18.5 - 24.9 kg/m²
Overweight	25.9 - 29.9 kg/m²
Obesity	≥30 kg/m²
Class 1 obesity	30.0 - 34.9 kg/m²
Class 2 obesity	35.0 - 39.9 kg/m²
Class 3 obesity	≥40 kg/m²

Lack of time and more important issues/concerns to discuss during the clinical encounter are the two most common reasons HCPs may not institute a discussion about weight with their patients.[9] This is a dilemma since compelling data from the National Health and Nutrition Examination Survey (NHANES) show that patients whose weight problem was diagnosed and who were told of their weight status by their HCP were significantly more likely to perceive themselves as overweight, attempt to lose weight,[10] and report a 5% weight loss over the year.[11]

There is no clearly established method for raising the topic of weight with patients; however, due to its sensitivity, words matter (Table 2.2). The approach HCPs use to broach this potentially sensitive topic may influence how patients react emotionally and cognitively to the discussion and advice provided.[12] Language used by the provider sets the stage for the interaction. The reason for this concern is that the word "obesity" is a highly charged, emotive term. It has a significant pejorative meaning for many patients, leaving them feeling judged and blamed when labeled as such. This is not the case when patients are told that they have other chronic diseases such as diabetes or hypertension. Patients prefer that clinicians use more neutral words such as "weight, excess weight, BMI, or unhealthy weight" compared with more stigmatizing terms such as "obesity, morbid obesity, or fatness." Asking permission to have the discussion is recommended as the first "A" in a modified 5 A's framework for counseling that is directed toward obesity (the 5 A's framework is discussed in more detail in Chapter 7).

STRUCTURING THE ENCOUNTER

Taking an Obesity-Focused History

Similar to any other presenting problem, the "history of present illness" (HPI) is an important and required section of the medical history when evaluating obesity as a distinct medical problem. The HPI includes the following:

- The changes in health that led the patient to seek medical attention, including a clear, chronological explanation of the patient's symptoms.
- Information relevant to the chief complaint, including answers to questions of *what, when, how, where, which, who,* and *why.*
- Information that informs the provider on the sequential development of the underlying pathologic process.

However, providers have not traditionally learned how to conduct an obesity-focused HPI. The two overarching features of an obesity history are to take a *life course perspective* and a *patient-centered* approach. The *life*

TABLE 2.2 Broaching the Topic of Obesity: Putting the Conversation Into Words

The following phrases are examples of provider dialogue:

- *I am concerned about your weight and would like to talk with you about it. Is that ok?*
  - Asking permission demonstrates respect for the patient and should foster a more therapeutic patient-provider relationship.
- *Monitoring your weight is as important as measuring your blood pressure and heart rate. I have noticed that your weight is up from last year. Is this a good time to talk to you about your weight? Has anything been going on that may have contributed to the weight gain?*
  - Identifying body weight as a clinical marker similar to other familiar and routine measurements places weight in a medical context.
- *I think that some of your medical concerns (e.g., shortness of breath, knee pain, heartburn, diabetes, hypertension, sleep disorder) may be related to your weight. What do you think?*
  - Remark relates the patients' current health concerns to their weight and assesses their insight into the problem.
- *What do you know about the risks of being overweight? Do you think that your weight is contributing to your health problems?*
  - The open-ended question inquires about the patient's understanding about medical problems that are obesity-related.

Follow-up questions to assess motivation, readiness, and barriers to initiating a weight management program, and a more detailed weight history may follow these broaching remarks. Additional questions may include the following:

- *What aspects of your weight would you like to talk about?*
- *What is hard about managing your weight?*
- *How does your weight affect you?*
- *Would you be interested in talking about options for working on your weight?*
- *Do you have some thoughts about things you might want to do to address your weight?*
- *Can I be of any help to you in how you might work on your weight?*
- *How motivated do you feel (0-10) to make long-term changes in your diet and physical activity?*

If the patient is not interested or ready to talk about weight, the healthcare professional can either gently probe the reasons why and/or acknowledge the patient's response or not pursue the topic further during this encounter. However, if clinically indicated, it is important to revisit weight at a follow-up visit.

Adapted from American Medical Association. Talking about weight with your patients. *Accessed February 28, 2020. https://northwestern.cloud-cme.com/assets/northwestern/pdf/ Obesity%202018%20talking-about-weight-kushner.pdf*

course perspective suggests that various biological, psychosocial, and cognitive factors throughout life influence health and disease risk.[13] This perspective is consistent with the complex nature of obesity. *Patient-centered* approach is defined as "providing care that is respectful of and responsive to individual patient preferences, needs, and values and ensuring that patient values guide all clinical decisions."[14] Information from the history should address the following six general questions:

1. *What factors contribute to the patient's obesity?*
2. *How is the obesity affecting the patient's health?*
3. *What is the patient's level of risk regarding obesity?*
4. *What are the patient's goals and expectations?*
5. *Is the patient motivated and engaged to enter a weight management program?*
6. *What kind of help does the patient need and want?*

Weight History

Many of the elements of an obesity-focused history are included in an expanded social history that includes diet, physical activity, sleep habits, stress, etc. and the Review of Systems section. However, the skill of how to obtain a weight history and how to use it in developing individualized care plans is generally new to providers. The mnemonic "OPQRST" is commonly used for ascertaining the patient's chief complaint and HPI and can be adapted for taking a weight history. The mnemonic stands for onset, precipitating events, quality of life/health, remedy, setting, and temporal pattern.[15] Examples of questions that can be used to explore these features are provided in Table 2.3.

These six probing areas provide a contextual understanding of how and when patients gained weight, what management efforts were employed, and the impact of body weight on their health. The mnemonic is not intended to be used in a prespecified order of questions, rather it was developed as a technique to prompt recall of important information to cover during the history. A more efficient method to obtain much of this information is to ask patients to complete a previsit questionnaire that can be reviewed during the encounter. An example of a self-completed questionnaire is shown in Figure 2.2. From a practical point of view, a questionnaire can be given to patients at the end of a routine visit to be completed at home in anticipation of a return visit where obesity will be the central focus of the

TABLE 2.3 Using the Mnemonic "OPQRST" to Take the Weight History	
	SAMPLE QUESTIONS
Onset	"When did you first begin to gain weight?" "Have you struggled with your weight since childhood?" "Do you remember how much you weighed in high school, college, early 20s, 30s, 40s?" "Did the weight gain begin when you started taking a new medication?"
Precipitating	"What life events led to your weight gain, e.g., college, long commute, marriage, divorce, financial loss, depression, illness, etc.?" "How much weight did you gain with pregnancy?" "How much weight did you gain when you stopped smoking?" "How much additional weight did you gain when you started insulin?"
Quality of life	"At what weight did you feel your best?" "What is hard to do at your current weight?" "How does your weight affect how you feel and function?"
Remedy	"What have you done or tried in the past to control your weight?" "Have you made any changes to your diet?" "Have you made any changes to your physical activity?" "Have you taken any medications to help control your weight?" "What is the most successful approach you tried to lose weight?" "What do you attribute the weight loss to?" "What caused you to regain your weight?" "What are the biggest challenges in maintaining your weight?"
Setting	"What was going on in your life when you last felt in control of your weight?" "What was going on when you gained your weight?" "What role has stress played in your weight gain?" "How important is social support or having a buddy to help you?" "Do you currently have social support from your family and friends to help you manage your weight?"
Temporal pattern	"What is the pattern of your weight gain?" "Did you gradually gain your weight over time, or is it more cyclic (yo-yo)?" "Are there large swings in your weight, and if so, what is the weight change?" "What was your lightest weight and heaviest weight as an adult?"

Reprinted from Kushner RF, Batsis JA, Butsch WS, et al. Weight history in clinical practice: The state of the science and future directions. Obesity. 2020;28:9-17.

encounter. Having patients reflect on these issues will save time and facilitate a more productive and therapeutic patient visit.

An additional technique is to ask patients to graph their weight changes over time, inserting life events or treatments that they feel were temporally related to weight changes[16] (Figure 2.3). Patients are then asked to reflect on and discuss their weight journey. This activity allows patients an opportunity to express any underlying burden, frustration, struggle, stigma, or shame that may have been associated with trying to manage body weight. Similar to the previsit questionnaire, this exercise is most useful if accomplished ahead of a visit that is dedicated to obesity care. If the weight history is conducted properly, patients will feel validated and acknowledged regarding their weight journey, while the clinician should feel more empathetic and informed to provide meaningful and practical patient-centered treatment.

Medication History

A thorough medication history should always be taken to uncover possible drug-induced weight gain as well as for medications interfering with weight loss. This is called iatrogenic weight gain. Table 2.4 provides a list of medications that are associated with a gain of body fat. Medications should always be considered when there is a change in the trajectory of body weight coincident with starting a new drug. The most common offenders are neuroleptics, antidiabetic agents, steroids, and antidepressants.[17] A list of medications that promote weight gain along with alternatives is also shown in Chapter 8 on Pharmacotherapy.

Taking a Comprehensive Social History

In addition to obtaining a weight history, other elements of the social history that are important for understanding the cause of weight gain include diet, physical activity, sleep patterns, and stress. This information can be largely obtained by using a standard patient questionnaire that assesses social determinants of health related to weight or by conducting a structured patient interview. More in-depth information about diet and physical activity will be covered in Chapters 5 and 6.

Diet History

It is important to review patients' eating habits—what, when, and where they eat; who shops and cooks for the

1. What is the least you have weighed as an adult (21 years and older)? _____

2. What is the most you have weighed as an adult, not including pregnancy (21 years and older)? _____

3. At what ages have you been overweight? *(Check all that apply)*

☐ Childhood (under 12 years old)   ☐ Middle adulthood (40 to 65 years old)

☐ Adolescence (12 to 18 years old)   ☐ Late adulthood (65 years and older)

☐ Early adulthood (18 to 40 years old)

4. What was the cause of your weight gain? *(Check all that apply)*

☐ Genetics   ☐ Menopause

☐ Unhealthy diet   ☐ Quitting smoking

☐ Not enough physical activity   ☐ Medications

☐ Pregnancy   ☐ Depression/grief/stress

☐ Medical problem   ☐ I don't know

5. What are your concerns about excess weight?

_____

_____

6. What methods have you tried to lose weight in the past? *(Check all that apply)*

☐ Nothing   ☐ Commercial diet programs

☐ Keeping track of the food I eat   ☐ Working with a registered dietitian

☐ Counting calories   ☐ Weight-loss medication

☐ Exercise   ☐ Weight-loss surgery (bariatric)

☐ Specific eating plans (Atkins/keto,
   South Beach, Zone, etc.)

7. What was your greatest amount of weight loss, and what strategies did you use to lose weight at that time?

_____

_____

8. What are your barriers to losing weight and/or keeping it off?

_____

_____

9. Please list what you typically eat and drink for meals and snacks. Please provide as much detail as you can (portion size, method of preparation, etc.)

Meal	Foods and beverages that I usually eat
Breakfast	
Snack	
Lunch	
Snack	
Dinner	
Snack	

FIGURE 2.2 (Continued)

10. Do you normally plan your meals and snacks? *Circle* **YES** *or* **NO**

11. Please check a box to tell us how often you eat or drink the following.

	Never	Once a week	Several times per week	Every day
Fast food				
Fruits and vegetables				
Any sugared drink (soda, juice, sweet tea, sports drinks)				

12. How may we help you manage your weight and eating habits? *(Check all that apply)*

☐ Diet and nutrition education   ☐ Stress-induced eating education

☐ Portion control education   ☐ Binge-eating education

☐ Meal planning education   ☐ Food preparation education

How many hours per day are you sitting? _____

13. Do you track your activity or your total calories burned on a device? *Circle* **YES** *or* **NO**

   If **YES**, what is your usual daily activity level (steps, minutes, distance)?

   _____

14. How many minutes per week do you do physical activity (such as brisk walking)?

   _____

15. Do you exercise (swim, bike, run, or use a cardio machine)? *Circle* **YES** *or* **NO**

   If **YES**, what do you do and how often?

   _____

   _____

16. Do you do strength training? *Circle* **YES** *or* **NO**

   If **YES**, how many times per week? _____

17. What barriers stand in your way of increasing your physical activity? *(Check all that apply)*

☐ Time limitations   ☐ Access to equipment or safe environment

☐ Lack of enjoyment   ☐ Lack of peer or family support

☐ Physical limitations   ☐ I don't know

18. Are you interested in any of the following assistance options? *(Check all that apply)*

☐ Weight-loss handouts/books   ☐ Health psychologist consultation

☐ Weight-loss websites   ☐ Weight-loss medication

☐ Commercial weight-loss program   ☐ Bariatric surgery

☐ Registered dietitian consultation ☐ I am not ready for assistance at this time

19. If you are interested in assistance, what is your preferred method of support? *(Check all that apply)*

☐ In-person consultation   ☐ In-person classes

☐ Phone call consultation   ☐ Online seminars

FIGURE 2.2 Weight management pre-visit questionnaire.

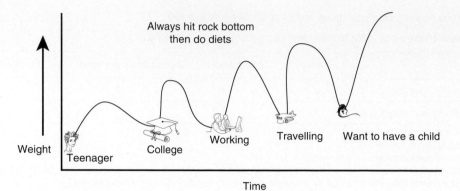

FIGURE 2.3 Weight history—life events graph. Using a weight (vertical line) and time (horizontal line) diagram, patients are asked to graph their weight over time and note any life events or treatments that may have impacted their weight. Patients may also include their weight (lb) on the vertical axis. In this example, the patient noted several life course milestones that both prompted and disrupted multiple diet attempts. Her interest in losing weight is to have a healthy pregnancy.

home; portion sizes; snacking; beverage intake; etc. This information provides a sense of overall dietary intake and nutritional knowledge that is used to target specific dietary behaviors.

TABLE 2.4 Drugs That Promote Weight Gain

CATEGORY	MEDICATION
Neuroleptics	Thioridazine, haloperidol, olanzapine, quetiapine, risperidone, clozapine
Antidiabetic agents	Insulin, sulfonylureas, thiazolidinediones
Steroid hormones	Glucocorticoids, progestational steroids, and contraceptives
Tricyclic antidepressants	Amitriptyline, nortriptyline, imipramine, doxepin
Monoamine oxidase inhibitors	Phenelzine
Selective serotonin reuptake inhibitors	Paroxetine
Other antidepressants	Mirtazapine, duloxetine
Anticonvulsants	Valproate, carbamazepine, gabapentin, pregabalin, vigabatrin
Antihistamines	Cyproheptadine
Beta-blockers and alpha-blockers	Propranolol, doxazosin

Adapted from Apovian CM, Aronne LJ, Bessesen DH, et al. Pharmacological management of obesity: an Endocrine Society clinical practice guideline. J Clin Endocrinol Metab. *2015;100(2):342-362.*

A dietary history can be obtained either by having the patient fill out a short questionnaire while in the waiting room or assessed as part of the patient interview. A useful and convenient technique is to ask the patient to describe a typical day. To get a complete sense of dietary intake in the previous 24 hours, it is helpful to review the patient's report and then confirm that there were no other sources of calories (e.g., drinks, snacks between meals).

Assuming yesterday was a typical day for you, to the best of your ability please tell me what you ate and drank since midnight the day before yesterday till midnight yesterday?

If yesterday was not a typical day, can you relate what you ate on a typical day within the past 3 days?

This open-ended and nonjudgmental approach allows patients to describe their dietary pattern without guilt, shame, or embarrassment.

Assessing for Eating Disorders

Screening for disordered eating should be part of the obesity assessment since it allows the provider to make appropriate referral and impacts treatment decisions. The DSM diagnostic criteria for the most common disorder—binge eating disorder (BED)—is displayed in Table 2.5. Binge eating occurs in only about 3% of the general population, but it is found in approximately 5% to 30% of persons with obesity.[19] The following two questions can be used to screen for BED in primary care:

Do you consume an amount of food that is substantially larger than what others would eat under comparable circumstances within a certain period of time?

Do you feel a sense of loss of control over eating during these times?

Patients who endorse symptoms or criteria for BED (or other eating disorders) should be considered for referral to a mental HCP by using shared decision-making.

TABLE 2.5 DSM-5 criteria for diagnosis of Binge Eating Disorder (DSM-5)

A. Recurrent episodes of binge eating. An episode of binge eating is characterized by both of the following:

1. Eating, in a discrete period of time (e.g., within any 2-hour period), an amount of food that is definitely larger than most people would eat during a similar period of time and under similar circumstances.
2. A sense of lack of control over eating during the episode (e.g., a feeling that one cannot stop eating or control what or how much one is eating).

B. The binge-eating episodes are associated with three (or more) of the following:

1. Eating much more rapidly than normal.
2. Eating until feeling uncomfortably full.
3. Eating large amounts of food when not feeling physically hungry.
4. Eating alone because of feeling embarrassed by how much one is eating.
5. Feeling disgusted with oneself, depressed, or very guilty afterward.

C. Marked distress regarding binge eating is present.

D. Binge eating occurs, on average, at least once a week for three months.

E. The binge eating is not associated with the recurrent use of inappropriate compensatory behavior as in bulimia nervosa and does not occur exclusively during the course of bulimia nervosa or anorexia nervosa.

Specify if:

In partial remission: After full criteria for binge-eating disorder were previously met, binge eating occurs at an average frequency of less than one episode per week for a sustained period of time.

In full remission: After full criteria for binge-eating disorder were previously met, none of the criteria have been met for a sustained period of time.

Specify current severity:

The minimum level of severity is based on the frequency of episodes of binge eating (see below). The level of severity may be increased to reflect other symptoms and the degree of functional disability.

Mild: 1-3 binge-eating episodes per week.

Moderate: 4-7 binge-eating episodes per week.

Severe: 8-13 binge-eating episodes per week.

Extreme: 14 or more binge-eating episodes per week.

TABLE 2.6 Practical Assessment of Physical Activity

- What is the most physically active thing you do in the course of the day? (examples may include walking as needed, walking the dog, stair climbing, house or yard work, exercising)
- How do you spend your working day and leisure time?
- What types of physical activity do you enjoy? How often do you do them?
- How many hours of TV do you watch every day? How many hours are you at a computer or desk every day?
- Are you *currently exercising regularly*?
- If answer yes (ask the following questions):
  - How many days per week do you exercise?
  - How many minutes per exercise session?
  - What type of activity do you engage in?
  - What is the intensity of your exercise? Low, moderate, or vigorous
- If answer no (ask the following questions):
  - How do you feel about/what are your thoughts on initiating/are you ready to initiate physical activity?
  - What are the barriers to initiating physical activity for you (i.e., access to gym, access to safe environment, injuries, or physical limitations)?
  - What are the benefits of physical activity for you?
  - Describe your previous experiences with exercise?
- Do you have any negative feelings about exercise or had any bad experiences with exercise?
- Do you have a support system to encourage you to exercise or exercise with you?
- How much time are you able to commit to exercise?

Physical Activity

Assessment of the patient's current and past level of physical activity can be accomplished by asking a set of question as shown in Table 2.6. These set of questions provide information on how active patients are in daily movement, level of sedentariness, whether they engage in any form of exercise, and perceived barriers. The information is then used to formulate a treatment plan. Alternatively, the Exercise is Medicine (https://exerciseismedicine.org/) initiative recommends two "vital sign" questions that can be used for all patients seen in primary care:

1. On average, how many days per week do you engage in moderate to strenuous exercise (like a brisk walk)? ___ days
2. On average, how many minutes do you engage in exercise at this level? ___ minutes

Total minutes per week of physical activity (multiply #1 by #2) _____ minutes per week

More expanded information on physical activity as a treatment modality is found in Chapter 6.

TABLE 2.7 Practical Assessment of Sleep

- What time do you usually go to bed?
- What time do you usually wake up in the morning?
- Do you fall asleep within 30 minutes of lying on the bed?
- How many times do you wake up at night?
- What is the reason you wake up at night?
- Do you feel well rested in the morning?
- How many times have you used sleep aids in the past month?

Sleep Patterns

Recent data have shown that compared with normal sleep, short sleep duration (<6 hours of sleep) is associated with a significant increase in deaths due to all causes[20] and an absolute increase of 37% for diabetes, 17% for hypertension, 16% for cardiovascular disease, and 38% for obesity. Although the mechanisms are uncertain, sleep restriction is associated with alterations in appetite regulation, sympathetic nervous system overactivity, insulin sensitivity, and changes in circadian rhythms.[21] Based on these data, "sleep health" has emerged as a new concept that contains multiple domains of sleep characteristics, including regularity, duration, timing, efficiency, and satisfaction.[22] In a 2018 random national sample poll of 1,010 US adults, sleep was ranked fourth among the top five items that were most important to responders.[23] The first three were fitness/nutrition, work, and hobbies/interests. Sleep can be assessed by asking the questions listed in Table 2.7.

Assessment of sleep in patients with obesity should also include screening for obstructive sleep apnea (further discussed in Chapter 4). A simple tool for this is the "STOP-BANG" screening, listed below. Any patient who has three of the following eight criteria should be tested for sleep apnea. Any patient with five of the eight criteria is considered to be high risk for having sleep apnea.

S = snoring (loud enough to be heard through closed doors)

T = tiredness (pathologic daytime sleepiness "would you fall asleep riding as a passenger in a car for up to an hour?")
O = observed apneas (patient's bed partner witnesses cessation of breathing during sleep)
P = blood pressure (diagnosis of hypertension)
B = BMI (≥ 35 kg/m^2)
A = age (≥ 50)
N = neck circumference (high risk is ≥ 17 for men and ≥ 16 for women)
G = gender (male)

Stress

Stress is a common experience in modern day life. In the Gallup 2019 Global Emotions Report, the majority of Americans (55%) said they had experienced stress during a lot of the day, and nearly half (45%) said they felt worried a lot.[24] In the 2019 Stress in America survey,[25] around 6 in 10 adults identified work (64%) and money (60%) as significant sources of stress, making them the most commonly mentioned personal stressors. Stress contributes to obesity, in part, due to activation of the hypothalamic/pituitary/adrenal axis, resulting in elevated cortisol levels. Patients also commonly report "stress or emotional eating" as a learned coping response.[26] The 10-item Perceived Stress Scale is one of the best validated instruments for screening, but because of its length, the abbreviated Perceived Stress Scale-4 is a better alternative in clinical settings[27] (Table 2.8). Identification of a high level of stress may prompt a more thorough evaluation for mood disorders or referral to a mental health professional.

Review of Systems

Since obesity can affect every organ system, the review of systems section of the medical history should be comprehensive. Table 2.9 displays a list of diseases or conditions that are associated with obesity. With the exception of hypothyroidism, polycystic ovarian syndrome (PCOS), and Cushing syndrome which may be considered secondary causes of obesity, all of the conditions listed in

TABLE 2.8 Practical Assessment of Stress

PERCEIVED STRESS SCALE 4

For each of the four questions, a range of scores is assigned based from 0 = never to 4 = very often.
Reverse scores for questions 2 and 3 like this: 0 = 4, 1 = 3, 2 = 2, 3 = 1, 4 = 0.
Now add up scores for each item to get a total score which varies between 0 and 16.
Higher scores indicative of higher perceived stress.

_____ 1. In the last month, how often have you felt that you were unable to control the important things in your life?
_____ 2. In the last month, how often have you felt confident about your ability to handle your personal problems?
_____ 3. In the last month, how often have you felt that things were going your way?
_____ 4. In the last month, how often have you felt difficulties were piling up so high that you could not overcome them?

Modified from Cohen S, Kamarck T, Mermelstein R. A global measure of perceived stress. J Health Soc Behav. 1983;24:385-396.

the table represent manifestations of the disease burden of obesity. The evaluation of many of these conditions will be further discussed in Chapter 4.

TABLE 2.9 Obesity-Related Organ Systems Review

Cardiovascular	Respiratory
Hypertension	Dyspnea/deconditioning
Congestive heart failure	Obstructive sleep apnea
Cor pulmonale	
Varicose veins	Obesity hypoventilation syndrome, also known as Pickwickian syndrome
Pulmonary embolism	Asthma
Coronary artery disease Atrial fibrillation	**Gastrointestinal**
Endocrine	Gastroesophageal reflux disease
Metabolic syndrome	Nonalcoholic fatty liver disease
Type 2 diabetes	Cholelithiasis
Dyslipidemia	Hernias
Polycystic ovarian syndrome	Colon cancer
Cushing syndrome	
Hypogonadism/erectile dysfunction	
Musculoskeletal	**Genitourinary**
Hyperuricemia and gout	Urinary stress incontinence
Immobility	Obesity-related glomerulopathy
Osteoarthritis (knees and hips)	Breast and uterine cancer
Low back pain	Pregnancy complications
Carpal tunnel syndrome	
Psychological	**Neurologic**
Depression/low self-esteem	Stroke
Body image disturbance	Idiopathic intracranial hypertension
Internal stigmatization	Meralgia paresthetica

TABLE 2.9 Obesity-Related Organ Systems Review (Continued)

Integument	Dementia
Striae distensae	
Stasis pigmentation of legs	
Lymphedema	
Cellulitis	
Intertrigo, carbuncles	
Acanthosis nigricans	
Acrochordons (skin tags)	
Hidradenitis suppurativa	

PHYSICAL EXAMINATION

The physical examination process for patients with obesity should focus on several special features as listed in Table 2.10.[28]

Most of these elements are routinely performed when conducting an adult comprehensive physical examination with the exception of measuring waist circumference. In addition to BMI, which is used to screen for and categorize obesity, the risk of overweight and obesity is independently associated with excess abdominal (visceral) fat. Current guidelines recommend that waist circumference be measured in patients with a BMI of 25 kg/m² to <35 kg/m².[3] Measurement of abdominal girth is not a difficult procedure and only takes a few seconds (Figure 2.6). The threshold for excessive abdominal fat is clinically defined as a waist circumference ≥102 cm (≥40 inches) in men and ≥88 cm (≥35 inches) in women. Similar to BMI, ethnic and racial differences exist for these thresholds and are lower for Asian populations[29] (Table 2.11). Persons with waist circumferences exceeding these limits should be urged more strongly to pursue weight reduction since it categorically increases disease risk for each BMI class for developing hypertension, type 2 diabetes, coronary artery disease, stroke, and total mortality. Such individuals may have the metabolic syndrome, a name for the group of cardiometabolic risk factors that cluster together (blood pressure, glucose, and lipids) and increase the risk for their respective conditions.

Measuring Blood Pressure

Another examination feature that is important for patients with obesity is to use a proper blood pressure cuff size to avoid "miscuffing." A bladder cuff that is not the appropriate width for the patient's arm circumference will cause a systematic error in blood pressure measurement. The error in blood pressure measurement is larger when the cuff is too small relative to the patient's arm circumference

TABLE 2.10 Physical Examination of the Patient With Obesity: Domains of Special Interest

DOMAIN	WHAT TO EXPECT	WHAT TO DO
Vital signs	Body mass index (BMI) requires accurate measurement of weight and height Miscuffing wide arm circumferences leads to spurious blood pressure readings	Have scales with wide base and weight limit >350 lb; use wall mounted stadiometer if possible Have large blood pressure cuffs available
Head and neck	Crowded oropharynx may suggest obstructive sleep apnea Patients may have insulin resistance	Use Mallampati score I to IV (Figure 2.4) to describe the pharynx Examine the neck and axillae for acanthosis nigricans (Figure 2.5)
Abdomen	Upper body fat distribution signifies increased risk for metabolic syndrome	Have paper or plastic tape measure available to measure waist circumference (if BMI 25 – <35 kg/m^2) Examination of the abdominal skin
Cardiovascular	Patients may have peripheral edema and venous status of the lower extremities	Check for pitting edema and examine the lower extremities with socks removed
Skin	Patients with excessive skinfolds are prone to develop carbuncles, furuncles, and fungal infections Bruising and purplish striae >1 cm may signify Cushing syndrome	Examine all skinfolds, particularly under the breasts and abdominal panniculus

Adapted from Silk AW, McTigue KM. Reexamining the physical examination for obese patients. J Am Med Assoc. *2011;305:193-194.*

than when it is too large—a situation commonly encountered among patients with obesity. It has been demonstrated that the most frequent error in measuring blood pressure is miscuffing with undercuffing large arms accounting for 84% of the miscuffings.[30] The ideal cuff should have a bladder length that is 80% and a width that is at least 40% of arm circumference (a length-to-width ratio of 2:1). Therefore, a large adult cuff (16 × 36 cm) should be chosen for patients with mild to moderate obesity (or arm circumference 14 to 17 inches) while an adult thigh cuff (16 × 42 cm) will need to be used for patients whose arm circumferences are greater than 17 inches. In patients who have very large circumferences with short

upper arm length, blood pressure can be measured from a cuff placed on the forearm and listening for sounds over the radial artery (although this may overestimate systolic blood pressure, whereas the diastolic pressure decreases).

Measuring Body Fat

Although it would likely be advantageous to measure body fat mass directly since obesity is defined as "an abnormal or excessive fat accumulation that presents a risk to health,"[2]

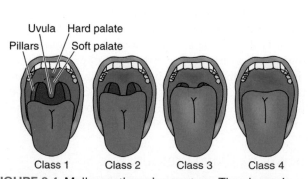

FIGURE 2.4 Mallampati scoring system. The airway is classified according to the structures seen, as follows: class I, soft palate, fauces, uvula, pillars; class II, soft palate, fauces, uvula; class III, soft palate, base of uvula; class IV, soft palate not visible at all. (Reprinted from Dimick JB, Upchurch GB Jr, Sonnenday CJ, Kao LS. *Clinical Scenarios in Surgery.* 2nd ed. Wolters Kluwer; 2018.)

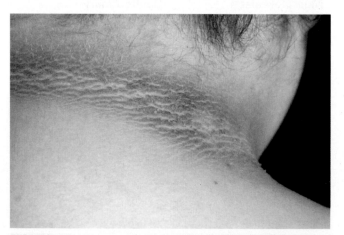

FIGURE 2.5 Acanthosis nigricans is a skin condition characterized by areas of dark, velvety discoloration in body folds, and creases affecting the neck, the armpits, groin, navel, forehead, and other areas. The affected skin can become thickened. It is commonly associated with insulin resistance. (Reprinted from Baranoski S, Ayello EA. *Wound Care Essentials.* 5th ed. Wolters Kluwer; 2020.)

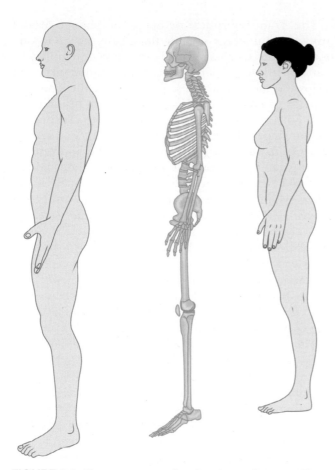

FIGURE 2.6 Measurement of waist circumference. To measure waist circumference, locate the upper hip bone and the top of the right iliac crest. Place a measuring tape in a horizontal plane around the abdomen at the level of the iliac crest. Before reading the tape measure, ensure that the tape is snug, but does not compress the skin, and is parallel to the floor. The measurement is made at the end of a normal expiration. Adapted from NHLBI Obesity Education Initiative Expert Panel on the Identification, Evaluation, and Treatment of Obesity in Adults (US). *Clinical Guidelines on the Identification, Evaluation, and Treatment of Overweight and Obesity in Adults: The Evidence Report*. Bethesda, MD: National Heart, Lung, and Blood Institute; 1998.

it is not routinely performed in the office setting due to cost and impracticality. The two most accurate methods used largely for research purposes are dual-energy X-ray absorptiometry, or DXA, and air displacement plethysmography using a BodPod device.[31] DXA is a noninvasive test that is most often ordered to measure bone mineral density for assessment of osteoporosis. By applying a computerized program, DXA can also be used to measure body composition, determining total body fat percentage, total fat mass, and fat-free mass. The BodPod uses whole-body densitometry to determine body fat and fat-free mass. This technique has replaced the traditional method of underwater weighing. In contrast to these methods, bioelectrical impedance analysis (BIA) is a device that is cheaper, portable, and more practical for the office setting. It is, however, less accurate than the other methods.

TABLE 2.11 Ethnic Specific Values for Waist Circumference (cm)

COUNTRY/ETHNIC GROUP	MALE	FEMALE
North American	≥102 cm	≥88 cm
European	≥94 cm	≥80 cm
South Asian/Chinese	≥90 cm	≥80 cm
Japanese	≥85 cm	≥90 cm
Ethnic South and Central Americans	Use South Asian recommendations	Use South Asian recommendations
Sub-Saharan Africans	Use European data	Use European data
Eastern Mediterranean and Middle East (Arab) populations	Use European data	Use European data

Modified from Alberti KG, Zimmet P, Shaw J. Metabolic syndrome—A new world-wide definition. A Consensus Statement from the International Diabetes Federation. Diabet Med. *2006;23:469-480.*

BIA uses a weak alternating electric current that flows through the body and the voltage is measured in order to calculate impedance (electrical resistance) of the body. After entering the patient's height and weight, a prediction equation estimates the volume of the electrolyte-rich total body water and thus body fat and lean mass. If BIA is used as part of the assessment process, it is important to use the manufacturer's standard measurement protocol that includes patient instructions since hydration status, exercise, skin temperature, and meal times can influence impedance readings. Although reference ranges will vary by age, race, and ethnicity, a healthy range of body fat for men is typically defined as 8% to 19%, while the healthy range for women is 21% to 33%.

LABORATORY ASSESSMENT

Laboratory testing should be based on patient risk and consistent with current screening guidelines for other medical conditions. These tests represent an objective measurement which complements history taking and clinical evaluation.[32] A reasonable screening panel (ideally fasting, for assessment of diabetes screening and for triglycerides) for all patients consists of the following:

- Chemistry profile that includes glucose, liver, and kidney function
- Thyroid function test (TSH)

- Lipid profile

Additional tests to be obtained if clinically indicated may include a glycosylated hemoglobin (HbA1c), uric acid, complete blood count, index of inflammation (hs-CRP), and 25-hydroxyvitamin D. Further diagnostic procedures will be dictated by clinical history and may include a sleep study for assessment of obstructive sleep apnea, electrocardiogram or a cardiac stress test to assess for underlying cardiovascular disease, endocrine investigations for Cushing syndrome (in the presence of easy bruising, wide purple striae, proximal muscle weakness, unexpected osteoporosis especially in a man, new acne, and a change in facial appearance), PCOS, or FibroScan to assess for hepatic fibrosis (see Chapter 4 for further evaluation of medical comorbidities).

ASSESSING PATIENT'S READINESS TO CHANGE BEHAVIOR

After completing the history and physical examination, the next essential part of the initial evaluation is determining the patient's interest and readiness for engaging in weight management. Initiating change when the patient is not ready often leads to frustration and may hamper future efforts. Patients who are ready and have thought about the benefits and difficulties of weight management are more likely to succeed.

The NHLBI's Practical Guidelines for readiness recommend that HCPs assess patient motivation and support, stressful life events, psychiatric status, time availability, and constraints, as well as appropriateness of goals and expectations to help establish the likelihood of lifestyle change.[33] It is not enough to simply ask a patient, "*Are you ready to lose weight?*" Inquiring about readiness necessitates a more in-depth assessment of the patient and his/her environment. Readiness can be viewed as the balance of two opposing forces: motivation, or the patient's desire to change, and resistance, or the patient's resistance to change.[34] It is important to remember that most patients are ambivalent about changing long-standing lifestyle behaviors, fearing that it will be difficult, uncomfortable, or depriving. One helpful method to begin a readiness assessment is to "anchor" the patient's interest and confidence to change on a numerical scale. To measure this, simply ask the patient, "*On a scale from 0 to10, with 0 being not important and 10 being very important, how important is it for you to lose weight at this time?*" and "*Also on a scale from 0-10, with 0 being not confident and 10 being very confident, how confident are you that you can lose weight at this time?*"[35] This is a very useful exercise to initiate further dialogue such as, "*What would it take to increase your confidence score from a 4 to a 7?*" This anchoring technique is a key element of motivational interviewing.[35]

The Transtheoretical or Stages of Change Model proposes that at any specific time, patients are in one of the six discreet stages of change: precontemplation, contemplation, preparation, action, maintenance, and relapse.[36] Assessing which stage of change the patient is in helps to tailor the advice and intensity of intervention. For example, if the patient is in the precontemplation stage regarding weight control ("*I'm not really interested in losing weight at this time*"), the appropriate action would be to provide information about health risks and benefits of weight loss and encourage taking action when ready. A reasonable response would be: "*Would you like to read some information about the health aspects of obesity?*" In contrast, if the patient is in the contemplation stage ("*I need to lose weight but with all that's going on in my life right now, I'm not sure I can*"), a reasonable action would be to help resolve ambivalence and discuss barriers. Here the HCP can respond by saying: "*Let's look at the benefits of weight loss, as well as what you may need to change.*"

There are known determinants of whether a patient is likely to institute behavioral changes. Whitlock et al.[37] define certain change-predisposing attributes that typically lead to behaviors that promote weight loss. Assessing these qualities during the patient interview helps determine a ready candidate for lifestyle modification. Although it is unlikely that every patient will display all seven qualities, they provide a useful benchmark for assessment. These patients:

- Strongly want and intend to change for clear, personal reasons
- Face a minimum of obstacles to change
- Have the requisite skills and self-confidence to make a change
- Feel positively about change and believe it will result in meaningful benefit
- Perceive the change as congruent with self-image and social group norms
- Receive encouragement and support to change from valued persons

These patient-specific features are assessed by assimilating information gathered during the encounter or asked directly to the patient.

SUMMARY

Obesity may be the most significant medical problem that healthcare providers will face over the coming decades. Clinicians need to aggressively address this chronic disease, providing both preventive and therapeutic care. Performing a detailed initial assessment, including an obesity-focused history, physical examination, and selected laboratory and diagnostic tests is fundamental to the process of care.

CLINICAL HIGHLIGHTS

- Although obesity is clinically defined as a BMI of ≥30 kg/m², BMI does not directly measure body fat or assess presence of weight-related complications. Patients should not be treated solely based on their BMI. Rather, they need to be evaluated and treated according to their overall risk, an assessment that is completed by performing a comprehensive medical history and physical examination.
- Broaching the topic of obesity with patients is often the first step in the evaluation process. Unlike other chronic medical conditions such as diabetes, hypertension, or arthritis, using the word "obesity" often carries negative connotations of laziness, lack of will power, and sloth. Using empathetic neutral terms such as "excess weight, unhealthy weight, or weight" in the conversation will support a more therapeutic dialogue.
- Due to multiple pathophysiological pathways, the disease burden of obesity can affect every organ system. A comprehensive *review of systems* should be taken on all patients presenting with obesity to uncover any symptoms, diseases, or conditions that may be related to excess adiposity. Sharing this information with the patient is a useful educational technique to discuss the link between excess weight and medical problems and the importance of engaging in weight management.
- Physical examination of the patient with obesity encompasses several additional features that are important in the diagnosis and assessment of burden of the disease. Measurement of weight, height, and waist circumference (for patients with a BMI of 25 kg/m² to <35 kg/m²) is important to categorize the disease. Use of a properly fitting blood pressure cuff is necessary to avoid "miscuffing" leading to a spurious blood pressure measurement. Careful examination of skinfolds is important to assess for areas of infection.

WHEN TO REFER?

- Patient requires a more in-depth evaluation of obesity and associated medical burden. Referral to an obesity medicine specialist
- Patient has an eating disorder or psychiatric condition and needs additional assessment and treatment. Referral to a mental healthcare provider
- After assessing and advising about need to treat, have option of referring to an intensive professional or commercial weight management program if indicated
- Patient desires additional dietary education and counseling. Referral to a registered dietitian nutritionist

CASE STUDIES

Discussion of Case Study 1

Using an obesity-centric approach, the patient's presenting medical problems of hypertension, dyslipidemia, GERD, and arthritis of knees can be considered as comorbid conditions of obesity and weight gain. An additional comorbid condition diagnosed on laboratory testing is prediabetes. Along with an elevated waist circumference measured on physical examination, he meets all five components of the metabolic syndrome, thus placing him at higher risk for development of type 2 diabetes and cardiovascular disease. Based on his height and weight, his calculated BMI is 34.4 kg/m² which is considered class I obesity. Contributors to his weight gain include excessive caloric intake, reduced physical activity, family history of obesity, and possibly long-term use of a beta-blocker. The topic of excess weight should be broached with the patient, beginning with asking permission to have the discussion and assessing his understanding of obesity and interest in engaging in weight management. Next steps and treatment recommendations will be based on his readiness to change.

CASE STUDY 2

A 38-year-old woman was asked to return for a visit that is dedicated to further assess her obesity. On her last visit, she stated, "I am tired of being fat. I need more help. I have gained 15 lbs. over the past year and this needs to stop." You asked her to complete a previsit questionnaire and weight history—life events graph in preparation of returning for a visit that would be solely focused on her weight. Medical history is notable for hypothyroidism and depression. The patient is divorced and is raising a 17-year-old daughter. She works full time as legal assistant. Family history is significant for her mother who is suffering from dementia and a brother with bipolar disorder. Medications are levothyroxine 75 µg/day and duloxetine 30 mg/day.

On physical examination, height is 66 inches, weight 200 lb, blood pressure 130/86, heart rate 88, BMI 32.6 kg/m², and waist circumference 95 cm. The remainder of examination is unremarkable. Laboratory tests are significant for fasting glucose 98 mg/dL, total cholesterol 200 mg/dL, triglycerides 150 mg/dL, LDL cholesterol 122 mg/dL, HDL cholesterol 48 mg/dL, and TSH 1.02 mIU/L.

Discussion of Case Study 2

You review the completed previsit questionnaire and body weight life events graph to guide the weight history.

Weight Management Previsit Questionnaire

1. What is the least you have weighed as an adult (21 years and older)? <u>130lbs</u>

2. What is the most you have weighed as an adult, not including pregnancy (21 years and older)? <u>200 lbs</u>

3. At what ages have you been overweight? *(Check all that apply)*

   ☐ Childhood (under 12 years old)   ☐ Middle adulthood (40 to 65 years old)

   ☐ Adolescence (12 to 18 years old)   ☐ Late adulthood (65 years and older)

   ☑ Early adulthood (18 to 40 years old)

4. What was the cause of your weight gain? *(Check all that apply)*

   ☐ Genetics   ☐ Menopause

   ☑ Unhealthy diet   ☐ Quitting smoking

   ☑ Not enough physical activity   ☐ Medications

   ☑ Pregnancy   ☑ Depression/grief/stress

   ☐ Medical problem   ☐ I don't know

5. What are your concerns about excess weight?

   <u>I don't like the way my body looks. I am disgusted with myself for not being able to keep the weight off</u>

6. What methods have you tried to lose weight in the past? *(Check all that apply)*

   ☐ Nothing   ☑ Commercial diet programs

   ☑ Keeping track of the food I eat   ☐ Working with a registered dietitian

   ☐ Counting calories   ☐ Weight-loss medication

   ☑ Exercise   ☐ Weight-loss surgery (bariatric)

   ☑ Specific eating plans (Atkins/keto, South Beach, Zone, etc.)

7. What was your greatest amount of weight loss, and what strategies did you use to lose weight at that time?

   <u>Lost 30 lbs on Weight Watchers</u>

8. What are your barriers to losing weight and/or keeping it off?

   <u>Trying to deal with taking care of my mother who has dementia. Working full time and raising my daughter. I am stressed and turn to food to feel better.</u>

9. Please list what you typically eat and drink for meals and snacks. Please provide as much detail as you can (portion size, method of preparation, etc.)

Meal	Foods and beverages that I usually eat
Breakfast	Skip
Snack	Donut and coffee in the office (snack bar)
Lunch	Turkey sandwich with chips and diet soda
Snack	A few cookies or candy
Dinner	Spaghetti with tomato sauce, or order in
Snack	Ice cream bar

10. Do you normally plan your meals and snacks? *Circle* **YES** *or* ✓ **NO**

11. Please check a box to tell us how often you eat or drink the following.

	Never	Once a week	Several times per week	Every day
Fast food			✓	
Fruits and vegetables		✓		
Any sugared drink (soda, juice, sweet tea, sports drinks)				✓

12. How may we help you manage your weight and eating habits? *(Check all that apply)*

☑ Diet and nutrition education   ☑ Stress-induced eating education

☐ Portion control education   ☐ Binge-eating education

☐ Meal planning education   ☐ Food preparation education

How many hours per day are you sitting? <u>6</u>

13. Do you track your activity or your total calories burned on a device? *Circle* **YES** *or* ✓ **NO**

   If **YES**, what is your usual daily activity level (steps, minutes, distance)?

   _____

14. How many minutes per week do you do physical activity (such as brisk walking)?
   <u>70</u>

15. Do you exercise (swim, bike, run, or use a cardio machine)? *Circle* **YES** *or* ✓ **NO**

   If **YES**, what do you do and how often?

   _____

   _____

16. Do you do strength training? *Circle* **YES** *or* ✓ **NO**

   If **YES**, how many times per week? _____

17. What barriers stand in your way of increasing your physical activity? *(Check all that apply)*

☑ Time limitations   ☐ Access to equipment or safe environment

☑ Lack of enjoyment   ☐ Lack of peer or family support

☐ Physical limitations   ☐ I don't know

18. Are you interested in any of the following assistance options? *(Check all that apply)*

☐ Weight-loss handouts/books   ☑ Health psychologist consultation

☐ Weight-loss websites   ☑ Weight-loss medication (??)

☐ Commercial weight-loss program   ☐ Bariatric surgery

☐ Registered dietitian consultation   ☐ I am not ready for assistance at this time

19. If you are interested in assistance, what is your preferred method of support? *(Check all that apply)*

☑ In-person consultation   ☐ In-person classes

☐ Phone call consultation   ☐ Online seminars

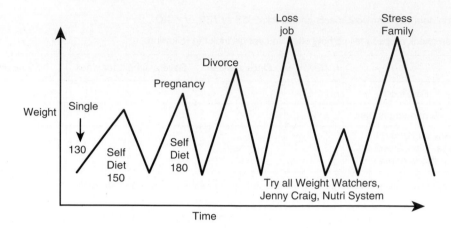

You note that she has experienced a progressive weight cycling pattern due to several life events, including pregnancy, divorce, loss of a job, and more recently, family stress. She has also participated in multiple commercial weight management programs, losing up to 30 lb following Weight Watchers. Her current weight of 200 lb is her heaviest body weight. She attributes the weight gain to an unhealthy diet, limited physical activity, and stress. The latter factor, along with limited time, is a major concern. Her current diet is characterized as unstructured, unplanned, and calorie dense. There is limited intake of fruit and vegetables. She engages in very low amounts of physical activity and is sedentary for 6 hours/day. She feels that a visit with a registered dietitian and health psychologist would be beneficial and has questions about the use of antiobesity medications. You classify her as having mild, class I obesity with upper body fat distribution based on her enlarged waist circumference. She is ready to engage in weight management and is looking for additional assistance.

All of this information is obtained and reviewed within the first 10 minutes of the visit. The remainder of time can be used to provide supportive language, such as "*Thank you for being so open about your weight history. I can ensure you that the issues you are struggling with are common and I can see why maintaining a healthy weight has been difficult. Referral to a dietitian and health psychologist to address healthy eating, planning, quick meal preparation, and stress eating makes a lot of sense. I can refer you to my colleagues.*" It would also be beneficial to ask the patient to start tracking her diet for self-monitoring, engage in shared decision-making about her ideas for healthier snack and meal options, and suggest a calorie goal of 1,200 to 1,500 kcal/day in anticipation of seeing a dietitian. You can also suggest that she stands up every hour at work to reduce sedentary time and increase her daily walking time. Lastly, you can review the indications and benefits of using antiobesity medications and gauge her interest (obesity pharmacotherapy is reviewed in Chapter 8).

QUIZ QUESTIONS

1. A 36-year-old woman makes an appointment as a new patient. She is concerned about gaining 15 lb (6.8 kg) over the past 10 years. On history, you learn that she has experienced several major life events over this time that have included marriage, two pregnancies, relocation to the suburbs, and starting paroxetine for depression. She also states that her mother and sister suffer from obesity. On examination, her body mass index is 31 kg/m². The remainder of examination is unremarkable. What is the next best step?

   A. Educate her about the health risks of weight gain and obesity.
   B. Recommend stopping the antidepressant medication since it is the likely cause of the weight gain.
   C. Inquire about the weight of her two children since obesity has a genetic contribution.
   D. Ask her what she thinks may have contributed to the weight gain.
   E. Provide diet and physical activity counseling.

   Answer: D. *Although answers A through D are reasonable responses, it is most important to first assess the patient's perceptions and understanding about her own weight gain. Answer E would not be appropriate at this time since it should be preceded by diet and physical activity history.*

2. During the physical examination of a 48-year-old man with class II obesity (body mass index 36.5 kg/m²) and upper body fat distribution (waist circumference 42 inches), you obtain a blood pressure measurement of 146/94 mm Hg on the right arm using an adult size cuff. He has been sitting for 5 minutes and both feet are resting on the floor. He does not have a history of hypertension. What assessment can be made about his blood pressure, and what is the next appropriate step?

   A. Accurate but needs to be repeated in the right arm
   B. Spuriously high and needs to be retaken using a large adult cuff
   C. Spuriously high and needs to be retaken at the level of the wrist
   D. Inaccurate and needs to be repeated after another 5 minutes of resting
   E. Accurate and a new diagnosis of hypertension should be added to problem list

   Answer: B. *A bladder cuff that is not the appropriate width for the patient's arm circumference will cause a systematic error in blood pressure measurement. This is called miscuffing. A large adult cuff (16 × 36 cm) should be chosen for patients with mild to moderate obesity (or arm circumference 14 to 17 inches).*

REFERENCES

1. Hales CM, Fryar CD, Carroll MD, et al. Trends in obesity and severe obesity prevalence in US youth and adults by sex and age. 2007-2008 to 2015-2016. *J Am Med Assoc.* 2018;319(16):1723-1725.

2. World Health Organization. *Obesity.* https://www.who.int/topics/obesity/en/

3. Jensen MD, Ryan DH, Apovian CM, et al. 2013 AHA/ACC/TOS guidelines for the management of overweight and obesity is adults: a report of the American College of Cardiology/American Heart Association Task Force on practice guidelines and the Obesity Society. *Circulation.* 2014;129(25 suppl 2):S102-S138.

4. Mayer VA. Screening for and management of obesity in adults: U.S. Preventive Services Task Force recommendation statement. *Ann Intern Med.* 2012;157:373-378.

5. Di Angelantonio E, Bhupathiraju SN, Wormser D, et al; The Global Mortality Collaboration. Body-mass index and all-cause mortality: individual-participant-data meta-analysis of 239 prospective studies in four continents. *Lancet.* 2016;388:776-786.

6. Ross R, Neeland IJ, Yamashita S, et al. Waist circumference as a vital sign in clinical practice: a consensus statement from the IAS and ICCR working group on visceral obesity. *Nat Rev Endocrinol.* 2020;16(3):177-189.

7. WHO Expert Consultation. Appropriate body-mass index for Asian populations and its implications for policy and intervention strategies. *Lancet.* 2004;363(9403):157-163.

8. Garvey WT, Mechanick JI, Brett EM, et al. American Association of Clinical Endocrinologists and American College of Endocrinology comprehensive clinical practice guidelines for medical care of patients with obesity. *Endocr Pract.* 2016;22(7):842-884.

9. Kaplan LM, Golden A, Jinnett K, et al. Perceptions of barriers to effective obesity care: results from the national ACTION study. *Obesity.* 2018;26:61-69.

10. Post RE, Mainous AG, Gregorie SH, et al. The influence of physician acknowledgement of patients' weight status on patient perceptions of overweight and obesity in the United States. *Arch Intern Med* 2011;171:316-321.

11. Pool AC, Kraschnewski JL, Cover LA, et al. The impact of physician weight discussion on weight loss in US adults. *Obes Res Clin Pract.* 2014;8:e131-e139.

12. *Talking about weight with your patients.* American Medical Association. Accessed February 28, 2020. https://northwestern.cloud-cme.com/assets/northwestern/pdf/Obesity%202018%20talking-about-weight-kushner.pdf

13. Kuh D, Ben-Shlomo Y, Lynch J, Hallqvist J, Power C. Life course epidemiology. *J Epidemiol Community Health.* 2003;57(10):778-783.

14. Institute of Medicine, (US) Committee on Quality of Health Care in America. *Crossing the quality chasm: a new health system for the 21st century.* National Academies Press (US); 2001.

15. Kushner RF, Batsis JA, Butsch WS, et al. Weight history in clinical practice: the state of the science and future directions. *Obesity* 2020;28:9-17.

16. Kushner RF, Ryan DH. Assessment and lifestyle management of patients with obesity. Clinical recommendations from systematic reviews. *J Am Med Assoc.* 2014;312(9):943-952.

17. Apovian CM, Aronne LJ, Bessesen DH, et al. Pharmacological management of obesity: an endocrine Society clinical practice guideline. *J Clin Endocrinol Metab.* 2015;100(2):342-362.

18. *Diagnostic and Statistical Manual of Mental Disorders, Fifth Education,* American Psychiatric Association; 2013.

19. Brownley KA, Berkman ND, Peat CM, et al. Binge-eating disorder in adults: a systematic review and meta-analysis. *Ann Intern Med.* 2016;165:409-420.

20. Itani O, Jike M, Watanabe N, Kaneita Y. Short sleep duration and health outcome: a systematic review, meta-analysis, and meta-regression. *Sleep Med* 2017;32:246-256.

21. Reutrakul S, Van Cauter E. Sleep influences on obesity, insulin resistance, and risk of type 2 diabetes. *Metabolism.* 2018;84:56-66.

22. Hale L, Troxel W, Buysse DJ. Sleep health: an opportunity for public health to address health equity. *Annu Rev Public Health.* 2020;41:81-99.

23. *2018 Sleep in America Poll.* National Sleep Foundation. Accessed January 19, 2020. https://www.sleepfoundation.org/press-release/national-sleep-foundations-2018-sleep-american-poll-shows-americans-failing

24. *Gallop poll stress.* Accessed March 4, 2020. https://news.gallup.com/poll/249098/americans-stress-worry-anger-intensified-2018.aspx

25. American Psychological Association. *Stress in America: Stress and Current Events.* Stress in America™ Survey; 2019. Accessed January 19, 2020. https://www.apa.org/news/press/releases/stress/2019/stress-america-2019.pdf

26. McEwen BS, Wingfield JC. The concept of allostasis in biology and biomedicine. *Horm Behav.* 2003;43:2-15.

27. Cohen S, Kamarck T, Mermelstein R. A global measure of perceived stress. *J Health Soc Behav.* 1983;24:385-396.

28. Silk AW, McTigue KM. Reexamining the physical examination for obese patients. *J Am Med Assoc.* 2011;305:193-194.

29. Alberti KG, Zimmet P, Shaw J. Metabolic syndrome – A new world-wide definition. A Consensus statement from the international diabetes federation. *Diabet Med.* 2006;23:469-480.

30. Pickering TG, Hall JE, Apple LJ, et al. Recommendations for blood pressure measurement in humans and experimental animals. Part 1: blood pressure measurement in humans. A statement for professionals from the subcommittee of professional and public education of the American Heart association council on high blood pressure research. *Circulation.* 2005;111(5):697-716.

31. Lemos T, Gallagher D. Current body composition measurement techniques. *Curr Opin Endocrinol Diabetes Obes.* 2017;24(5):310-314.

32. Schutz DD, Busetto L, Dicker D, et al. European practical and patient-centred guidelines for adult obesity management in primary care. *Obes Facts.* 2019;12:40-66.

33. National Heart, Lung, and Blood Institute (NHLBI), North American Association for the Study of Obesity (NAASO). *Practical Guide to on the Identification, Evaluation, and Treatment of Overweight and Obesity in Adults.* National Institutes of Health; 2000. NIH Publication number 00-4084.

34. Katz DL. Behavior modification in primary care: the pressure system model. *Prev Med.* 2001;32:66-72.

35. Britt E, Hudson SM, Blampied NM. Motivational interviewing in health settings: a review. *Patient Educ Couns.* 2004;53:147-155.

36. Prochaska JO, Velicer WF. The transtheoretical model of health behavior change. *Am J Health Promot.* 1997;12(1):38-48.

37. Whitlock EP, Orleans CT, Pender N, Allan J. Evaluating primary care behavioral counseling intervention: an evidence-based approach. *Am J Prev Med.* 2002;22(4):267-284.

3

ASSESSMENT AND STAGING: IDENTIFICATION AND EVALUATION OF THE HIGH-RISK PATIENT

W. Timothy Garvey

CASE STUDY

A 55-year-old woman makes an appointment after being told that her fasting glucose was elevated on a worksite screening test. She has also recently noted increased shortness of breath on exertion, daytime lethargy, and low back pain. Past medical history is significant for hypertension, hypercholesterolemia, depression, and obesity. Medications include enalapril 20 mg/day, atenolol 100 mg/day, atorvastatin 40 mg/day, and paroxetine 40 mg/day.

She is single, lives alone, and likes her work as a paralegal but is guarded in social settings because of her weight. In high school, she weighed 105 lb. She lost her fiancé to an auto accident when she was 26 years of age, quit exercising, started overeating, and began showing signs of depression. She gained weight progressively until she sought help in the Weight Watchers program at the age of 50 years and lost 10 lb. However, she regained the weight due to an inability to change her lifestyle. She feels that paroxetine helps her depression, but she still lacks confidence in her ability to lose weight by changing her lifestyle. In particular, she gets hungry at night and engages in excessive snacking while watching television. She relies on fast food for lunch and often picks something up for dinner on her way home from work. She does not engage in regular exercise but she does enjoy walking her dog.

On examination, her weight = 228 lb, height = 64 inches, body mass index (BMI) = 39.1 kg/m^2, waist circumference = 38 inches, blood pressure (BP) = 144/91, heart rate (HR) = 88. The remainder of the examination is unremarkable. Laboratory tests show a fasting glucose = 118 mg/dL, HbA1c = 6.2%; lipids (mg/dL): total cholesterol = 189, low-density lipoprotein cholesterol (LDL-c) = 105, high-density lipoprotein cholesterol (HDL-c) = 42, triglycerides 194; alanine transaminase (ALT) = 95 U/L, aspartate transaminase (AST) = 34 U/L; complete blood count (CBC), creatinine, and electrocardiogram (ECG) are normal. Polysomnography done to evaluate daytime lethargy shows an apnea-hypopnea index (AHI) of 25.

CLINICAL SIGNIFICANCE

Optimal obesity care requires individualized assessment and treatment plans involving medical evaluation, a multidisciplinary team, resources for lifestyle therapy, access to medications and surgical procedures, and long-term management. However, the impact of excess adiposity on health varies widely and not all patients require intensive interventions. Like other chronic diseases, the complications of obesity are responsible for impairing health and quality of life. The presence and severity of complications vary widely among patients, and this necessitates an evaluation of complications as a guide to developing care plans and treatment goals.[1,2] Risk assessment and disease staging allow the clinician to match the aggressiveness of interventions to disease severity. More aggressive treatments can then be employed in those at high risk in a manner that optimizes effectiveness, safety, health benefits, and cost effectiveness.

An additional aspect underscores the need to individualize the treatment plan rather an employing a "one size fits all" approach. Optimal therapy entails behavior change regarding caloric intake and physical activity. A personalized treatment plan must, therefore, take into account each patient's capability for adherence to a lifestyle intervention based on personal and cultural preferences and psychological, social, and environmental factors. Interventions that do not take these factors into account are likely to lead to a poorer outcome. Accordingly, the diagnostic evaluation of obesity must provide clinical data that address psychosocial, behavioral, and environmental factors in addition to the presence of complications and their impact on quality of life. The diagnosis of overweight and obesity as well as risk stratification and determination of which treatment approaches are appropriate has historically been based on the American Heart Association (AHA) and World Health Organization (WHO) guidelines which exclusively use BMI and waist circumference. The use of new clinical staging systems that take into account other characteristics besides simply BMI provides the opportunity for healthcare providers (HCPs) to match and prioritize treatments to individuals with obesity depending upon the severity and complications of their disease.

KEY COMPONENTS OF THE PATIENT EVALUATION AND OVERALL VIEW

Figure 3.1 illustrates the clinical findings and considerations required for identifying high-risk patients with obesity. These assessments evaluate the impact of the disease on health and identify factors that place patients at risk of poor clinical outcomes. Of critical importance are findings pertaining to the risk, presence, and severity of obesity-related complications, since these complications confer morbidity and mortality and indicate that obesity is having an adverse impact on health.

Obesity is a chronic disease with opportunities for primary, secondary, and tertiary prevention. Primary prevention prevents the development of obesity in the first place and can involve health education and changing the built environment. With the development of excess adiposity but prior to emergence of complications, clinicians are in a secondary prevention mode of treatment with the goal of preventing further weight gain and the emergence of complications. Once obesity

complications are present, this signifies that the degree of adiposity regardless of the BMI level is sufficient to impair the health of the patient. The HCP is then in a tertiary prevention mode when weight loss therapy must be sufficient to prevent further disease deterioration and treat the complications. For this reason, there is an emphasis on complications that can be prevented or ameliorated with weight loss. Since the purpose of treatment is to improve the health and quality of life of the patient, the goal of weight loss therapy is to achieve sufficient weight loss to result in clinically meaningful improvements in complications and/or a reduction in the risk of complications. There are several straightforward and useful approaches to stage the severity of obesity based on the presence and severity of complications discussed below.[1,3] For the most part, these approaches use objective clinical criteria for the diagnosis of complications and assessment of the severity of complications.

In addition to the objective clinical assessment of obesity complications, it is important to assess the degree of symptom formation and functional impairment regarding complications, and the extent to which these symptoms worsen quality of life. Patients with degenerative osteoarthritis who have similar changes on knee x-ray could exhibit marked differences in the severity of symptoms as a consequence of this complication. Therefore, it is also important to assess the subjective severity of symptoms and the degree to which these symptoms adversely impact function and quality of life. These considerations are analogous to patient-reported outcomes and indicate complication severity according to the patient's experience.

Finally, the HCP must assess aggravating factors that place the patient at risk for poor outcomes. These can include medications prescribed for various purposes that promote weight gain, as well as "psychological overlay" including stigmatization, poor self-esteem, depression, or binge eating disorder, which can predominate as causes of decreased quality of life. In many patients, these factors must be incorporated into a personalized treatment approach or addressed specifically if the weight loss intervention is to be successful. Social and environmental determinants of obesity can also present obstacles to effective treatment and must be addressed in an individualized care plan. It is important to gauge

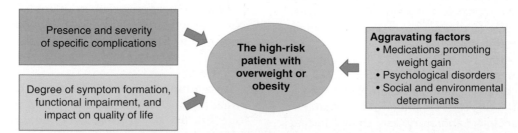

FIGURE 3.1 Identification of the high-risk patient with overweight or obesity.

factors such as personal and cultural preferences for food and physical activity, the built environment with access to unprocessed food or exercise facilities, support systems, and health literacy in developing effective lifestyle prescriptions.

These aspects of the patient evaluation will be described in more detail; however, two points are salient at this juncture. First, while these evaluations are required to identify high-risk patients, it is important to understand that this is part of the clinical assessment for all patients in treating obesity as a disease. All patients should be examined for disease complications, the impact of these complications on quality of life, and aggravating factors in devising personalized and effective treatment plans. Second, it will become clear that this does not entail an extraordinary effort on the part of the HCP outside of a standard intake evaluation consisting of an obesity-focused history, review of systems (ROS), physical examination, and appropriate laboratory tests. Like diabetes, obesity is a metabolic disease that can systemically affect multiple organ systems and involves lifestyle and behavioral change as components of therapy. The evaluation should be considered as a standard of care for medical management of obesity. The evaluation is required for the staging of all patients across the full spectrum of disease risk and severity and provides the basis for rational selection of treatment modality and intensity and for establishing goals and desired treatment outcomes.

THE DIAGNOSTIC EVALUATION OF OBESITY

Anthropometric and Clinical Components of the Diagnosis

The initial evaluation of patients with obesity was discussed in Chapter 2. Key components of the assessment are reviewed here with a focus on staging the severity of obesity and providing individualized care.

The Anthropometric Component

The identification of the high-risk patient with obesity begins with the diagnostic evaluation, which has both anthropometric and clinical components,[4] as shown in Figure 3.2. The anthropometric component is largely satisfied by BMI as outlined in the AHA guidelines. The anthropometric component of the diagnosis of "obesity" is applied to adults with BMI of ≥30 kg/m² and "overweight" with BMI 25 to 29.9 kg/m², while epidemiological data justify the lower cutoffs of BMI 23 to 24.9 kg/m² as overweight and BMI of ≥25 kg/m² as the definition of obesity in many Southeast Asian populations.[5] Waist circumference measurements provide additional information regarding fat distribution and cardiometabolic disease risk, as well as a simple measure to monitor weight loss progress that can be shared with patients.

The limitations of BMI as a measure of body fat are described in Chapter 2. Other technologies that can be used to practically measure adipose tissue mass and % body fat include bioelectric impedance plethysmography, air displacement plethysmography, and dual-energy X-ray absorptiometry (DEXA), although they are not in general use in primary care settings. Body fat percentage cut points for obesity have been proposed as 25% and 35% for men and women, respectively.[6] In most patients, an elevated BMI with clinical confirmation of excess adiposity will suffice.

The Clinical Component

While the use of BMI categories to stage patients with overweight and obesity has been useful, a major shortcoming of focusing exclusively on BMI and waist circumference is that these measures do not provide specific information about the impact of excess adiposity on the health of the patient. As with any chronic disease, complications confer morbidity and mortality and adversely affect health. For this reason, the diagnostic evaluation of obesity extends beyond the anthropometric measure

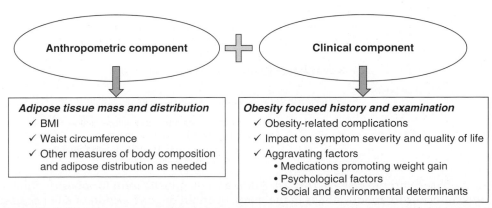

FIGURE 3.2 The diagnostic evaluation of patients with obesity has both anthropometric and clinical components. BMI, body mass index.

of BMI to include a clinical component. The clinical component of the diagnosis involves a full medical history and examination that assess the risk, presence, and severity of complications and establishes the degree to which an increase in adipose mass affects the patient's health. The development of weight-related complications varies markedly among patients at any given BMI level.[1] While the likelihood of weight-related complications generally increases as a function of progressive obesity, there can be a poor correlation between BMI and the emergence of complications. Patients with obesity need not have weight-related complications and can be free of increased risk for certain disease-related morbidity and mortality. On the other hand, patients with comparable degrees of excess adipose tissue can develop multiple cardiometabolic and biomechanical complications in a manner that is independent of the increased BMI. Thus, the clinical evaluation can provide the basis for the identification of the high-risk patient and disease staging. Since weight loss will ameliorate or prevent many weight-related complications, the clinical component of the diagnosis also helps guide the intensity and modality of treatment and helps inform the end points of therapy.

Adiposity-Based Chronic Disease

The diagnosis of obesity based only on BMI has led to confusion among the lay public and healthcare professionals regarding significance of obesity and the appreciation of obesity as a chronic disease.[4] This is primarily because BMI conveys little information about complications associated with excess adiposity that adversely affect health. Furthermore, the term obesity carries with it stigma that can generate negative perceptions

about the personal character of patients, generating guilt, depression, and shame. The bias and uncertainty regarding health implications help perpetuate factors that limit access of patients to effective therapy. Adiposity-based chronic disease (ABCD) has been proposed as a diagnostic term that conceptualizes obesity as a chronic disease associated with complications, considers the pathophysiological basis of the disease, and avoids the stigmata, ambiguity, differential use, and multiple meanings of the term obesity.[7,8] This term alludes to what we are treating and why we are treating it. As illustrated in Figure 3.3, the phrase "adiposity-based" is used because the disease is primarily due to abnormalities in the mass, distribution, and/or function of adipose tissue. The phrase "chronic disease" is apropos because the disease is lifelong, associated with complications that confer morbidity and mortality, and has a natural history that offers opportunities for primary, secondary, and tertiary prevention. Abnormalities in adipose tissue mass predispose to biomechanical complications, and defects in the function and distribution of adipose tissue lead to cardiometabolic disease complications as well as other health problems. The new diagnostic term provides a conceptual basis that can help inform and structure the evaluation and diagnosis of patients with obesity, as well as identifying high-risk patients suffering from disease complications. The term ABCD underscores the principle that the diagnostic evaluation of obesity as a disease will require both anthropometric and clinical components. Finally, ABCD is a new disease coding and classification system that has been proposed as an alternative to the current International Classification of Diseases (ICD) paradigm, which provides rational implications for diagnosis, disease staging, treatment, and billing for medical services.[9]

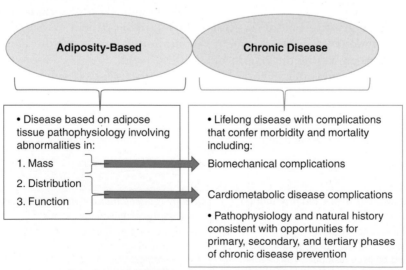

FIGURE 3.3 Adiposity-based chronic disease (ABCD). ABCD as a diagnostic term for obesity signifies: (1) "what we are treating" which relates to abnormalities in the mass, distribution, or function of adipose tissue, and (2) "why we are treating it" as a chronic disease which is to prevent or ameliorate obesity complications that confer morbidity and mortality and impair the quality of life.

History, Physical Examination, and Clinical Laboratory

Consistent with general standards of clinical care, patients with the disease of obesity require an initial medical evaluation with history, ROS, physical examination, and laboratory testing. In addition to a generalized clinical assessment, these components are adapted in specific ways to evaluate the impact of excess adiposity on health and to obtain information needed to develop a personalized care plan. Details of the comprehensive evaluation process are discussed in Chapter 2.

Aggravating Factors

In the context of the high-risk patient, certain aspects of the evaluation deserve emphasis. A care plan that is not individualized places the patient at risk of poor outcomes due to nonadherence, and this requires that key pieces of information be obtained during the initial evaluation. This includes personal and cultural preferences for diet and physical activity in formulating lifestyle prescriptions. In addition, certain aggravating factors exacerbate obesity and should be accounted for in a personalized management plan, as shown in Table 3.1. These factors are unique to each patient in the natural history of their disease and are critically important in designing personalized approaches for effective treatment. There are three general categories of aggravating factors: medications that promote weight gain, psychological and psychiatric factors, and social and environmental determinants of health.[9] In many patients, treatment will not be successful unless these issues are addressed and incorporated into a personalized therapeutic plan.

Medications that can promote weight gain should be identified and consideration given to possibly discontinuing these or substituting them with a weight neutral alternative (see Chapter 8 on Pharmacotherapy). Psychological factors can also contribute to obesity and mitigate against successful treatment outcomes unless these issues are addressed directly as a component of the care plan. Depression, anxiety, stress, stigmatization, and binge eating should be assessed as contributors to obesity on an individual basis. Specific interventions including counseling, medications, or referrals that address psychological factors may be required to assure optimal effectiveness of lifestyle and medical therapy.

Social and environmental determinants of obesity can directly impact the feasibility and effectiveness of the care plan, and it is important to be aware of these factors and act to minimize their adverse impact on successful treatment. Poor health literacy, limited access to healthcare facilities, and absence of insurance impair

TABLE 3.1 Aggravating Factors and Social and Environmental Determinants		
	FACTORS AFFECTING INDIVIDUALIZED CARE PLAN	**POSSIBLE INTERVENTIONS**
Medications	Examples: insulin, TZDs, sulfonylureas; β-adrenergic receptor blockers; antipsychotics; certain antidepressants; antiepileptics; glucocorticoids	• Assess the need for offending medication • Substitute with weight neutral alternative

Psychological/ psychiatric factors	• Depression
	• Anxiety disorder
	• Psychosis
	• Binge eating disorder
	• Night eating syndrome
	• Stigmatization
	• Stress
		• Psychological screening
		• Counseling
		• Referral
		• Medications
		  • Antidepressants
		  • Anxiolytics
		  • Antiobesity medications to address cravings

Social and environmental determinants	• Behaviors • Cultural factors • Time management • Access to unprocessed foods • Physical activity resources • Work related • Health literacy • Access to clinics/hospitals • Economic status • Health insurance	• Motivational interviewing • Counseling (personal and family) • Dietitian referral • Education • Social work referral • Information regarding community resources

TZDs, thiazolidinediones.

the empowerment of patients for self-care and the availability of evidence-based treatments. Lack of access to unprocessed and healthy foods or outlets for physical activity can reduce the effectiveness of prescriptions for lifestyle therapy. Behavioral attributes, cultural preferences, work patterns, and time management issues can also impede therapeutic success if not identified and addressed. Solutions to address these social and environmental determinants can involve culturally appropriate education and lifestyle modifications, individualized counseling, and referrals to social workers, registered dietitian nutritionist (RDN), and community resources.

Obesity Due to Overt Etiologic Influences and Genetic Abnormalities

Most patients with obesity have idiopathic or common type disease without an overt etiologic cause. Idiopathic obesity arises from the interaction of over 900 identified susceptibility genes,[10] each conferring a small relative disease risk, which then interact with each other and with biological, environmental, and behavioral factors unique to each individual. However, HCPs should be aware that a minority of patients will have obesity that can be directly attributed to identifiable causal influences. While obesity due to overt causal influences is less common, these patients may require specific modalities of therapy and attention to specific patterns of complications. These include genetic mutations or chromosomal abnormalities producing forms of monogenic or syndromic obesity. Table 3.2 lists features of the medical history, family history, and physical findings that can provide a clue as to whether a genetic form of obesity may be present. Other patients with overt causal inferences may have obesity arising from or aggravated by endocrine disease or disability/immobility. The HCP should be alerted to hallmark findings in the history and physical examination that portend the presence of these disease processes, as shown in Table 3.2. This is critical in evaluating and identifying high-risk patients and has direct implications regarding the development of effective therapeutic interventions. Patients with overt causes of obesity may need to be referred to geneticists, endocrinologists, or rehabilitation medicine specialists for subspecialty care.

IDENTIFICATION AND STAGING OF THE HIGH-RISK PATIENT WITH OBESITY

Complications of Obesity/ABCD

The presence and severity of obesity complications constitute the basis for the identification of the high-risk patient. Many complications of obesity can be ameliorated or reversed by weight loss.[1] The treatable complications

comprise three pathophysiological categories, namely, biomechanical, cardiometabolic, and abnormalities involving sex steroids. Since these complications confer morbidity and impair health, the goal of therapy is to achieve sufficient weight loss to treat and reverse these complications in the management of obesity as a disease. Other complications are not responsive to weight loss therapy. An example is gall stones which can be exacerbated by weight loss. Another example is depression that occurs with increased frequency in patients with obesity. While depression may improve during therapy, the beneficial effects are largely not related to the degree of weight loss and might be explained as a function of increased contact and care by healthcare professionals.[1] For this reason, depression, binge eating, stigmatization, poor self-esteem, and other psychological disorders are considered as aggravating factors that can drive weight gain and need to be addressed in developing effective individualized care plans, sometimes requiring specific treatment (Table 3.1).

Within the context of the ABCD staging system,[7] biomechanical complications arise due to an increase in adipose tissue mass and produce impairment in mechanical function including obstructive sleep apnea, obesity-hypoventilation syndrome, osteoarthritis of knee or hip, urinary stress incontinence, gastroesophageal reflux disease, pain syndromes, and immobility/disability. Cardiometabolic complications arise due to abnormalities in the distribution and function of adipose tissue and a pathophysiological process that produces both end-stage metabolic and vascular sequela.[11] The progression of cardiometabolic complications begins with insulin resistance, progresses to the high-risk states of metabolic syndrome (MetS) and pre-diabetes, and then culminates in type 2 diabetes (T2D), nonalcoholic steatohepatitis (NASH), cardiovascular disease (CVD), or all three in single individuals. Dyslipidemia is characterized by increased triglycerides, decreased HDL-c, and increased concentration of atherogenic small dense LDL particles without necessarily an overall increase in LDL-c. Obesity exacerbates insulin resistance and can propel cardiometabolic disease progression toward T2D and CVD.[11] Thus, beyond simple increases in adipose tissue mass causing biomechanical complications, abnormalities in adipose tissue function and distribution are causally involved in the pathogenesis of cardiometabolic complications in obesity.[7] An additional category of complications involves sex steroids leading to abnormal gonadal function and infertility in patients with polycystic ovary syndrome, female infertility, and male hypogonadism.

Table 3.3 lists obesity complications by organ system that HCPs should evaluate in the management of high-risk patients with obesity. The table delineates symptoms, physical examination findings, and clinical laboratory relevant to each complication. In some

TABLE 3.2 Underlying Causes of or Aggravating Factors Causing Obesity		
CAUSE OF OBESITY	**SPECIFIC DISORDER**	**SIGNS AND SYMPTOMS**
Monogenic or syndromic	Prader-Willi syndrome	• Onset in childhood • Strong family history • Infertility/hypogonadism • Delayed or absent puberty • Short stature or macrosomia • Intellectual disability • Behavior problems • Unexplained organ system defects (e.g., heart, kidney) • Visual or olfactory impairment • Dysmorphic features (e.g., face, digits)
	MC4R deficiency	
	Leptin deficiency	
	Leptin receptor deficiency	
	POMC deficiency	
	Alström syndrome	
	Bardet-Biedl syndrome	
	Beckwith-Wiedemann syndrome	
	WAGR-O syndrome (BDNF deficiency)	
	Wilson-Turner syndrome	
Aggravating endocrine disorders	Hypothyroidism	• Cold intolerance, lethargy, weakness • Constipation • Delayed reflexes • Bradycardia
	Hypercortisolism	• Weakness, poor concentration • Bruising and purple striae • Acne, moon facies • Thin skin and central fat redistribution
	Hypothalamic/CNS injury	• Lethargy • Decreased libido • Polyuria
Aggravated by disability	Immobilization	• Muscle weakness • Gait abnormality • Disability evident on presentation
	Neuromuscular disease or injury	
	Movement disorder	
Idiopathic/common type		• Most common • Diagnosis of exclusion • No identifiable causal influence

BDNF, brain-derived neurotrophic factor; CNS, central nervous system POMC, pro-opiomelanocortin, WAGR-O, Wilms tumor, aniridia, genitourinary anomalies, and mental retardation and obesity.

instances, further testing beyond the intake evaluation may be necessary for the diagnosis and assessing the severity of individual complications.

Disease Staging and the High-Risk Patient

In addition to identification of complications, it is also important to assess their severity, impact on quality of life, and aggravating factors (Table 3.1) that place the patient at high risk for poor disease outcomes unless these factors are taken into account in formulating the treatment plan.

While several staging systems have been proposed, two have emerged as particularly useful for assessing overall disease severity. The American Association of Clinical Endocrinologists (AACE) Obesity Guidelines advocate a simple and clinically useful paradigm,[1] as illustrated in Figure 3.4. Each complication is evaluated for severity and impact on the patient's health. Stage 0 is identified when no complication is present; stage 1, if any and all complications are mild-moderate; or stage 2, if at least one complication is severe. The adjudication of a complication as mild-moderate versus severe is based on criteria unique to each complication and,

TABLE 3.3 Examination, Review of Systems (ROS), and Laboratory Findings for the Identification of Weight-Related Complications

ORGAN SYSTEM	ROS	EXAMINATION	LABORATORY FINDING	COMPLICATION	FURTHER TESTING
Anthropometric Component of the Diagnosis of Obesity					
Adipose tissue		BMI, waist circumference Exclude: muscularity, edema, sarcopenia, solid tumor mass, lipodystrophy		• **Increased adipose tissue mass**	Impedance plethysmography, DEXA scan
Clinical Component of the Diagnosis of Obesity					
Diabetes	Symptoms of hyperglycemia	Foot examination	Fasting glucose, HbA1c	• **Prediabetes**	HbA1c 5.7%-6.4% or fasting glucose 100-125 mg/dL
				• **Diabetes**	HbA1c ≥ 6.5% or fasting glucose ≥126 mg/dL
Insulin resistance		Waist circumference, blood pressure, acanthosis nigricans	Fasting glucose, lipid panel	• **Metabolic syndrome** • **Dyslipidemia** • **Hypertension**	Non-HDL-c or apoB-100 may further define risk; ambulatory BP monitoring
Liver		Enlarged liver, firm liver edge	LFTs, NASH biomarker scoring	• **NAFLD** • **NASH**	Ultrasound, consider referral, biopsy
Cardiovascular	Chest pain, syncope, orthopnea, SOB, claudication, stroke/TIAs	Heart examination, ABI, carotid auscultation, edema	ECG	• **CAD** • **CVD** • **PVD** • **CHF**	Stress test, imaging, arteriography, or ultrasound, consider referral
Pulmonary	Fatigue, snoring, poor sleep, SOB, poor exercise tolerance	Neck circumference, lung examination (wheezing, rales)		• **Obstructive sleep apnea** • **Asthma**	Polysomnography (clinical laboratory or home testing), spirometry, consider referral
Endocrine	Lethargy, weakness, skin changes, hair loss, trouble concentrating, acne, decreased libido, cold intolerance	Skin and hair abnormalities, pigmented striae, fat distribution, proximal muscle weakness, abnormal muscle reflexes, abnormal thyroid		• **Hypothyroidism** • **Hypercortisolism** • **Hypopituitarism** • **Hypothalamic/ CNS injury**	Hormone testing, endocrine gland imaging, consider referral
Sex steroids	Oligomenorrhea, infertility	Hirsutism	Testosterone, estradiol LH/ FSH	• **PCOS** • **Infertility**	Imaging of ovaries, consider referral

TABLE 3.3 Examination, Review of Systems (ROS), and Laboratory Findings for the Identification of Weight-Related Complications (Continued)

ORGAN SYSTEM	ROS	EXAMINATION	LABORATORY FINDING	COMPLICATION	FURTHER TESTING
Musculoskeletal	Joint pain, limited motion	Swelling, crepitus		• **Osteoarthritis**	Radiographic imaging
Gastrointestinal	Heartburn, abdominal pain	Abdominal tenderness	LFTs	• **GERD** • **Cholelithiasis/ cystitis**	Endoscopy, esophageal motility study, abdominal imaging, consider referral
Urinary tract	Stress incontinence			• **Urinary stress incontinence**	Urine culture, consider referral, urodynamic testing
Psychological	Depressed, suicidal ideation, anxiety, stigmatization, binge eating, drugs, and alcohol			• **Depression Anxiety disorder Psychosis Binge eating syndrome, Night eating syndrome Stigmatization Stress**	Validated questionnaires, psychological testing and evaluation, consider referral
Impaired functional capacity	Impaired activities of daily living, immobility	Weakness, paralysis, limited motion		• **Immobilization** • **Neurological disease/injury**	Functional testing may be helpful

ABI, ankle-brachial index; BMI, body mass index; BP, blood pressure; CAD, coronary artery disease; CHF, congestive heart failure; CNS, central nervous system; CVD, cardiovascular disease; DEXA, dual-energy X-ray absorptiometry; ECG, electrocardiograph; GERD, gastroesophageal reflux disease; HDL-c, high-density lipoprotein cholesterol; LFT, liver function tests; LH/TSH, luteinizing hormone/follicle-stimulating hormone; NAFLD, nonalcoholic fatty liver disease; NASH, nonalcoholic steatohepatitis; PCOS, polycystic ovary syndrome; PVD, peripheral vascular disease; SOB, shortness of breath; TIA, transient ischemic attack.

in many instances, will depend upon clinical judgment together with objective findings and quantitative measures. In addition to severity determined by physical findings or objective laboratory measures, an important question is the degree to which the complication affects subjective symptom formation, patient-reported outcomes, impaired function, and adverse impact on quality of life. Since weight loss is well documented as an effective treatment for most obesity complications, patients with severe disease based on clinical findings and/or symptomatology can be treated more aggressively with weight loss therapies to improve health. Thus, the AACE staging approach provides guidance for the selection of therapeutic modality and intensity (Figure 3.4).

A recent proposal for a medically actionable coding system for obesity provides examples of potential criteria designating disease severity for specific obesity-related complications, with the provision that actual criteria are determined by data and expert opinion relevant to each complication.[9] Clinical judgment is required in staging disease severity based on both the interpretation of objective clinical measurements and the degree to which complications impair quality of life.

The Edmonton Obesity Staging System is another useful staging approach that evaluates the medical, psychological, and functional impact of obesity in aggregate and proposes five stages ranging from no limitations to severe impairment (Figure 3.5).[3] Stage 0 reflects no disease complications, psychological symptoms, or functional limitations. Stage 1 indicates subclinical factors and mild physical and psychological impairments that do not require medical intervention for obesity, and these patients should be managed using other preventive options.[13] Stage 1 includes patients with prehypertension, prediabetes, MetS, and elevated liver enzymes. In stage 2, patients have established obesity complications, such as T2D, obstructive sleep apnea, or osteoarthritis, requiring medical intervention together with moderate psychological or functional limitations. Stage 3 indicates significant end-organ damage, for example, CVD events or diabetes

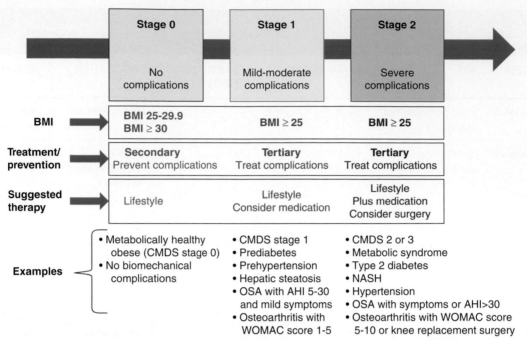

FIGURE 3.4 Staging the severity of obesity using the AACE clinical practice guidelines. AHI, apnea-hypopnea index; BMI, body mass index; CMDS, cardiometabolic disease staging; NASH, nonalcoholic steatohepatitis; OSA, obstructive sleep apnea; WOMAC, Western Ontario and McMaster Universities Osteoarthritis Index and is a patient-reported outcome measure for osteoarthritis registering pain, stiffness, and function.[12]

complications, significant psychological symptoms (major depression, suicidality), and impairment of well-being. Stage 4 represents disabling and end-stage disease. Clearly, these classifications also have implications regarding the intensity of treatment for obesity.

Special consideration must be given to staging patients with cardiometabolic disease before they develop the end-stage manifestations of T2D, CVD, and NASH. These conditions exert a huge burden on patient suffering and social costs and can be prevented

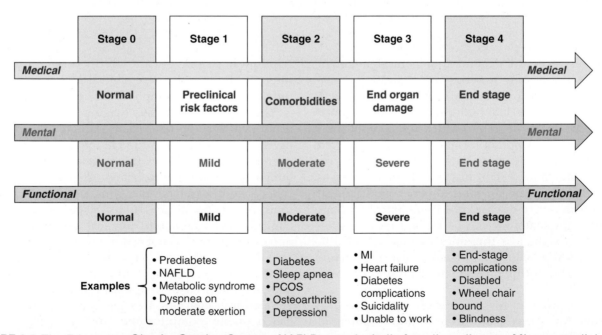

FIGURE 3.5 The Edmonton Obesity Staging System. NAFLD, nonalcoholic fatty liver disease; MI, myocardial infarction; PCOS, polycystic ovary syndrome. (Adapted from Sharma AM, Kushner RF. A proposed clinical staging system for obesity. *Int J Obes (Lond).* 2009;33(3):289-295.)

TABLE 3.4 The Cardiometabolic Disease Staging System for Prediction of Diabetes in Patients With Overweight or Obesity

STAGE	CRITERIA	SPECIFICATIONS
0	No risk factors	Metabolically healthy obese
1	One or two risk factors	Waist, blood pressure, triglycerides, HDL-c
2	Metabolic syndrome or prediabetes	Only one of the following: metabolic syndrome or IFG or IGT
3	Metabolic syndrome plus prediabetes	Two or more of the following: metabolic syndrome, IFG, IGT
4	T2DM and/or CVD	End-stage cardiometabolic disease

CVD, cardiovascular disease; HDL-c, high-density lipoprotein cholesterol; IFG, impaired fasting glucose; IGT, impaired glucose tolerance; T2DM, type 2 diabetes mellitus.
Adapted from Guo F, Moellering DR, Garvey WT. The progression of cardiometabolic disease: validation of a new cardiometabolic disease staging system applicable to obesity. Obesity. 2014;22:110-118.

via weight loss. Patients with overweight/obesity at high risk for these end-stage manifestations of cardiometabolic disease have prediabetes, MetS, hepatic steatosis, and prehypertension. These early indications of cardiometabolic disease are quite common; for example, 34.5% of adults in the US NHANES sample population have prediabetes.[14] Given the large pool of at-risk patients with MetS and/or prediabetes, it is not feasible to treat all patients with obesity aggressively using structured lifestyle interventions and obesity medications. However, the risk for developing the end-stage manifestations of T2D, CVD, and NASH varies greatly, and this presents opportunities for identifying and targeting patients at higher risk for more aggressive interventions.

One approach HCPs can simply and accurately stage patients for risk of future diabetes is referred to as Cardiometabolic Disease Staging (CMDS) (Table 3.4).[15,16] This framework uses quantitative data readily available to HCPs treating obesity to stratify risk of progression to T2D. Using MetS traits (Table 3.5), namely values for waist circumference, blood pressure, fasting glucose, triglycerides, and HDL-c, HCPs can stratify risk of progression to T2D over 40-fold among patients with overweight/obesity, as shown in Figure 3.6. The lowest risk stratum consists of patients with overweight/obesity who have no MetS traits and represent metabolically healthy obesity. However, having one or two traits, or meeting criteria for MetS or prediabetes but not both, confers progressively higher risk for future diabetes.

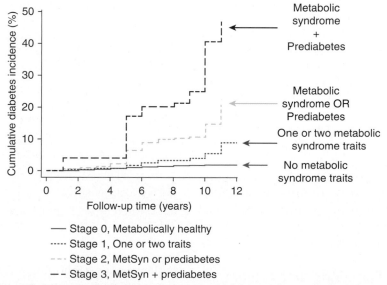

FIGURE 3.6 Cumulative risk of developing diabetes among patients with overweight or obesity. Validation of the prediction of incident diabetes in the CARDIA Study cohort. (Modified from Guo F, Moellering DR, Garvey WT. The progression of cardiometabolic disease: validation of a new cardiometabolic disease staging system applicable to obesity. *Obesity.* 2014;22:110-118.)

TABLE 3.5 ATP III Criteria for Metabolic Syndrome (Must Have at Least Three of These Five Risk Factors)

RISK FACTOR	DEFINING LEVEL
1. Waist	≥40 in (102 cm) men
	≥35 in (88 cm) women
2. Triglycerides	≥150 mg/dL (1.7 mmol/L)
3. HDL-c	<40 mg/dL (1.03 mmol/L) men
	<50 mg/dL (1.29 mmol/L) women
4. Blood pressure	≥130/≥85 mm Hg
5. Fasting glucose	≥100 mg/dL (5.6 mmol/L)

ATP III, Adult Treatment Panel III; HDL-c, high-density lipoprotein cholesterol.

The highest risk stratum consists of patients who meet criteria for both prediabetes and MetS. For patients in high-risk stratum, weight loss effectively prevents progression to diabetes with a lower "number-needed-to-treat" and with a superior benefit/risk ratio.[17] Given the rising personal and social cost of diabetes, clinicians and healthcare systems can use this strategy to identify patients with obesity at high risk for diabetes and employ more aggressive interventions in those patients who will most benefit.

Despite the wide variation in diabetes risk among patients with insulin resistance, prediabetes, or MetS, all these patients would be classified as Edmonton stage 1 (subclinical factors).[3,13] CMDS and the AACE system provide more discrimination of risk in this large pool of patients with cardiometabolic disease risk factors. Patients in CMDS risk stratum 0 (no traits) would be AACE stage 0 (no complications); CMDS stratum 1 (one or two traits) would be AACE stage 1 (mild-moderate risk); and CMDS strata 2 (MetS or prediabetes) and risk stratum 3 (MetS plus prediabetes) would be AACE stage 2 (severe risk of diabetes). Thus, the AACE staging would call for concerted efforts at weight loss therapy in the higher risk strata of patients. Clinics or healthcare systems could develop policy to aggressively treat high-risk patients with CMDS strata 2 or 3 to prevent diabetes in order to augment benefit/risk of the intervention and with greater cost effectiveness. With these assessments, HCPs can target higher risk patients, among the large number of patients with obesity, with more aggressive weight loss therapies to prevent diabetes.

Symptom Formation, Functional Impairment, and Quality of Life

In addition to the identification of complications and objective clinical measures for rating severity, it is important to assess the degree of symptom formation related to complications and the impact these have on quality of life. These subjective factors can vary among patients independent of objective measures of disease severity. For example, a patient who has a formal sleep study that objectively demonstrates moderate obstructive sleep apnea may be asymptomatic and without psychological or metabolic sequela and could be evaluated as AACE stage 1. Others with the similar scores may experience debilitating symptoms of poor sleep, fatigue, depression, poor productivity, and diminished ability to enjoy life. The sleep apnea in these latter patients could be clinically assessed as severe or stage 2 based on these symptoms. Thus, pronounced symptom formation adversely affecting quality of life can warrant more aggressive interventions.

Patient-reported outcomes indicate how each patient experiences obesity and its complications.[18] The HCP should query the patient regarding severity of symptoms that specifically arise from individual complications, for example, symptoms listed in the ROS in Table 3.3. HCPs can ascertain this information with their own series of questions (see sample questions to assess quality of life) or self-report questionnaires that address relevant issues: physical functioning and activities of daily living (walking, bending over, bathing, and dressing), energy level and outlook on life, emotional impact of obesity (self-image, self-esteem and confidence, depression, anxiety), interest in sexual activity, productivity at work, and comfort level for social interactions.

Sample Questions to Assess Patient-Reported Outcomes and Impact of Obesity on Quality of Life

Patients can address each of these points individually using a 5-point scale:

1. Physical functioning and activities of daily living (walking, bending over, bathing, and dressing)
2. Energy level and outlook on life
3. Emotional impact of obesity (self-image, self-esteem and confidence, depression, anxiety)
4. Interest in sexual activity
5. Productivity at work
6. Comfort level for social interactions

Many patients following weight loss therapy may experience less pain, greater mobility, enhanced self-esteem and confidence, a greater degree of comfort in social settings, higher energy and productivity, and renewed interest in life. These factors can account for the greatest increments in quality of life and can be the most rewarding part of treatment for both patient and the HCP.

SUMMARY: THE HIGH-RISK PATIENT AND THERAPEUTIC IMPLICATIONS

As with most illnesses, the HCP must assimilate and interpret a range of data in order to formulate a personalized treatment plan for obesity with interventions and treatment goals effectively designed for each patient. The diagnostic evaluation and disease staging needed to identify high-risk patients provide this information for all patients with obesity, as illustrated in Figure 3.7.

The dual aspects of the diagnostic evaluation, the anthropometric and clinical components, provide the information needed for disease staging. First, patients with obesity due to overt causal influences (e.g., genetic forms, endocrine disorders, and immobility) are identified distinct from the much larger numbers of patients with common-type obesity. Second, consistent with the ABCD diagnostic term, the evaluation confirms the presence of abnormalities in the mass, distribution, and function of adipose tissue and the presence and severity of obesity complications that confer morbidity and mortality.[7] The severity of these complications are used to stage the severity of the disease and its impact on the patient's health. The AACE Obesity Guidelines staging[1] or Edmonton staging approach[3] can be used to globally assess disease severity, and CMDS can be used to stratify the large number of patients with overweight/obesity for differential risk of future diabetes. Thus, the staging uniquely corresponds to each individual patient

and reflects the complication burden with an emphasis on complications that can be reversed or improved with weight loss.

Staging has clear implications for guiding decisions regarding the mode and intensity of treatment. Using the AACE Obesity Guidelines approach,[1] uncomplicated overweight or obesity (stage 0) warrants secondary prevention strategies designed to prevent further weight gain and/or to promote weight loss with the goal of preventing the emergence of complications. A structured lifestyle intervention may be appropriate at this stage. Once complications develop, it is evident that the excess adiposity is adversely affecting the health of the patient irrespective of the BMI class, and a more intensive approach to management is indicated. Tertiary prevention/treatment is then required to achieve sufficient weight loss with the goals of ameliorating the complications and preventing further deterioration due to the disease. In patients with mild to moderate complications (stage 1), consideration should be given to combined lifestyle and antiobesity medications as needed to ameliorate the specific complications present. For moderate to severe complications (stage 2), the addition of pharmacotherapy is appropriate and bariatric surgery should be considered in selected patients. Thus, the diagnostic framework that combines a measure of adiposity and an assessment of the presence and severity of weight-related complications is actionable in that it aids in therapeutic decisions. This is consistent with the "complications-centric" approach to obesity management as advocated by the AACE.[1,2] This medical approach to treatment of obesity as a disease employs

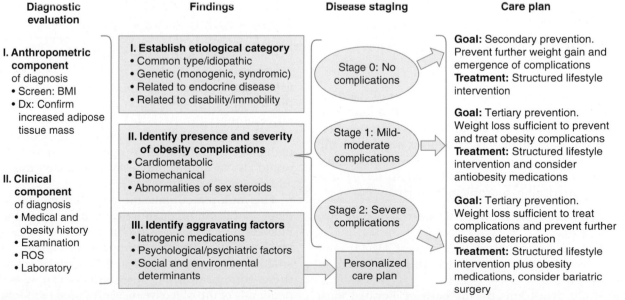

FIGURE 3.7 Diagnostic evaluation and disease staging: implications regarding therapy. Staging provides a guide for selecting the modality and intensity of therapy as well as treatment goals. BMI, body mass index; ROS, review of systems.

weight loss therapy to treat or prevent weight-related complications as the primary end point of therapy over a singular focus on the degree of weight loss per se.

However, there are additional considerations in identifying high-risk patients. First, aggravating factors place the patient at high risk of poor outcomes unless these factors are primarily addressed. These include medications that promote weight gain, psychological disorders that might require counseling or other therapy, and social and environment determinants of health that limit accessibility to evidence-based interventions or the ability to adhere to lifestyle prescriptions.[9] In addition, the HCP must make clinical judgments regarding the impact of the disease on symptomatology and quality of life. Symptomatology can vary among patients with similar complication severity assessed by objective measures, and this must be taken into account in assessing the adverse impact on health and quality of life. Thus, identification of the high-risk patient with obesity requires both objective measures and findings, patient-reported outcomes, as well as clinical judgment.

It should be clear from this discussion that obesity is a chronic disease that can exert a heavy burden of suffering. The care of patients requires a medical model that addresses the impact of the disease on health and the development of individualized treatment plans based on diagnostic evaluation and disease staging. In particular, it is important to identify the high-risk patient for more aggressive interventions in a manner that enhances the benefit/risk ratio. Treatment that takes into account the medical consequences of obesity allows the opportunity to more effectively manage obesity as a disease.

CASE STUDY

Discussion

Diagnosis

Regarding the **anthropometric component** of the diagnosis, it is clear that the patient has class II obesity with a BMI of 39 kg/m^2 and an elevated waist circumference. The **clinical component** of the diagnosis begins with the identification of obesity complications with an emphasis on those that can be treated by weight loss. These can be summarized in a problem list format:

1. Hypertension not at optimal control despite two medications.
2. Prediabetes, evident on the basis of HbA1c and confirmed by fasting glucose, both in the range of prediabetes.
3. Metabolic syndrome, on the basis of elevated waist circumference, blood pressure, triglycerides, and fasting glucose as well as reduced HDL-c.

4. Obstructive sleep apnea, with an AHI of 25 on polysomnography which is in the moderate range of severity.

The overall diagnosis is ABCD complicated by hypertension, prediabetes, metabolic syndrome, and obstructive sleep apnea. The patient had an elevated BMI that was confirmed to represent excessive adipose tissue since the patient did not exhibit high muscularity, edema, or other factors that could alter BMI independent of adipose mass. In the clinical component of the diagnosis of ABCD, the patient suffers from multiple **cardiometabolic complications** of obesity including prediabetes, metabolic syndrome, hypertension, and dyslipidemia, which are indicative of underlying insulin resistance and abnormalities in adipose tissue function and distribution. The patient also has a **biomechanical complication** attributable to an abnormality in adipose tissue mass, namely obstructive sleep apnea. Therefore, excess adiposity is clearly affecting the patient's health. The presence of an elevated ALT is possibly indicative of NASH as an additional cardiometabolic disease complication.

Staging

The severity of ABCD in this patient is AACE stage 2 based on the presence of multiple severe complications.[1] First, she qualifies for the diagnosis of both metabolic syndrome and prediabetes. This places the patient in the highest risk category of CMDS with 10-year risk of diabetes that is 40-fold higher than obesity without metabolic syndrome traits (i.e., the metabolically healthy obese), as shown in Figure 3.5. The Edmonton system stage for these complications would be preclinical stage 1 where patients are not targeted for medical management.[13] The AACE Guidelines and staging would instead strongly recommend aggressive weight management given this CMDS category to prevent progression to diabetes and improve CVD risk factors. Hypertension would also merit a severity category of AACE stage 2 with blood pressure not optimally controlled despite the use of two hypertension medications. Finally, the polysomnography AHI indicates moderate disease. However, as discussed below, symptom formation attributable to this complication (marked daytime lethargy) would also move this into a severe category due to the adverse impact on quality of life.

The multiple complications in this patient are all diagnosed based on quantitative clinical data. However, in assessing severity, it is also important to assess **symptom formation, functional impact, and quality of life**, analogous to patient-reported outcomes related to these complications. These aspects can vary independently of the objective measures used to identify the complications. The patient has daytime lethargy which can be attributed to the obstructive sleep apnea. The dyspnea on exertion could also be due to the mechanical effects of obesity in the absence of other causes such as congestive heart failure or lung disease. Thus, the increase in adipose tissue mass is impairing functionality and quality of life.

It is also important to assess **aggravating factors** that place the patient at high risk of poor outcomes unless these are accommodated in a personalized management plan. Aggravating factors include medications that promote weight gain, psychological factors, and the social and environmental determinants of health. First, the patient is on two medications that can exacerbate weight gain, atenolol and paroxetine. The atenolol could be replaced with a weight neutral selective beta blocker for hypertension (e.g., carvedilol) or a calcium channel blocker. Similarly, the paroxetine could be substituted for an antidepressant that is less likely to contribute to weight gain (e.g.,

venlafaxine or bupropion) perhaps in consultation with her psychiatrist. Aggravating factors also include the psychological overlay of obesity. In addition to depression, it is clear from the obesity-focused medical history that the patient experiences stigmatization being guarded in social settings and feelings of ineffectiveness regarding her ability to make changes in her life. Social determinants include the sedentary nature of employment and poor social support since she lives alone, does not have family living in her city, and few friends perhaps related to stigmatization. She does not do much cooking, picks up fast foods for many lunches and dinners, and has food cravings while watching television at night. Thus, the patient could benefit from psychological counseling and a dietitian referral.

The diagnostic evaluation and staging of this high-risk patient is summarized in Table 3.6.

TABLE 3.6 Disease Staging for the High-Risk Case Study Patient

COMPLICATION		AACE STAGE	RATIONALE
Cardiometabolic	Metabolic syndrome	AACE Stage 2	Meets criteria for both prediabetes and metabolic syndrome placing the patient in the highest CMDS risk stratum for future diabetes
	Prediabetes		
	Hypertension	AACE Stage 2	Blood pressure not at target despite two hypertension medications
Biomechanical	Obstructive sleep apnea	AACE Stage 2	The AHI at polysomnography consistent with moderate severity but symptom of marked daytime lethargy indicates that this complication should be treated at a higher level of severity

Aggravating Factors to Be Considered in Developing an Effective Treatment Plan

Category	Factor	Solution
Iatrogenic	Atenolol and paroxetine could contribute to obesity	Switch to calcium channel blocker for hypertension and bupropion or venlafaxine for depression
Psychological	Depression	Consider referral to psychologist; continue medication
	Nighttime food cravings	Antiobesity medication to blunt cravings; dietitian referral
	Stigmatization (guarded in social settings)	Consider referral to psychologist; counseling; education about obesity as a disease; motivational interviewing
	Feelings of ineffectiveness	
Social and environmental	Sedentary job (paralegal)	Engage in progressively longer walks with dog in the evening
	Reliance on fast food	Encouraged to have "dinner nights" with coworker taking turns several times per week to prepare dinner with leftovers for lunch on the next day. Dietitian referral

AACE, American Association of Clinical Endocrinologists; CMDS, Cardiometabolic Disease Staging.

Therapeutic Implications of Diagnosis and Staging

This patient has severe ABCD and aggressive management is warranted. Weight loss would be predicted to (1) prevent or delay progression to diabetes in this high-risk patient, (2) improve control of hypertension without the need to add an additional antihypertensive medication, (3) lower triglycerides and improve other CVD risk factors, and (4) improve sleep apnea with respect to both symptoms and the AHI. In patients with AACE stage 2, the guidance is to treat with lifestyle intervention plus an antiobesity medication and to consider bariatric surgery (Figure 3.5).[1] A relevant question is how much weight loss is needed to treat the patient's complications. For prevention of diabetes, 10% weight loss is superior to a 5% weight loss based on the Diabetes Prevention Program[19] and clinical trials with antiobesity medications.[20,21] In the Look AHEAD study, there was a "dose-dependent" improvement in comorbidities with weight loss, including ≥15% weight loss for lowering blood pressure and triglycerides in patients with type 2 diabetes.[22] Furthermore, 10% or more weight loss is needed to predictably improve the AHI in sleep apnea.[1] On balance, while a 5% weight loss produces meaningful health benefits, the HCP could aim for at least 10% weight loss in this patient, and this is something that can be obtained in many patients using lifestyle modification plus antiobesity medications. Medications would help address the patient's problems with food cravings in the evenings. Based on the information relevant to aggravating factors, the treatment plan should also include substitution of medications that promote weight gain with alternatives, motivational interviewing, and potentially referrals to a psychologist and dietitian.

CLINICAL HIGHLIGHTS

- Current staging systems that focus primarily on BMI and waist circumference to assess risks of excess adiposity do not allow treatment to be tailored to individual patients who vary in the degree to which weight affects their health and quality of life.
- The term adiposity-based chronic disease (ABCD) more accurately reflects the nature of the disease of obesity and carries less of a stigma.
- The clinical assessment should include not just anthropometric measures but a complete history, physical examination, and appropriate testing to look for aggravating factors, comorbid conditions, and how these variables impact quality of life.

- The AACE Clinical Practice Guidelines on the staging of obesity provide a framework for evaluating the patient with obesity that focuses on cardiometabolic disease risk and objective measures of comorbid conditions.
- The Edmonton Obesity Staging System incorporates the presence or absence of specific weight-related comorbidities and impacts of weight on quality of life to more completely characterize patients with obesity.
- The Cardiometabolic Disease Staging System can be used to more accurately assess an individual patient's risk for developing type 2 diabetes.
- The use of a more detailed assessment strategy will allow the HCP to tailor treatment to the specific needs of individual patients.

WHEN TO REFER

- To an obesity medicine specialist if uncomfortable, prescribing antiobesity medications.
- To subspecialists for advice, evaluation, treatment of specific obesity complications as needed; could include, for example, pulmonologist for obstructive sleep apnea, endocrinologists for diabetes or other endocrine disorders, hepatologist for NAFLD/NASH, or a geneticist for monogenic or syndromic obesity.
- To a bariatric surgeon for selected patients with severe complications, particularly when other weight loss efforts did not achieve therapeutic goals.

- To a psychologist or psychiatrist for depression, anxiety, disordered eating, stigmatization, low self-esteem/ineffectiveness, stress, or other conditions.
- To a previously defined RDN skilled in lifestyle therapy of obesity.
- To a trainer or physical therapist for physical activity prescription.
- To a physical therapist, occupational therapist, or rehabilitation specialist for impairments in function or mobility.
- To a social worker to address social and environmental issues such access to unprocessed foods, physical activity resources, poor health literacy, access to health care, lack of health insurance, or economic limitations.

QUIZ QUESTIONS

1. SJ is a 49-year-old woman who comes to see you for a variety of symptoms including marked fatigue, knee and back pain, urinary stress incontinence, gastroesophageal reflux unresponsive to H2 blocking therapy, and depression. Because of marked fatigue and joint pain, she feels she is no longer able to work at her job as a cashier at a local grocer. On review of systems, she says that her partner says that she snores and she reports AM headaches and daytime hypersomnolence. Her life situation is making her feel hopeless. On examination, she has a BMI = 38 kg/m², a blood pressure of 155/98, decreased range of motion at her knees, 2+ edema in her ankles, and a depressed affect. Her HbA1c = 7.5%; her ECG shows q waves inferiorly. What stage is she using the Edmonton Obesity Staging System?

   A. Stage 1
   B. Stage 2
   C. Stage 3
   D. Stage 4

   Answer: C. *The AHA and WHO guidelines would place this patient in the obese category. However, this classification system does not include factors reflecting either the presence of objective complications of obesity or the impact of weight and weight-related comorbidities on quality of life. This patient has been severely affected by her weight and associated conditions. She has osteoarthritis, has diabetes, may have had a previous MI, likely has sleep apnea, and is quite depressed. The value of the Edmonton staging system is that it focuses on both the presence of weight-related comorbidities and the impact that these comorbidities have on quality of life. A limitation of this system is that individuals will have features that put them in different stages, and it is not clear how some of the features are to be diagnosed for purposes of staging (osteoarthritis, heart failure). In addition, there are limited controlled data on the value of using this staging system in treatment decisions. However, it does reflect an effort to target therapy to those more affected by their weight. The patient described is stage 3 in the Edmonton system because she is unable to work and has evidence of a previous MI.*

2. JB is a 35-year-old man who comes to see you for help managing his weight. He currently has a BMI of 29 kg/m². His blood pressure is 125/81, and his waist circumference is 38″. His fasting glucose is 118 mg/dL, his HDL cholesterol is 38 mg/dL, and his fasting triglyceride level is 210 mg/dL. Which stage is he in the Cardiometabolic Disease Staging System for Prediction of Diabetes?

   A. Stage 1
   B. Stage 2
   C. Stage 3
   D. Stage 4

   Answer: C. *The Cardiometabolic Disease Staging System allows the HCP to assess an individual patient's risk for developing diabetes. JB has both impaired fasting glucose (prediabetes, >100 mg/dL) and metabolic syndrome (increased triglyceride level, reduced HDL cholesterol, and increased fasting glucose; 3/5 criteria are met). Even though his BMI puts him in the "overweight" category in the traditional AHA, his other laboratory tests suggest his risk of developing diabetes over the next 12 years is almost 40%. This risk can be substantially reduced with weight loss. This case demonstrates both the limitations of risk stratification based entirely on BMI and the value of considering cardiometabolic risk markers in determining what treatments might be appropriate.*

PRACTICAL RESOURCES

- AACE Obesity Resource for education and practice facilitation, and the AACE Algorithm for Medical Care of Patients with Obesity (obesity.aace.com)
- Obesity Medicine Association website, educational resources, and treatment recommendations (obesity-medicine.org)

- AACE Obesity Guidelines (www.aace.com/disease-state-resources/nutrition-and-obesity/guidelines)
- Gonzalez-Campoy JM, Hurley DL, Garvey WT, eds. *Bariatric Endocrinology*. Springer; 2019. ISBN 978-3-319-95653-4
- WOMAC score online calculator for assessing patient-reported outcomes for osteoarthritis (www.orthopaedicscore.com); click WOMAC at this site.

REFERENCES

1. Garvey WT, Mechanick JI, Brett EM, et al; Reviewers of the AACE/ACE Obesity Clinical Practice Guidelines. American Association of Clinical Endocrinologists and American College of Endocrinology clinical practice guidelines for comprehensive medical care of patients with obesity. *Endocr Pract.* 2016;22(suppl 3):1-203.

2. Garvey WT. New tools for weight loss therapy enable a more robust medical model for obesity treatment: rationale for a complications-centric approach. *Endocr Pract.* 2013;19:864-874.

3. Sharma AM, Kushner RF. A proposed clinical staging system for obesity. *Int J Obes (Lond).* 2009;33(3):289-295.

4. Garvey WT, Garber AJ, Mechanick JI, et al; on behalf of the AACE Obesity Scientific Committee. American Association of Clinical Endocrinologists and American College of Endocrinology position statement on the 2014 advanced framework for a new diagnosis of obesity as a chronic disease. *Endocr Pract.* 2014;20:977-989.

5. WHO Expert Consultation. Appropriate body mass index for Asian populations and its implications for policy and intervention strategies. *Lancet.* 2004;363(9403):157-163.

6. Gallagher D, Heymsfeld SB, Heo M, Jebb SA, Murgatroyd PR, Sakamoto Y. Healthy percentage body fat ranges: an approach for developing guidelines based on body mass index. *Am J Clin Nutr.* 2000;72:694-701.

7. Mechanick JI, Hurley DL, Garvey WT. Adiposity-based chronic disease as a new diagnostic term: American association of clinical endocrinologists and the American college of endocrinology position statement. *Endocr Pract.* 2017;23(3):372-378.

8. Fruhbeck G, Busetto L, Dicker D, et al. The ABCD of obesity: an EASO position statement on a diagnostic term with clinical and scientific implications. *Obes Facts.* 2019;12(2):131-136.

9. Garvey WT, Mechanick JI. Proposal for a scientifically correct and medically actionable disease classification system (ICD) for obesity. *Obesity (Silver Spring).* 2020;28(3):484-492.

10. Yengo L, Sidorenko J, Kemper KE, et al; GIANT Consortium. Meta-analysis of genome-wide association studies for height and body mass index in ~700000 individuals of European ancestry. *Hum Mol Genet.* 2018;27(20):3641-3649.

11. Mechanick JI, Farkouh ME, Newman JD, Garvey WT. Cardiometabolic-based chronic disease, adiposity and dysglycemia drivers: JACC state-of-the-art review. *J Am Coll Cardiol.* 2020;75(5):525-538.

12. Bellamy N, Buchanan WW, Goldsmith CH, Campbell J, Stitt LW. Validation study of WOMAC: a health status instrument for measuring clinically important patient relevant outcomes to antirheumatic drug therapy in patients with osteoarthritis of the hip or knee. *J Rheumatol.* 1988;15(12):1833-1840.

13. Accessed March 3, 2020. www.drsharma.ca/wp-content/uploads/edmonton-obesity-staging-system-tool.pdf

14. National Diabetes Statistics Report. 2020. *Centers for Disease Control and Prevention.* Accessed March 3, 2020. www.cdc.gov

15. Guo F, Moellering DR, Garvey WT. The progression of cardiometabolic disease: validation of a new cardiometabolic disease staging system applicable to obesity. *Obesity.* 2014;22:110-118.

16. Guo F, Garvey WT. Development of a weighted cardiometabolic disease staging (CMDS) system for the prediction of future diabetes. *J Clin Endocrinol Metab.* 2015;100(10):3871-3877.

17. Garvey WT, Guo F. Cardiometabolic disease staging predicts effectiveness of weight-loss therapy to prevent type 2 diabetes: pooled results from phase III clinical trials assessing phentermine/topiramate extended release. *Diabetes Care.* 2017;40(7):856-862.

18. Kolotkin RL, Ervin CM, Meincke HH, Højbjerre L, Fehnel SE. Development of a clinical trials version of the Impact of Weight on Quality of Life-Lite questionnaire (IWQOL-Lite Clinical Trials Version): results from two qualitative studies. *Clin Obes.* 2017;7(5):290-299.

19. Hamman RF, Wing RR, Edelstein SL, et al. Effect of weight loss with lifestyle intervention on risk of diabetes. *Diabetes Care.* 2006;29(9):2102-2107.

20. Garvey WT, Ryan DH, Henry R, et al. Prevention of type 2 diabetes in subjects with prediabetes and metabolic syndrome treated with phentermine and topiramate extended release. *Diabetes Care.* 2014;37(4):912-921.

21. Le Roux CW, Astrup A, Fujioka K, et al; SCALE Obesity Prediabetes NN8022-1839 Study Group. 3 years of liraglutide versus placebo for type 2 diabetes risk reduction and weight management in individuals with prediabetes: a randomised, double-blind trial. *Lancet.* 2017;389(10077):1399-1409.

22. Wing RR, Lang W, Wadden TA, Safford M, Knowler WC, Bertoni AG, Hill JO, Brancati FL, Peters A, Wagenknecht L; Look AHEAD Research Group. Benefits of modest weight loss in improving cardiovascular risk factors in overweight and obese individuals with type 2 diabetes. *Diabetes Care.* 2011;34(7):1481-1486.

COMANAGEMENT OF OBESITY-RELATED COMORBIDITIES: ASSESSMENT, TREATMENT, AND MONITORING

Sharon J. Herring, Keerthana Kesavarapu, Jessica Briscoe

CASE STUDY 1

Janice is a 54-year-old woman with a history of class 2 obesity (body mass index [BMI] 37 kg/m²), prediabetes, and nonalcoholic fatty liver disease (NAFLD) who presents to her primary care office for annual follow-up. She is concerned about developing type 2 diabetes (T2D) and cirrhosis and wants to learn more about how she can prevent complications from her higher body weight. She reports a diet high in simple carbohydrates and saturated fat. Her physical examination is unremarkable except for an elevated blood pressure reading of 165/95 mm Hg and darkening of the skin around her neck and in her axillae. HBA1C is 6.0%.

OVERVIEW

Nearly every organ system is affected by obesity. Cardiovascular disease (CVD) and its risk factors (diabetes, hypertension [HTN], and lipids) are the most commonly treated by primary care providers. Other complications, such as reproductive abnormalities in both men and women, also have huge impacts on health-related quality of life. Obstructive sleep apnea (OSA) and obesity hypoventilation syndrome (OHS) are common complications of obesity and are underdiagnosed. NAFLD is increasingly recognized as a common complication of obesity. Additionally, some mental health disorders such as depression and binge eating disorder (BED) have a complex, bidirectional relationship with obesity and need evaluation and treatment. Thus, comprehensive obesity care should include

evaluation for these weight-related conditions along with weight management using a combination of lifestyle/behavioral, pharmacologic, and surgical therapies. The degree of weight loss needed to ameliorate these conditions varies. This chapter covers the evaluation, management, and monitoring for each of the major complications of excess weight.

CLINICAL SIGNIFICANCE

Healthcare professionals (HCPs) play a critical role in the assessment and treatment of weight-related comorbidities in patients with obesity. Obesity is a leading risk factor for many of the chronic conditions that remain the leading causes of death among US adults.[1] Over 230 comorbidities and complications of obesity have been identified, with nearly every body system affected (Figure 4.1).[2] The net impact of the increased burden of disease associated with obesity is increased mortality.[3] Successful medical management of obesity will result in significant improvements in health outcomes,[4] and reductions in mortality occur with substantial weight losses from bariatric surgery.[5]

CARDIOVASCULAR COMPLICATIONS OF OBESITY

Hypertension

Assessment

Prevalence

The strong association between obesity and the risk of developing HTN is well documented in both men

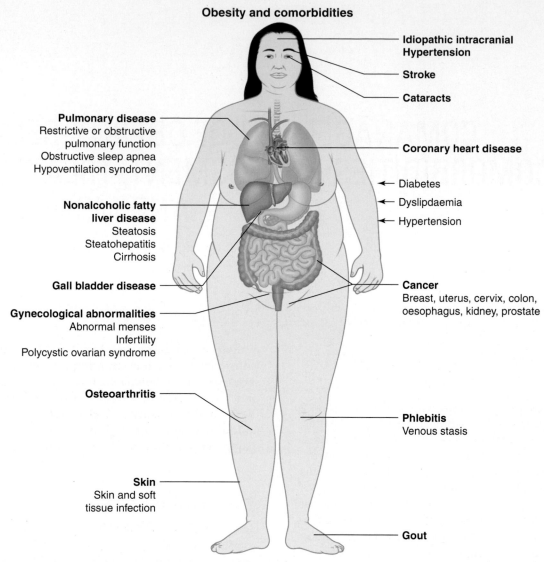

FIGURE 4.1 Obesity and its multiple comorbidities affecting many systems, organs, and tissues.

and women.[6] The Framingham Study demonstrated that persons in the highest BMI quintile had a 16 to 17 mm Hg higher systolic blood pressure and an 11 mm Hg higher diastolic blood pressure than persons in the lowest BMI quintile. In this study, a 10-pound weight gain was associated with a 4 mm Hg increase in systolic blood pressure.[7] Additionally, just over one-quarter of HTN cases were attributable to excess body weight.[8] Numerous mechanisms for the link between obesity and elevations in blood pressure exist and likely operate simultaneously, including low vascular reactivity, renal injury, hyperinsulinemia and insulin resistance, sleep-disordered breathing, the melanocortin pathway, and genetic susceptibility.[9]

Screening

According to the 2015 US Preventive Services Task Force Guidelines (USPSTF), annual blood pressure screening for HTN is recommended in adults aged 18 years or older who are overweight or obesity, first using office blood pressure measurements followed by confirmation with ambulatory blood pressure measurements.[10] For accurate in-office measurements, the American College of Cardiology (ACC) and American Heart Association (AHA) stress the use of the correct blood pressure cuff size (cuff bladder should encircle 80% or more of the patient's arm circumference), particularly in patients with excess adiposity, and no measurements over clothes. HCPs are advised to measure blood pressure in both arms and to use the higher reading; an average of two to three measurements taken on two to three separate occasions will minimize error and provide a more accurate estimate.[11]

Definition

In November 2017, the ACC and AHA released clinical practice guidelines for HTN in adults.[11] Although the definition of normal blood pressure remained the same as in JNC 7, the 2017 guideline replaced the term "prehypertension" with "elevated" and "stage 1 HTN" (Table 4.1). The upper end of prehypertension was reclassified as stage 1 HTN because adults with blood pressure in this range have an approximately twofold increase in CVD risk compared with adults having normal blood pressure. Randomized clinical trials demonstrated a reduction in CVD events with a systolic blood pressure below 130 mm Hg.[12]

Management

A variety of lifestyle modifications are beneficial in the treatment of HTN, including reduction of sodium intake, moderation of alcohol consumption, weight loss, increased physical activity, smoking cessation, and a diet rich in fruits, vegetables, legumes, and low-fat dairy products and low in snacks, sweets, meat, and saturated fat (Table 4.2).[11] Stage 1 HTN is particularly responsive to weight loss, sodium and alcohol restriction, and increased physical activity.[13] The Dietary Approaches to Stop Hypertension (DASH) trial demonstrated the benefit of this eating plan

for HTN (see Chapter 5, Dietary Treatment of Obesity, for additional details of the trial).[14]

Weight loss through caloric reduction is more important than selecting a diet with a specific macronutrient composition for blood pressure lowering. In general, the reduction in blood pressure with weight loss follows a dose-response effect (e.g., greater weight loss produces a greater reduction in blood pressure).[15] Antihypertensive agents are necessary if patients cannot achieve normal blood pressures with lifestyle modification. In general, beta blockers are thought to make weight reduction more difficult and should be considered as second-line agents for blood pressure control.

Coronary Artery Disease/Cerebrovascular Disease

Assessment

Prevalence

Obesity is associated with a number of physiologic and metabolic changes that contribute to increased cardiovascular morbidity and mortality, including insulin resistance and glucose intolerance, systolic and diastolic HTN, hypertriglyceridemia, reduced high-density lipoprotein–cholesterol (HDL-C), and increased systemic inflammation (e.g., C-reactive protein, interleukin-6 and tumor necrosis factor-alpha). There is consistent epidemiologic evidence for an association between obesity and coronary artery disease (CAD), particularly in individuals with increased abdominal adiposity, and significant CAD risk associated with obesity beginning as early as childhood.[16,17] A publication from the Framingham Heart Study suggested that obesity in middle-aged adults could account for as much as 23% of cases of CAD in men and 15% in women.[8] Obesity is additionally associated with an increased risk of stroke, and stroke risk is mitigated by weight loss.[18]

Screening

Most asymptomatic adults do not need routine screening for CAD/CVD. However, as described in the 2013 American Heart Association/American College of Cardiology/The Obesity Society (AHA/ACC/TOS) Guideline for the Management of Overweight and Obesity in Adults, patients with obesity should undergo risk assessment for cardiovascular risk factors, including lipids, blood pressure measurement, and fasting blood glucose. A waist circumference measurement is recommended for individuals with BMI 25 to 34.9 kg/m² to provide additional information on risk. It is unnecessary to measure waist circumference in patients with BMI ≥35 kg/m² because the waist circumference will likely be elevated and will add no additional risk information. Cut points of (≥88 cm [≥35 inches] for women and ≥102 cm [≥ 40 inches] for men) are indicative of

TABLE 4.1 Criteria for the Diagnosis of HTN[a]	
NORMAL	**LESS THAN 120/80 MM HG**
Elevated	Systolic between 120-129 and diastolic less than 80 mm Hg
Stage 1	Systolic between 130-139 or diastolic between 80-89 mm Hg
Stage 2	Systolic at least 140 or diastolic at least 90 mm Hg
Hypertensive Crisis	Systolic over 180 and/or diastolic over 120 mm Hg, with patients needing prompt changes in medication if there are no other indications of problems, or immediate hospitalization if there are signs of acute end organ damage

HTN, hypertension.

[a]Based on accurate measurements and average of at least 2 readings on at least 2 occasions. Adapted from Whelton PK, Carey RM, Aronow WS, et al. 2017 ACC/AHA/AAPA/ABC/ACPM/AGS/APhA/ASH/ASPC/NMA/PCNA guideline for the prevention, detection, evaluation, and management of high blood pressure in adults: a report of the American College of Cardiology/American Heart Association Task Force on Clinical Practice Guidelines. J Am Coll Cardiol. 2018;71(19):e127-e248.

TABLE 4.2 Lifestyle Modification and Its Effect on Blood Pressure and Treatment of Hypertension

	NONPHARMACOLOGIC INTERVENTION	DOSE	APPROXIMATE IMPACT ON SBP	
			HYPERTENSIVE	NORMOTENSIVE
Weight loss	Weight/body fat	Ideal body weight is best goal but at least 1 kg reduction in body weight for most adults who are overweight. Expect about 1 mm Hg for every 1 kg reduction in body weight	−5 mm Hg	−2/3 mm Hg
Healthy diet	DASH dietary pattern	Diet rich in fruits, vegetables, whole grains, and low-fat dairy products with reduced content of saturated and trans fat	−11 mm Hg	−3 mm Hg
Reduced intake of dietary sodium	Dietary sodium	<1,500 mg/d is optimal goal but at least 1,000 mg/d reduction in most adults	−5/6 mm Hg	−2/3 mm Hg
Enhanced intake of dietary potassium	Dietary potassium	3,500-5,000 mg/d, preferably by consumption of a diet rich in potassium	−4/5 mm Hg	−2 mm Hg
Physical activity	Aerobic	• 90-150 minutes/week • 65%-75% heart rate reserve	−5/8 mm Hg	−2/4 mm Hg
	Dynamic resistance	• 90-150 minutes/week • 50%-80% 1 rep maximum • Six exercises, three sets/exercise, 10 repetitions/set	−4 mm Hg	−2 mm Hg
	Isometric resistance	• 4 × 2 minutes (hand grip), 1 minute rest between exercises, 30%-40% maximum voluntary contraction, three sessions/week • 8-10 weeks	−5 mm Hg	−4 mm Hg
Moderation in alcohol intake	Alcohol consumption	In individuals who drink alcohol, reduce alcohol to • Men: ≤2 drinks daily • Women: ≤1 drink daily	−4 mm Hg	−3 mm Hg

DASH, Dietary Approaches to Stop Hypertension; SBP, systolic blood pressure.
Modified from Whelton PK, Carey RM, Aronowthe WS, et al. 2017 ACC/AHA/AAPA/ABC/ACPM/AGS/APhA/ASH/ASPC/NMA/PCNA guideline for the prevention, detection, evaluation, and management of high blood pressure in adults: a report of the American College of Cardiology/American Heart Association Task Force on Clinical Practice Guidelines. J Am Coll Cardiol. 2018;71(19):e127-e248.

increased cardiometabolic risk.[19] While there is little evidence to support routine exercise testing in asymptomatic adults, ACC/AHA guidelines suggest that exercise electrocardiogram (ECG) testing may be of benefit in patients with multiple risk factors for CAD in the following situations: as a guide to risk reduction therapy; men ≥45 years of age and women ≥55 years of age who are sedentary and planning to begin a vigorous exercise program; or patients who are involved in occupations linked to public safety.[20] If stress testing reveals an abnormal result, referral to a cardiologist and aggressive treatment is needed with secondary prevention measures (e.g., statin therapy, aspirin, tight blood pressure control). The use of computed tomography (CT) to obtain a coronary artery calcium (CAC) score may be useful to further risk stratify and to guide a discussion regarding statin therapy in adults at borderline (5% to < 7.5%) or intermediate (7.5% to < 20%) 10-year atherosclerotic cardiovascular disease (ASCVD) risk. Chapter 3 contains an in-depth discussion of how cardiovascular risk factors can be used to risk stratify patients with obesity.

Management

In adults who are overweight or have obesity with cardiovascular risk factors (HTN, hyperlipidemia, and hyperglycemia), lifestyle changes that produce even modest, sustained weight losses of 3% to 5% result in clinically meaningful reductions in triglycerides, blood glucose, HBA1C, and the risk of developing T2D. Greater amounts of weight loss will reduce blood pressure, improve low-density lipoprotein–cholesterol (LDL-C) and HDL-C, and reduce the need for medications to control blood pressure, blood glucose, and lipids as well as further reduce triglycerides and blood glucose.[19]

Observational studies suggest significant benefits of a Mediterranean diet on reduction in cardiovascular mortality—this diet is typically high in fruits, vegetables, whole grains, beans, nuts, and seeds, includes extra-virgin olive oil as an important source of monounsaturated fat, and allows low to moderate wine consumption. It generally includes low to moderate amounts of fish, poultry, and dairy products, but little red meat. In a meta-analysis of randomized trials, a Mediterranean diet reduced the risk of stroke compared with a low-fat diet (HR 0.60, 95% CI 0.45-0.80) but did not reduce the incidence of cardiovascular or overall mortality.[21] Data additionally support high-quality plant-based diets that include whole grains as the main form of carbohydrate, unsaturated fats as the predominate form of dietary fat, an abundance of fruit and vegetables, and adequate n−3 fatty acids as important components in preventing CVD.[22] Randomized trials support the use of vegetarian diets for weight loss.

Statin therapy may be necessary if 10-year ASCVD risk is ≥7.5%. Lipid-lowering therapy with statins reduces relative cardiovascular risk by approximately 20% to 30%

regardless of baseline LDL-C.[23] HCPs can quickly calculate ASCVD risk and need for medication management beyond lifestyle changes using the ASCVD Risk Estimator Plus from the ACC/AHA: http://tools.acc.org/ASCVD-Risk-Estimator-Plus/#!/calculate/estimate/.

METABOLIC DISORDERS OF OBESITY

Prediabetes/Diabetes Mellitus Type 2

Assessment

Prevalence of Prediabetes and T2D in Populations With Obesity

The prevalence of both diabetes and obesity have continued to rise from 1999/2000 to 2013/2014 using the most recent NHANES data.[24] More than 88% of people with T2D have overweight or obesity with 26% of adults being overweight, 44% having obesity, and 18% having severe obesity.[25] The risk of T2D rises with increasing body weight, with the prevalence of T2D being three to seven times higher in those with obesity than normal weight adults. Obesity-associated insulin resistance, particularly in patients with visceral adiposity, is the primary mechanism of T2D in populations with obesity.

Symptoms and Physical Examination Findings Associated With Insulin Resistance

Patients may complain of symptoms from hyperglycemia, which include polydipsia, polyuria, polyphagia, fatigue, nausea/vomiting, and abdominal pain, or symptoms from microvascular complications, such as sensory loss (peripheral neuropathy) and vision changes (retinopathy). Physical examination should include a comprehensive foot examination observing for skin integrity, foot deformities, ulcerations, pedal pulses for peripheral arterial disease, and a 10 g monofilament examination for sensation. Skin changes seen in T2D include acanthosis nigricans, which is defined as dark, coarse, and thickened skin commonly located at the back of the neck, and acrochordons (skin tags), defined as small, soft, pedunculated, and benign skin tumors found on the neck, axilla, or groin. These lesions are a sign of insulin resistance and impaired carbohydrate metabolism.[26]

Screening

Testing for prediabetes and T2D in asymptomatic individuals should be considered in adults of any age who have overweight or obesity (BMI ≥25 kg/m² or ≥23 kg/m² in Asian Americans) and who have one or more additional risk factors for diabetes (Table 4.3). As per the USPSTF, all adults aged 40 to 70 years should be screened at least once for prediabetes and T2D.

TABLE 4.3 Risk factors for Testing for Diabetes or Prediabetes in Asymptomatic Adults

1. First-degree relative with diabetes
2. High-risk race/ethnicity (e.g., African American, Latino, Native American, Asian American, and Pacific Islander)
3. History of cardiovascular disease
4. Hypertension
5. Dyslipidemia (HDL cholesterol level < 35 mg/dL and/ or a triglyceride level >250 mg/dL)
6. Polycystic ovary syndrome
7. Other clinical conditions associated with insulin resistance

Modified from American Diabetes Association. Standards of Medical Care in Diabetes-2019 Abridged for Primary Care Providers. Clin Diabetes. 2019;37(1):11-34.

TABLE 4.4 Criteria for Diagnosing Prediabetes and Diabetes

	PREDIABETES	DIABETES
HBA1C[c]	5.7%-6.4%[a]	≥6.5%
FPG[c]	100-125 mg/dL (5.6-6.9 mmol/L)[a]	≥126 mg/dL (7.0 mmol/L)
OGTT[c]	150-199 mg/dL (7.8-11.0 mmol/L)[a]	≥200 mg/dL (11.1 mmol/L)
RPG[b]		≥200 mg/dL (11.1 mmol/L)

Modified from American Diabetes Association. Standards of Medical Care in Diabetes-2019 Abridged for Primary Care Providers. Clin Diabetes. 2019;37(1):11-34. FPG, fasting plasma glucose; OGTT, oral glucose tolerance test; RPG, random plasma glucose.
[a]For all three tests, risk is continuous, extending below the lower limit of the range and becoming disproportionately greater that the higher end of the range.
[b]Only diagnostic in a patient with classic symptoms of hyperglycemia or hyperglycemic crisis.
[c]Test requires two abnormal test results prior to establishing diagnosis of diabetes.

Definition of Prediabetes and Diabetes

Diabetes and prediabetes may be diagnosed based on plasma glucose, with either fasting plasma glucose (FPG) or 2-hour plasma glucose (2-h PG) value during a 75-g oral glucose tolerance test (OGTT), or using the HBA1C criteria (Table 4.4). Unless there is a clear clinical diagnosis of diabetes in the case of hyperglycemic crisis, classic symptoms of hyperglycemia, or random plasma blood glucose >200 mg/dL, diagnosis requires two abnormal test results.

Management

Prediabetes

The goal of management of prediabetes is prevention or delay in progression to diabetes. The Diabetes Prevention Program (DPP) demonstrated that weight loss achieved through intensive lifestyle modifications can prevent or delay the onset of T2D. In the DPP, the relative incidence of diabetes was reduced by 58% over 3 years in participants randomized to intensive lifestyle intervention.[27] The lifestyle intervention arm ran over 1 year. During the first 6 months, patients met weekly for 1 hour to learn about eating healthy, adding physical activity, dealing with stress, coping with challenges, and getting back on track. During the subsequent 6 months, patients focused on sticking to new habits. Follow-up in the Diabetes Prevention Program Outcomes Study has shown a sustained reduction in the rate of developing T2D, by 34% at 10 years and 27% at 15 years.[16]

Given these findings, the American Diabetes Association (ADA) recommends referral of patients with prediabetes to an intensive lifestyle intervention program modeled on the DPP, with goals to achieve and maintain 7% loss of body weight and to increase moderate intensity physical activity to at least 150 minutes/ week. The Center for Medicare and Medicaid Services (CMS) covers the DPP with no patient out-of-pocket cost, if patients meet the criteria and if the HCP uses ICD-10 diagnosis codes for prediabetes or abnormal blood glucose without diabetes. These programs are readily available in the community (e.g., YMCA).

Based on intervention trials, eating patterns that may be helpful for prediabetes include a Mediterranean eating plan and/or a low-calorie, low-fat eating plan, as was employed in the DPP.[28] For diabetes prevention, the emphasis should be on whole grains, legumes, nuts, fruits, and vegetables and minimal refined and processed foods.[29] Red meats and sugar-sweetened beverages are associated with an increased risk of T2D.[29]

Physical activity, as modeled in the DPP, should be encouraged with at least 150 minutes/week of moderate-intensity activities, such as brisk walking and resistance training.[27,30] This allows for improvement in insulin sensitivity.[30] These findings also extend to prevention of gestational diabetes mellitus.[31]

Lifestyle intervention may be supplemented with pharmacotherapy. Metformin for prevention of diabetes mellitus type 2 (DM2) should be considered in those with prediabetes who are at high risk for progression, especially those with BMI ≥35 kg/m², those aged <60 years, and women with prior gestational diabetes (ADA recommendations). In the DPP, participants randomized to metformin had a 31% relative reduction in incidence of T2D vs. control. Long-term use of metformin may be associated with vitamin B12 deficiency, and annual measurement should be performed.

Diabetes

The goal of managing diabetes is to achieve glycemic control and prevent and/or reduce progression of microvascular and macrovascular complications. The Look AHEAD trial, a 12-year multicenter randomized trial of patients with T2D, found that meaningful weight loss (≥5%) achieved with lifestyle intervention led to improved glycemic control and a decrease in antihyperglycemic medications use.[32]

Nutrition therapy plays an integral role in the treatment of T2D and should be done in collaboration with a registered dietitian nutritionist (RDN). Dietary plans created and delivered by an RDN are associated with improvements in glycemic control with HBA1C decreases of 0.3% to 2% in those with DM2.[33]

There is no ideal percentage of macronutrient distribution (fat, carbohydrate, and protein) that is suited for all people with obesity and T2D. Meal plans should be individualized, keeping total calorie count low. Studies of reduced calorie interventions show reductions in HBA1C of 0.3% to 2.0% in adults with T2D, as well as reductions in medication doses and improvement in quality of life.[34]

Carbohydrate Restriction

Data examining the ideal amount of carbohydrate intake is inconclusive. Monitoring carbohydrate intake and the resulting blood glucose response is key to improving postprandial glucose control, regardless of weight loss. The quality of carbohydrates consumed also is important. Specifically, carbohydrate foods with a high glycemic index (rate of breakdown and absorption) lead to higher postprandial blood glucose, compared to carbohydrate foods with lower glycemic index.

The role of low-carbohydrate diets (<130 g/day, compared to 150 to 175 g for a macronutrient balanced but calorie-restricted eating plan) in T2D remains unclear. Some studies show that lowering glycemic load (i.e., reducing both the glycemic index of carbohydrates consumed, as well as overall carbohydrate intake) lowers HBA1C by 0.2% to 0.5%.[35] Studies longer than 12 weeks report no significant influence of glycemic index on HBA1C independent of weight loss. Very-low-carbohydrate or ketogenic diets (<50 g/day) have shown similar weight loss after 1 year, as compared with more balanced eating plans.

Fat Restriction

The ideal total dietary fat content for people with obesity and T2D is inconclusive. The types of fat as well as the quantity of fats appear to play an important role in achieving metabolic goals. As described above, eating a Mediterranean-style diet rich in monounsaturated and polyunsaturated fats and avoiding saturated fats can improve glucose metabolism and lower CVD risk.

Physical Activity

Similar to prediabetes, 150 minutes or more of moderate- to vigorous-intensity aerobic activity, spread over at least 3 days/week, with two sessions per week of resistance training on nonconsecutive days, is recommended by the ADA. Shorter durations of vigorous intensity or interval training may be sufficient for younger and more physically fit individuals. Data suggest that the additive benefit of aerobic and resistance exercise improves insulin sensitivity and lowers HBA1C by 0.66% even without a change in BMI.[36] More recent research has focused on improving glucose control by interrupting prolonged sitting (sedentary time) with short bouts of physical activity.

Because of the progressive nature of T2D, lifestyle changes may not be enough over time to maintain euglycemia. Many patients with T2D will require pharmacotherapy. Currently there are 10 approved classes of agents for diabetes management (Table 4.5). A patient-centered approach should be taken to guide use of pharmacologic agents considering comorbidities, risk of hypoglycemia, cost/health plan formularies, and side effects.

When considering glucose-lowering agents for patients with obesity and with T2D, medications promoting weight loss or that are weight neutral should ideally be chosen immediately after metformin (Table 4.5). Agents with weight loss effects include biguanides, SGLT2 inhibitors, and GLP-1 agonists. Metformin is the preferred initial pharmacologic agent.[37] Once initiated at 500 mg once daily, metformin should be titrated to maximum tolerated dose (assuming normal renal function). Patients with T2D and coexisting chronic kidney disease (CKD) or CAD should be initiated on SGLT2 inhibitors or GLP-1 receptor agonists, as these classes of medications have been shown to decrease the risk of progression of CKD and/or CVD. Insulin should be considered if there is evidence of ongoing catabolism (weight loss), if symptoms of hyperglycemia are present, or when HBA1C (≥10%) or blood glucose levels (>300) are very high. Combination drug therapy should be considered in those newly diagnosed with diabetes who have an HBA1C >1.5% above target.

Monitoring

If results of diabetes screening tests are normal, repeat testing is recommended at a minimum of 3-year intervals. If patients have results near the margins of diagnostic threshold, the HCP should follow the patient closely and repeat the assay in 3 to 6 months. Patients with diabetes on medications should be reevaluated at regular intervals (3 to 6 months), with dose adjustments based on HBA1C findings. Patients with prediabetes should be tested yearly for development of diabetes. Women who are diagnosed with gestational diabetes mellitus (GDM) should have lifelong testing at least every 3 years.

TABLE 4.5 Drug-specific and Patient Factors to Consider When Selecting Antihyperglycemic Treatment in Adults With DM2

	HYPOGLYCEMIA	EFFECT ON WEIGHT	CARDIOVASCULAR EFFECTS		ORAL/SQ	RENAL EFFECTS	OTHER
			ASCVD	CHF		PROGRESSION OF CKD	
Biguanide: Metformin	No	Modest weight loss	Potential benefit	Neutral	Oral	Neutral	Gastrointestinal side effects B12 deficiency
SGLT-2 inhibitors: Canagliflozin Empagliflozin Dapagliflozin Ertugliflozin	No	Loss	Benefit	Benefit	Oral	Benefit	FDA black box: Risk of amputation (canagliflozin)
GLP-1 agonists: Liraglutide Semaglutide Exenatide ER Dulaglutide	No	Loss	based on agent	Neutral	SQ	Benefit	FDA black box: thyroid C-cell tumors. GI side effects
DPP-4 inhibitors: Saxagliptin Alogliptin Sitagliptin Linagliptin	No	Neutral	Neutral	Risk	Oral	Neutral	Risk of acute pancreatitis
Thiazolidinediones: Pioglitazone	No	Gain	Benefit	Risk	Oral	Neutral	FDA black box: CHF
Sulfonylureas: Glyburide Glipizide Glimepiride	Yes	Gain	Neutral	Neutral	SQ	Neutral	Injection site reactions
Insulin	Yes	Gain	Neutral	Neutral	SQ	Neutral	Higher risk of hypoglycemia with human insulin vs. analogs

ASCVD, atherosclerotic cardiovascular disease; CHF, congestive heart failure; CKD, chronic kidney disease; DM2, diabetes mellitus type 2; ER, extended release; FDA, U.S. Food and Drug Administration; GI, gastrointestinal; SQ, subcutaneous.
Modified from American Diabetes Association. 9. Pharmacologic approaches to glycemic treatment: standards of medical care in diabetes-2019. Diabetes Care. 2019;42(suppl 1);S90-S102.

Polycystic Ovary Syndrome

Assessment

Using the Rotterdam criteria, a diagnosis of polycystic ovary syndrome (PCOS) can be made if two of the three following criteria are met: (1) androgen excess, (2) ovulatory dysfunction, or (3) polycystic ovaries.[38] Disorders that mimic the clinical features of PCOS including thyroid disease, prolactin excess, and congenital adrenal hyperplasia should be excluded with measurement of thyroid-stimulating hormone (TSH), serum prolactin, and serum 17-hydroxyprogesterone.[38] Patients with more severe phenotypes may benefit from more extensive evaluation to exclude other causes.

Androgen excess can present as hirsutism (65% to 75%), excessive terminal hair that appears in a male pattern, acne (14% to 25%), or male pattern hair loss.[39] Biochemical testing with total and/or free testosterone level may show elevated androgen levels; however, testosterone levels differ during time of day, by age, and by medications and are not specific for PCOS but rather hyperandrogenism. Notably, in women with PCOS, obesity and insulin resistance signified by acanthosis nigricans and skin tags is often present.

On initial visit, a comprehensive menstrual history should be taken to identify infertility (25% to 40%) and oligo or anovulation (70% to 90%), the latter which manifests as frequent bleeding at intervals <21 days or infrequent bleeding at intervals ≥35 days. Biochemical testing with midluteal phase progesterone may help in diagnosis if bleeding appears to be regular. Polycystic ovaries can be documented if ultrasound shows 12 or more follicles 2 to 9 mm in diameter and/or an increased ovarian volume ≥10 mL in either ovary.[38]

Women with PCOS are at increased risk of pregnancy complications including gestational diabetes, preterm delivery, and preeclampsia. These findings are exacerbated in the setting of obesity. Prior to pregnancy, assessment of BMI, blood pressure, and glucose tolerance with an OGTT are recommended.

Prevalence

Obesity is a common finding in women with PCOS and between 40% and 80% of women with PCOS are reported to have overweight or obesity.[40] Insulin resistance is a common finding in both PCOS and obesity. Women with PCOS have increased central fat, waist circumference, and waist-hip ratio compared to BMI-matched control women.[40]

Management

PCOS and Weight Management

Weight loss, accomplished via lifestyle modification, use of medications, or bariatric surgery, is recommended as a first-line therapy for women with obesity and PCOS.

While randomized controlled trials are limited, weight loss (5% to 10%) in women with obesity and PCOS has been shown to normalize hyperandrogenemia, improve hirsutism, improve menstrual function, and improve pregnancy outcomes.[38] The response to weight loss is variable, with not all individuals having restoration of ovulation or regular menses.

Lifestyle Therapy

The Endocrine Society recommends calorie-restricted diets and exercise therapy in management of women with PCOS who have overweight or obesity.[38] There are no large randomized trials of exercise alone or in combination with dietary intervention to improve weight loss among those with obesity and PCOS. While weight loss is helpful in patients with PCOS and obesity, it is not helpful in treating PCOS in normal-weight women.

Pharmacotherapy

Metformin is the first-line therapy for women with PCOS presenting with cutaneous manifestations (acne or hirsutism) and obesity or glucose intolerance who fail lifestyle modification. The reader is referred elsewhere for a detailed review of the pharmacologic treatment of PCOS.[38]

Infertility and Hypogonadism

Obesity can impair reproduction in both males and females, resulting in infertility in couples attempting to conceive. Reproductive disturbances are more common in women with obesity, regardless of PCOS status, and include menstrual cycle abnormalities and ovulatory dysfunction. Higher rates of menstrual irregularity exist in females with obesity compared to leaner women.[41] Even with normal menstrual cycles, hormonal changes such as decreased luteinizing hormone (LH) pulse frequency, prolonged folliculogenesis, and decreased luteal progesterone lower the chance of conception within 1 year of stopping contraception.[42]

Ovulatory dysfunction due to excess estrogen downregulating gonadotropin hormone secretion is commonly seen in obesity. The relative risk of anovulatory infertility increases at a BMI of 25 kg/m² with the highest risk at BMI over 27 kg/m² and those with increased abdominal fat. Pregnancy loss also is linked with obesity in women with PCOS.

For males who have obesity, not all experience infertility. However, those that do, have lower sperm quality (count, concentration and motility) and impaired erectile function. Surveys suggest the prevalence rates of hypogonadism are as high as 45% to 57% among men with obesity. There is a bidirectional relationship between obesity and hypogonadism. Obesity increases levels of leptin, insulin, proinflammatory cytokines, and estrogen that can cause a defect at the level of the hypothalamus resulting in hypogonadotropic hypogonadism. The resulting hypogonadism may worsen obesity by lowering lean body mass (thus, adversely affecting energy expenditure).

Male obesity resulting in hypogonadism is diagnosed in men who meet all of the following criteria: (1) BMI ≥ 30 kg/m^2, (2) clinical signs and symptoms of hypogonadism including low libido, erectile dysfunction, fatigue, decreased concentration, reduced body hair, small testes, gynecomastia, and low bone mineral density, and (3) biochemical hypogonadism showing either primary or secondary hypogonadism.

Total testosterone levels should be measured in the morning and repeated on two occasions, preferably 4 weeks apart. Men with close to or below the low normal range of total testosterone should have free testosterone drawn as obesity is associated with altered sex hormone binding globulin. Serum LH, follicle-stimulating hormone (FSH), and prolactin levels should be measured to differentiate between primary and secondary hypogonadism.

Management

Preconception counseling should be offered to all couples with obesity to discuss reproductive consequences of excess weight. Weight management should include dietary modification, increased physical activity, and behavioral interventions with a role for pharmacotherapy and bariatric surgery for those that fail lifestyle modification.

Women with obesity wishing to conceive should be enrolled in a weight management program with the goals of decreasing preconception weight and weight gain in pregnancy and achieving long-term weight reduction. Weight reduction in women with obesity and anovulatory infertility improves the rate of pregnancy with return of ovulatory function. Delaying pregnancy in order to optimize weight should be balanced with declining fertility due to age.

Current recommendations include weight loss of 7% of body weight with calorie restriction and increased exercise to 150 minutes/week of moderate-intensity activity.[43] Pharmacotherapy to improve ovulatory function or alternative methods of conception is not routinely recommended based on BMI in women with obesity.

Similarly, men with obesity that lose 15% of body weight have improvements in erectile function and biochemical markers of hypogonadism including total testosterone, free testosterone, and LH.[44] Of note, the degree of weight loss required for improvement (15%) is higher for male hypogonadism, compared to other weight-related conditions.[44]

Current recommendations in men include a low-calorie, high-protein diet with personalized dietary counseling and increased physical activity. Achievement of these targets can induce positive changes in hormonal profile and body composition. Physical activity, specifically aerobic exercise, can increase LH and testosterone production and help recover erectile function in this population. Additionally, exercise augments the effect and durability of testosterone replacement therapy during and after cessation of medication use.[44,45]

For men whose testosterone level does not normalize with weight loss, testosterone therapy should be considered. Testosterone should be administered to men with symptoms and signs of low testosterone and consistently low serum total testosterone levels to induce and maintain secondary sex characteristics and correct symptoms of testosterone deficiency. In healthy men with obesity and androgen deficiency symptoms and testosterone deficiency, testosterone therapy improves erectile dysfunction and testosterone levels. In men with obesity and hypogonadism, testosterone replacement therapy may be helpful in preserving lean body mass.

Testosterone therapy is not recommended in men planning to conceive, as exogenous testosterone can suppress spermatogenesis and cause testicular atrophy. Additionally, testosterone therapy should be avoided in those with prostate cancer, elevated PSA or increased risk or presence of prostate or breast cancer, and comorbidities including untreated OSA, uncontrolled heart failure, myocardial infarction, or stroke within the last 6 months or thrombophilia, all of which are commonly seen in obesity.

RESPIRATORY DISEASES OF OBESITY

Obstructive Sleep Apnea

Assessment

Prevalence of OSA in Populations With Obesity

OSA is a breathing disorder characterized by narrowing of the upper airway that impairs normal ventilation during sleep. Obesity alters sleep quantity and quality via multiple mechanisms including alterations in upper airway structure from fatty tissue accumulation. This leads to narrowing of the upper respiratory muscles resulting in apnea and recurrent nighttime hypoxia. The converse is also true: those with OSA are at risk for worsening obesity. Untreated OSA and insufficient sleep are linked to weight gain through multiple mechanisms including loss of lean muscle mass and neurohormonal changes leading to increased appetite. The prevalence of OSA is high (77%) in patients with obesity undergoing bariatric surgery.[46] Relative to stable weight, a 10% weight gain predicts a sixfold increase in the odds of developing moderate to severe sleep-disordered breathing (SDB).[47]

Screening for OSA

The USPSTF does not recommend screening asymptomatic adults despite having risk factors for OSA unless they are symptomatic.[48] A preoperative sleep clinic evaluation is recommended to evaluate for OSA in patients undergoing bariatric surgery.

Symptoms and Physical Examination Findings

A comprehensive sleep history should include evaluation for snoring, witnessed apnea, impaired cognition, gasping or choking at night, unrefreshing sleep, and excessive daytime fatigue, nocturia, morning headaches, and sleepiness not explained by other factors. Potential screening questionnaires and prediction tools to identify high risk patients include the Epworth sleepiness scale (ESS), the STOP-BANG Questionnaire, and the Berlin Questionnaire (Table 4.6). These tests have low levels of accuracy making them poor diagnostic tools but good at quickly identifying those who might benefit from referral for home sleep apnea testing (HSAT) described below.[52]

Physical examination should note presence and severity of obesity (by BMI) and signs of upper airway narrowing including neck circumference (≥17 inches in men, ≥16 inches in women), presence of retrognathia, macroglossia, tonsillar hypertrophy, elongated/ enlarged uvula, high-arched/narrow hard palate, and/ or overjet. A Mallampati score can also be used as a visual assessment of the distance from the tongue base to the roof of the mouth.

Diagnosis of OSA

Polysomnography (PSG) is the standard diagnostic test for the diagnosis of OSA in adult populations in whom there is concern for OSA based on screening sleep evaluation.[53] Uncomplicated adult patients with signs and symptoms that indicate risk of moderate to severe OSA should have an overnight PSG performed in a sleep laboratory or a HSAT.

The HSAT, an alternative for those unable to present to a sleep laboratory, is more accurate in identifying patients who have a high pretest likelihood of moderate to severe OSA.[53] Patients with significant cardiopulmonary disease, potential respiratory muscle weakness due to a neuromuscular condition, history of stroke, chronic opioid medication use, severe insomnia, or symptoms of other sleep disorders should chose PSG over HSAT.[53] A split-night diagnostic protocol, which allows for diagnosis and positive airway pressure (PAP) titration, should be favored over full-night diagnostic protocol, which only allows for diagnosis.

TABLE 4.6 OSA Screening Questionnaires and Prediction Tools		
BERLIN QUESTIONNAIRE[49]	**EPWORTH SLEEPINESS SCALE**[50]	**STOP-BANG**[51]
Are there changes in weight? **Category 1:** Do you snore? Snoring loudness Snoring frequency Has snoring bothered others? Frequency of witnessed apnea? **Category 2:** Morning fatigue? Frequency of morning fatigue Have you fallen asleep at the wheel? **Category 3:** History of hypertension BMI ≥30 mg/m²	How likely are you to doze off or fall asleep in the following situations, in contrast to feeling tired (0-3)? 1. Sitting and reading 2. Watching TV 3. Sitting, inactive in public place 4. As a passenger in a car for an hour without break 5. Lying down to rest in the afternoon when circumstances permit 6. Sitting and talking to someone 7. Sitting quietly after a lunch without alcohol 8. In a car, while stopped for a few minutes in the traffic	Do you **snore** loudly? Do you feel **tired**, fatigued, or sleepy during the daytime? Has anyone **observed** you stop breathing or choking/gasping during sleep? Do you have high blood **pressure**? **BMI** ≥ 35 mg/m² **Age** ≥ 50 years old **Neck** size (male ≥ 17 inches, females ≥ 16 inches) **Gender** = Male
High risk: If there are two or more categories where the score is positive	**High risk:** A score of ≥10	**High risk:** Yes to five to eight questions Yes to more than two STOP questions + male gender or BMI ≥ 35 kg/m² or neck circumference

BMI, body mass index; OSA, obstructive sleep apnea.

Both the PSG and the HSAT quantify the apnea hypopnea index (AHI), which is required to diagnose OSA. Apnea is the complete obstruction of airflow, and hypopnea is the partial obstruction of airflow. Both must last 10 seconds. The AHI is then calculated by adding the sum of apnea and hypopnea episodes and dividing by the total sleep time. An AHI ≥5 events/hour associated with typical symptoms of OSA, or an obstructive AHI ≥15 events/hour even without symptoms is diagnostic for OSA.[53] OSA severity is defined as mild for AHI ≥5 and <15, moderate for AHI ≥15 and <30, and severe for AHI ≥30/hour.

Management

Role of Weight Loss in OSA

Weight reduction leads to improvement in OSA. A 10% weight loss predicted a 26% decrease in the AHI.[47] Given extensive data, weight loss is encouraged for all patients with OSA and obesity through dietary changes, exercise, pharmacotherapy, or bariatric surgery.[54] There is no one specific meal plan that has shown to be most successful.

PAP, Oral Appliances, and Surgery

Treatment should be delivered using a multidisciplinary care team that includes a sleep specialist and a referring HCP. The goal of treatment includes the resolution of clinical signs and symptoms of OSA and normalization of AHI as well as the nighttime oxyhemoglobin saturation.[53]

Medical therapy for OSA includes PAP, delivered as continuous (CPAP), bilevel with an enhanced ventilatory component (BIPAP), or auto titrating (APAP). PAP can be applied through a nasal, oral, or oronasal interface during sleep.[53] Use of oral appliances (mandibular advancement device) can be considered for patients with mild OSA. Some patients may be candidates for upper airway surgery to relieve upper airway obstruction. Bariatric surgery has a 40% remission rate of OSA related to the amount of weight loss and should be considered as an adjunct to first-line therapies for OSA.

Monitoring

Monitoring OSA (e.g., Once Diagnosed With OSA, Role for Repeating Sleep Study and How Often)

To ensure satisfactory therapeutic benefit from upper airway surgical treatments, oral appliances, and substantial weight loss or gain, insufficient clinical response to CPAP, or recurrence of symptoms despite good initial response, follow-up PSG is recommended. In patients on CPAP whose symptoms continue to be resolved, follow-up testing is not needed. Patients with positive symptomatic response can be monitored using questionnaires (e.g., ESS as described above). After initial PAP setup, long-term follow-up is indicated yearly and as needed to troubleshoot mask, machine, or usage problems.

Obesity Hypoventilation Syndrome

Assessment

Obesity induces increased demand on the respiratory system requiring increased oxygen demand, decreased diaphragmatic motility, upper airway obstruction, and oxygen desaturation. Loss of the compensatory mechanisms to maintain adequate ventilation leads to OHS. The prevalence of OHS rises with BMI.

OHS is the most severe form of obesity-induced respiratory compromise and leads to high mortality, chronic heart failure, pulmonary HTN, and hospitalization due to acute on chronic hypercapnic respiratory failure.[55] There is an overlap between OSA and OHS with approximately 90% of patients with OHS having coexisting OSA, typically severe. Multiple studies have reported a prevalence of OHS between 8% and 20% in patients with obesity, particularly in patients with BMI greater than 34 kg/m².[56]

Patients with OHS typically have severe obesity and also have typical signs and symptoms similar to OSA including dyspnea, daytime sleepiness, fatigue, nocturia, loud snoring, witnessed apneas, as well as mild hypoxemia during waking hours and/or significant hypoxemia during sleep. Many patients are undiagnosed and untreated. They often present to the hospital with acute on chronic hypercapnic respiratory failure.

Testing is recommended in patients with obesity and SDB, the latter defined as either (1) the presence of any apneas or hypopneas or (2) insufficient ventilation during sleep. OHS is defined by the combination of obesity, SDB, and awake daytime hypercapnia.[55] Hypercapnia is defined as an awake resting Pa_{CO_2} >45 mm Hg via an arterial blood gas.[55] Hypoxia seen on pulse oximetry or elevated serum bicarbonate levels (>27 mmol/L) seen on laboratory work can also suggest OHS. Patients with abnormal Pa_{CO_2} should undergo PSG to diagnose hypoventilation and identify optimal PAP settings.

Management

For patients with OHS, marked sustained weight loss of 25% to 30% of actual body weight is needed to achieve meaningful reduction of hypoventilation. While lifestyle changes should be recommended, this magnitude of weight loss is most likely achieved with bariatric surgery.

PAP with CPAP or BIPAP is the mainstay of therapy for OHS to reverse the awake hypoventilation. Clinicians should monitor these patients closely for the first 2 to 3 months after initiating PAP therapy. Inadequate clinical response, insufficient improvement in gas exchange using Pa_{CO_2}, or continued hospital admissions for acute-on-chronic hypercapnic respiratory failure can suggest treatment failure. If treatment failure occurs on CPAP, after ensuring treatment adherence, transition patients to BIPAP.

GASTROINTESTINAL DISORDERS OF OBESITY

Gastroesophageal Reflux Disease

Assessment

Definition of GERD and Prevalence in Obesity

Gastroesophageal reflux disease (GERD) is common in the general population, defined as symptoms or complications from reflux of gastric contents into the esophagus and oral cavity.[57] Common symptoms include heartburn, regurgitation, chronic cough, and dyspepsia. The prevalence of GERD in the general population is estimated to be 10% to 20%, and current literature suggests a two- to threefold increase in severe reflux symptoms among persons with obesity, with stronger associations of symptoms in women, elevated waist circumference, and white race.[57]

Physiology of GERD in Obesity

Multiple mechanisms have been proposed to describe the increase in acid reflux in obesity. Mechanical mechanisms include increased intragastric pressure as a result of visceral fat, increased prevalence of hiatal hernias in individuals with obesity, and increased pressure gradient across the gastroesophageal junction with associated increased frequency of transient lower esophageal sphincter relaxation.[58] Abnormalities of the motility of the GI tract are also associated with obesity, including esophageal peristaltic dysfunction, higher fasting gastric volume, and reduced satiation.[59] Additionally, visceral fat is recognized as metabolically active, producing adipocytokines which can increase GERD symptoms or GERD-related sequelae such as erosive esophagitis and Barrett esophagus.[58]

Evaluation

GERD is a clinical diagnosis; patients can be treated empirically if they have typical symptoms of heartburn and regurgitation. However, patients with chest pain as a symptom should have an appropriate cardiac evaluation ruling out primary cardiac etiologies of symptoms. Otherwise, a trial of a proton pump inhibitor (PPI) can be initiated and monitored. Patients with obesity undergoing evaluation for bariatric surgery with GERD should be considered for GI evaluation for reflux preoperatively.[57]

Management

In patients with obesity, weight loss in addition to GERD lifestyle modification is an essential component of therapy. Avoidance of food triggers is critical; these include caffeine, spicy foods, chocolate, and foods with high fat content or acidity. Head of bed elevation and avoidance of meals 2 to 3 hours prior to sleeping are also recommended. A trial of PPI for 8 weeks can be initiated in patients with typical GERD symptoms, administered 30 to 60 minutes before their first meal. Patients with partial response can be titrated to twice daily dosing. Patients with no response or incomplete response to PPI should be referred to a gastroenterologist for further evaluation.[57]

Nonalcoholic Fatty Liver Disease and Nonalcoholic Steatohepatitis

Assessment

Definition and Prevalence of NAFLD in Obesity

The American Association for the Study of Liver Diseases (AASLD) defines NAFLD as evidence of hepatic steatosis on imaging or histology, without secondary causes of hepatic fat infiltration. NAFLD can be further subdivided into histologic classification: nonalcoholic fatty liver (NAFL), defined as ≥5% hepatic steatosis without hepatocellular injury, or nonalcoholic steatohepatitis (NASH), defined as ≥5% hepatic steatosis with inflammation and hepatocellular injury.[60]

The global prevalence of NAFLD is increasing with similar rate of rise as the prevalence of obesity. NAFLD is estimated to affect approximately 25% of the global population; this increases to 57% to 74% in obesity (BMI ≥30 kg/m^2) and >90% in severe obesity (BMI ≥40 kg/m^2).[60]

Evaluation

The AASLD recommends against routine screening for NAFLD in patients with obesity given lack of cost effectiveness and ambiguity in diagnostic testing and therapy. However, a high index of suspicion for NAFLD should remain in patients with metabolic syndrome.

In patients with suspected NAFLD or imaging evidence of steatosis, other common causes of hepatic steatosis should be excluded. Secondary steatosis can be caused by significant alcohol consumption, Wilson disease, total parental nutrition, medications (mipomersen, lomitapide, amiodarone, methotrexate, tamoxifen, corticosteroids), and chronic hepatitis B or C. Additionally, other chronic liver diseases (e.g., autoimmune hepatitis) should be ruled out, especially in the setting of abnormal liver chemistries.[60]

It is important to investigate potential fibrosis in NAFLD patients given the risk of advanced fibrosis and cirrhosis. Normal or abnormal liver chemistries do not necessarily correlate with the presence of steatohepatitis or fibrosis. To determine the degree of inflammation and/or fibrosis in patients with NAFLD, liver biopsy remains the gold standard, although this test is not routinely performed due to cost and procedural risk. Noninvasive methods have been developed to estimate the degree of fibrosis including serum laboratory testing (FibroTest, Hepascore), validated scoring tests (NAFLD fibrosis score, FIB-4 index), and imaging. The NAFLD fibrosis score (NFS) uses age, BMI, platelet count, presence of diabetes, aspartate transaminase/alanine aminotransferase (AST/ALT) ratio, and albumin to estimate the degree of fibrosis (online scoring calculator: http://gihep.com/calculators/hepatology/nafld-fibrosis-score/). The FIB-4 index uses age, BMI, AST/ALT, and platelets to estimate fibrosis (online scoring calculator: http://gihep.com/calculators/hepatology/fibrosis-4-score/). Both scoring systems are reliable to predict advanced fibrosis (stage 3 bridging fibrosis and stage 4 cirrhosis). The above tests can be used in conjunction with specialized liver imaging modalities, ultrasound elastography, and MR elastography, which measure liver stiffness to predict degree of fibrosis.[60] A referral to hepatology should be made in patients who have high risk of fibrosis based on the NFS or the FIB-4.

Management

The mainstay of treatment is for NAFLD is lifestyle modification to produce weight loss. A 3% to 5% weight reduction can improve steatosis, and 7% to 10% reduction can improve NASH and fibrosis. Additionally, patients who qualify for bariatric surgery should be referred to a surgeon for evaluation for weight loss surgery. NAFLD patients have significant cardiovascular risk overlap and modifiable risk factors should be treated.

Gallbladder Disease

Assessment

Physiology of Gallstone Formation in Obesity

Obesity increases the risk of symptomatic gallstones, particularly in female patients with BMI ≥30 kg/m².[61] Increased gallstone formation is secondary to excess cholesterol secreted in bile, which is in turn due to increased body adiposity. Elevated concentrations of cholesterol in bile increase the propensity for stone formation.[62] Rapid weight loss as occurs following bariatric surgery or with very-low-calorie diets can also increase the risk for gallstone formation due to increased fat metabolism causing increased cholesterol excretion in bile.[62] The risk for gallstone formation is higher when patients have rapid and sustained weight loss (i.e., ≥1.5 kg/week for at least 4 weeks).[63]

Presentation and Evaluation

Patients with uncomplicated symptomatic gallstone disease typically present with sporadic episodes of postprandial pain, ~30 to 60 minutes after ingestion of a meal, particularly a high-fat meal. Pain is typically moderate to severe in intensity, lasting 1 to 5 hours, and localized to the right upper quadrant of the abdomen. Approximately 50% of patients may experience radiation to the right scapular tip (Collins sign). Initial evaluation should consist of laboratory studies (complete blood count, basic metabolic panel, liver function, and lipase) and abdominal ultrasound imaging. Leukocytosis, abnormal liver function, fever, or persistent pain may be signs of complicated gallstone disease such as cholecystitis, gallstone pancreatitis, choledocholithiasis, or cholangitis.

Management

Patients with uncomplicated symptomatic gallstone disease are typically managed conservatively with pain control with NSAIDs during episodes. In the long term, patients can be managed expectantly or referred for surgical evaluation to determine eligibility for laparoscopic cholecystectomy. Some patients who are not candidates for surgery may be candidates for ursodeoxycholic acid or extracorporeal shock wave lithotripsy.

MUSCULOSKELETAL DISEASES OF OBESITY

Osteoarthritis

Assessment

Prevalence of OA in Obese Populations

Joint pain is strongly associated with body weight, particularly affecting the knees, hips, and spine. Excess weight increases the mechanical stress on weight-bearing joints such as the knee and hip, allowing breakdown of cartilage. For every 11 lb weight gain, there is a 36% increased risk of developing OA.[64]

Women with BMI ≥25 kg/m² have nearly four times the risk of knee OA, and for men, the risk is five times greater.[64] Obesity is a modifiable risk factor for progression of arthritis, limitation, disability, reduced quality of life and for poor clinical outcomes after joint replacement.

Review of Symptoms and Physical Examination

Symptoms of OA can vary but predominantly include pain worse with joint use and relived by rest, stiffness (morning or inactivity-related), and locomotor restrictions.

On physical examination, inspection of the joints often shows swelling, deformity, and muscle wasting. Joint effusions, joint line tenderness, and periarticular tenderness can be palpated along with coarse crepitus, reduced range of motions, and weak local muscles with movement examination. OA involving the hip can cause pain felt in the groin, inner thigh, buttocks or even knees that limits dressing or putting on shoes. OA of the spine can impinge on nerves resulting in weakness, tingling, or numbness along the distribution of a nerve.

Role of Imaging in Diagnosis

Diagnosis of OA may be made without radiographic or laboratory investigations in the at-risk age group with typical symptoms and signs. Radiographic examination can be normal in OA and, therefore, should not routinely be used to establish a diagnosis of OA. Additional laboratory assessments could be considered if signs and symptoms suggest an autoimmune disorder.

Management

Weight Loss and OA

An 11-pound weight loss has been shown to result in a 50% relative drop in the risk of OA.[65] If persons with obesity lose enough weight to drop to the overweight category or overweight individuals lose enough weight to drop to the normal weight category, knee OA would drop by 22% and 35% in men and women, respectively.[66] Weight loss can improve symptoms by restoring function and quality of life, as well as decrease the need for total knee replacement.

Physical Activity in OA

All patients should be enrolled in an individualized exercise program. The current evidence does not recommend a specific exercise prescription but shows that exercise results in improvements in pain and functional limitations.[67] Specifically, balance exercises focusing on control and stabilizing body position have been shown to reduce the risk of falls.

Physical therapy is helpful for evaluating patients' ability to perform aerobic and/or resistance activities, to receive assistive devices, to instruct in joint protection techniques, and to educate on use of thermal agents for relief of pain and stiffness.[67] A walking aid may be warranted in patients with knee and/or hip OA to aid in ambulation, joint stability, or pain.[67]

Tibiofemoral knee braces and patellofemoral braces may provide benefit in joint stabilization and pain. Additionally, Kinesio Taping can be useful in patients with OA permitting range of motion while stabilizing the joint.[67]

Tai chi is strongly recommended for patients with knee or hip OA to improve strength and balance and for fall prevention.[67] While more data are required on yoga, acupuncture and cognitive behavioral therapy trials have demonstrated improvements in pain.

Pharmacotherapy

There are a variety of therapies available for OA management based on the joints involved and age of the patient. Large studies evaluating alternative therapies including glucosamine and chondroitin sulfate have failed to demonstrate clinical efficacy of these agents, and they are currently not recommended by the American College of Rheumatology. Pharmacotherapy options for OA include topical agents, acetaminophen, nonsteroidal anti-inflammatory agents, intra-articular steroid injections, tramadol, opiates, and adjunctive nonopiate therapies (e.g., duloxetine). Pharmacologic treatment options for OA are thought to be weight neutral.

Surgery

Patients with OA refractory to lifestyle management (weight loss, individualized exercise plan) and pharmacotherapy should be referred for evaluation for total joint arthroplasty. Orthopedists often require patients to meet various BMI cut-off criteria (typically BMI <40 kg/m²) to minimize complication rates. While older guidelines operate under the notion that higher BMI is a risk factor for complication rates, recent data suggest that pain relief and functional gain was similar in those with obesity compared to those without.[68] Randomized control trials are needed to remove strict institutional cutoffs.

MALIGNANCY

There is consistent evidence that higher amounts of body fat are associated with increased risk of at least 13 different types of cancer outlined in Figure 4.2. Excess weight is thought to account for 40% of all cancers diagnosed in 2014, affecting more than 630,000 people in the United States. The incidence of most cancers associated with overweight and obesity increased from 2005 to 2014, except for colorectal cancer. The higher risk for cancer per 1 kg/m² increase in BMI ranged from 1% each for thyroid and ovarian cancers to 9% for esophageal adenocarcinoma (Table 4.7).

Assessment

Physiology for Tumorigenesis in Obesity

Persons with obesity have chronic low-level inflammation that, over time, may lead to DNA damage.[70] Individuals with overweight/obesity are more likely to have conditions that cause chronic local inflammation that act as risk factors for certain cancers. For example, gastroesophageal reflux can result in Barrett esophagus and esophageal adenocarcinoma. Similarly, chronic gallbladder inflammation and a history of gallstones is a strong risk factor for gallbladder cancer, and NAFLD is a strong risk factor for hepatocellular cancer.[71]

Another mechanism suggested in the pathophysiology of tumorigenesis in obesity is hormone production by adipose tissue. Excess amounts of estrogen produced from fat confers an increased risk of developing breast, endometrial, and ovarian malignancies. Higher blood levels of insulin-like growth factor 1 (IGF-1) found in obesity can promote colon, kidney, and endometrial cancers. A number of other hormones may also be involved.

Screening for Cancer

There are no changes in cancer screening based on BMI. The USPSTF has screening guidelines for breast cancer, cervical cancer, and colorectal cancer (Table 4.8). They do not recommend screening for the remaining cancers in the asymptomatic general population or persons with overweight/obesity.

Management

How Does Weight Loss Impact Cancer Risk?

Weight loss has been shown to reduce cancer risk. When studying the bariatric surgery population, patients with obesity who underwent surgery and had a 20% reduction of BMI halved their cancer incidence. This protection in the postbariatric surgery population extends to patients with genetic predisposition to malignancy.[73] While there are limited large, prospective studies, evidence from observational studies show that lower weight gain during adulthood is associated with lower risk of colon cancer, kidney cancer, and postmenopausal breast cancer, as well as endometrial and ovarian cancers.[74]

Cancer Survivorship and Obesity

Obesity may worsen aspects of cancer survivorship including quality of life, cancer recurrence, cancer progression, and prognosis. For example, obesity is associated with increased risk of lymphedema in breast cancer survivors and incontinence in prostate cancer survivors treated with radical prostatectomy. Patients with higher baseline BMI in stage II-III rectal cancer

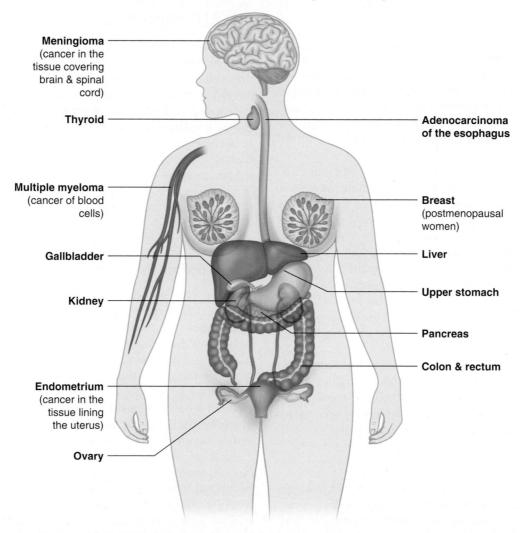

Cancers Associated with Overweight & Obesity

Meningioma (cancer in the tissue covering brain & spinal cord)

Thyroid

Multiple myeloma (cancer of blood cells)

Gallbladder

Kidney

Endometrium (cancer in the tissue lining the uterus)

Ovary

Adenocarcinoma of the esophagus

Breast (postmenopausal women)

Liver

Upper stomach

Pancreas

Colon & rectum

FIGURE 4.2 Cancers associated with overweight and obesity.

TABLE 4.7 Risk of Cancer in Populations With Overweight/Obesity

CANCER	% INCREASE IN RISK FOR CANCER PER 1 kg/m² INCREASE IN BMI
Esophageal adenocarcinoma	9
Gastric cardia cancer	4
Liver cancer	5
Pancreatic cancer	2
Colon and rectum	2
Gallbladder cancer	5
Breast (in postmenopausal women)	2
Ovarian cancer	1
Endometrial cancer	8
Kidney (renal cell carcinoma)	5
Thyroid	1
Meningioma	4
Multiple myeloma	2

BMI, body mass index.
Adapted from Steele CB, Thomas CC, Henley SJ, et al. Vital signs: trends in incidence of cancers associated with overweight and obesity – United States, 2005-2014. MMWR Morb Mortal Wkly Rep. 2017;66(39):1052-1058.

had increased risk of local recurrence. Patients with obesity undergoing colorectal laparoscopic procedures such as hemicolectomy are at high risk for open conversion. Obesity also has an impact on complications after abdominal cancer surgery, such as incisional and parastomal hernia development.

Chemotherapy Considerations

According to the American Society of Clinical Oncology guidelines, full body weight should be used when selecting cytotoxic chemotherapy doses, regardless of obesity status especially when the goal of treatment is cure.[75] Only certain agents should be given as fixed dosing (e.g., carboplatin, bleomycin, and vincristine).

There is pharmacodynamic and pharmacokinetic variability in patients with obesity. Chemotherapy dosing using adjusted body weight has shown increases in severe toxicity with anthracycline- and taxane-containing regimens. Herceptin administration has been shown to have increased cardiac toxicity in patients with obesity.[75]

TABLE 4.8 Society Cancer Screening Recommendations

United States Preventive Services Task Force (USPSTF) A and B Recommendations

Breast cancer screening	Screening mammography for women, with or without clinical breast examination, every 1-2 years for women aged 50 years or older. The decision to start screening mammography in women prior to age 50 years should be an individual one.
Cervical cancer screening	The USPSTF recommends screening for cervical cancer every 3 years with cervical cytology alone in women aged 21-29 years. For women aged 30-65 years, the USPSTF recommends screening every 3 years with cervical cytology alone, every 5 years with high-risk human papillomavirus (hrHPV) testing alone, or every 5 years with hrHPV testing in combination with cytology.
Colorectal cancer screening	The USPSTF recommends screening for colorectal cancer starting at the age of 50 years and continuing until the age of 75 years.

American Association for the Study of Liver Disease recommendations

Liver cancer screening*	The AASLD recommends abdominal ultrasound and/or AFP every 6 months for patients with cirrhosis from NAFLD based on laboratory test, imaging, or biopsy. No screening is recommended for noncirrhosis NAFLD.

AASLD, American Association for the Study of Liver Diseases; AFP, alpha-fetoprotein; NAFLD, nonalcoholic fatty liver disease.
*No screening is recommended for gastric cardia cancer, pancreatic cancer, or gallbladder cancer in the asymptomatic population.
Adapted from Heimbach JK, Kulik LM, Finn RS, et al. AASLD guidelines for the treatment of hepatocellular carcinoma. Hepatology. 2018;67(1):358-380.

There is some evidence that antiangiogenic agents such as bevacizumab might be less effective in patients with obesity. Excess adiposity is associated with increased circulating level of vascular endothelial growth factor, a regulator of tumor angiogenesis. This has been found in colorectal cancer, renal cell carcinoma, and ovarian cancer.

MENTAL HEALTH AND OBESITY

Depression

Assessment

Prevalence of Depression in Individuals With Obesity

Obesity and depression are known to have a reciprocal relationship, in that obesity notably increases the risk of major depressive disorder (MDD), and MDD also increases the risk of obesity. Patients with obesity and severe obesity were found to have 1.5 to 2 times increased prevalence of MDD. Women with BMI ≥35 kg/m² may have up to 5 times increased prevalence of MDD.[76]

Evaluation

Screening for depression is recommended in primary care settings. Several screening tools exist; the most commonly used screening tools are the patient health questionnaires (PHQ-9 and PHQ-2) (Table 4.9). The PHQ-2 is effective for ruling out depression, with 93% negative predictive value, but does not confirm the diagnosis. If the patient responds positively to either question on the PHQ-2, this should prompt further investigation with PHQ-9. Scores of 10 to 27 on the PHQ-9 suggest moderate to severe depression, and this diagnosis should then be confirmed by the *Diagnostic and Statistical Manual* (DSM) criteria for depression. Additionally, the PHQ-9 can be used for monitoring symptoms and response to therapy. HCPs should also rule out concurrent conditions that can mimic MDD, including anemia, hypothyroidism, infection, or metabolic derangements.[77]

Management

Given the reciprocal relationship of depression and obesity, therapy considerations should include mechanisms of weight loss in addition to mental health management via psychotherapy and pharmacotherapy.

Psychotherapeutic options include cognitive behavioral therapy (CBT) that is included within behavioral weight loss programs and interpersonal therapy. Multiple pharmacotherapeutic options exist; however, careful selection is imperative as many antidepressants can induce weight gain. Table 4.10 summarizes the weight effects of common classes of antidepressant medications.[78]

Binge Eating Disorder

Assessment

Definition of BED

BED is an eating disorder characterize by repeated episodes of binge eating (i.e., eating an abnormally large amount of food within a 2-hour window of time), without intentional corrective behaviors such as vomiting or laxative abuse.[79] Individuals with this disorder may report eating until uncomfortably full, eating when not physically hungry, and feelings of guilt/disgust associated with overeating. In the general population, the prevalence of BED is 2% to 5%; this increases to 5% to 30% in patients who are being evaluated for weight loss therapy.[79] Diagnosis can be made based on DSM-5 criteria, typically with referral to psychiatry for confirmation and management.

TABLE 4.9 Comparison of PHQ9 to PHQ2 Depression Screening Tests

PATIENT HEALTH QUESTIONNAIRE-9 (PHQ-9[B])	PATIENT HEALTH QUESTIONNAIRE-2 (PHQ-2[A])
Over the past 2 weeks, how often have you been bothered by any of the following problems? (0-Not at all, 1-Several days, 2-More than half the days, 3-Nearly every day)	
Little interest in doing things	Little interest in doing things
Feeling down, hopeless or depressed	Feeling down, hopeless or depressed
Trouble falling asleep or staying asleep, or sleeping too much	
Feeling tired or having little energy	
Poor appetite or overeating	
Feeling bad about yourself, feeling like a failure	
Trouble concentrating on things	
Moving or speaking slowly, or the opposite, restless and fidgety	
Thoughts that you would be better off dead, or thoughts of hurting yourself	

[a]PHQ-2: Score of >3 is positive, proceed with PHQ-9.
[b]PHQ-9: Scoring 1 to 4 = minimal depression; 5 to 9 = mild depression; 10 to 14 = moderate depression; 15 to 19 = moderately severe depression; 20 to 27 = severe depression.
Adapted from Maurer DM, Raymond TJ, Davis BN. Depression: screening and diagnosis. Am Fam Physician. 2018;98(8):508-515.

TABLE 4.10 Antidepressant Medications Effect on Weight

WEIGHT GAIN	WEIGHT NEUTRAL/LESS WEIGHT GAIN	WEIGHT LOSS
Tricyclics	SSRIs (Fluoxetine, Sertraline)	Bupropion
MAOIs		
SSRIs (Paroxetine)	SNRIs (Duloxetine, Venlafaxine)	
Mirtazapine		

MAOIs, monoamine oxidase inhibitors; SNRIs, serotonin norepinephrine reuptake inhibitors; SSRIs, selective serotonin reuptake inhibitors.
Adapted from Igel LI, Kumar RB, Saunders KH, Aronne LJ. Practical use of pharmacotherapy for obesity. Gastroenterology. 2017;152(7):1765-1779.

Management

BED is a complex disorder which requires a multidisciplinary approach to management, with goal of avoidance of binge episodes and weight loss. Lifestyle modifications including diet and exercise should be incorporated into an individualized treatment plan. CBT is the mainstay of therapy for patients with BED to correct negative eating behaviors and induce remission in 50% to 60% of cases. In conjunction with behavioral therapy, pharmacotherapy with antidepressants can help to induce and maintain remission. Selective serotonin reuptake inhibitors (SSRIs), bupropion, topiramate, and lisdexamfetamine are all used for the treatment of BED. The latter three agents may help to induce some weight loss. Lisdexamfetamine is a Schedule II controlled substance and should be used with caution due to addiction potential.

Night Eating Syndrome

Assessment

Definition of Night Eating Syndrome

Night eating syndrome (NES) is characterized by nighttime hyperphagia (≥25% of caloric intake after an evening meal) with recall of the event at least twice per week. Associated characteristics include insomnia, stress, depressed mood, and morning anorexia.[79,80] Additionally, these patients are noted to preferentially consume carbohydrates during nighttime meals. The prevalence of NES in the general population is approximately 1.5%; this increases to 8.9% to 14% in patients with obesity and up to 27% in severe obesity.[81]

CLINICAL HIGHLIGHTS

This chapter has reviewed the evaluation and treatment of the common medical and behavioral conditions that affect patients with obesity. Obesity is considered a chronic disease and also impacts nearly every other organ system in the human body. Some conditions (diabetes, HTN) result from the metabolic effects of excess weight, whereas others (OSA, osteoarthritis) result from the mechanical impacts. Major depressive disorder has a bidirectional relationship with obesity. The lifestyle changes and degree of weight loss required to improve each condition varies greatly. The chapter also outlines the optimal treatment for each condition to maximize weight loss and, subsequently, improvement in that disorder.

WHEN TO REFER

- CVD: High risk for CAD in a patient wanting to start a vigorous exercise program; abnormal exercise stress test.
- Diabetes: Hyperglycemia persisting despite combination drug therapy; complications of diabetes (renal disease, retinopathy).
- PCOS: Women with PCOS desiring fertility.
- OSA: Medical treatment with PAP therapy (pulmonary/sleep specialist) or surgical treatment (head and neck surgeon).
- Gastroenterology: GERD unresponsive to PPIs; NAFLD at high risk for fibrosis by screening calculator.
- Orthopedics: OA unresponsive to weight loss, exercise, and medical therapy.
- Psychiatry: Depression refractory to commonly used medications; BED.

Physiology and Management of NES in Obesity

It is postulated that patients with NES and obesity have chronotropic disruption, aberrations in circadian rhythms via imbalances in glucocorticoid and serotonergic systems which eventually lead to altered behavior and obesity.[80] Further studies are required to fully elucidate the relationship and understand the disease. SSRI therapy is being investigated as a treatment option; a small randomized study does show an induction of remission with use of sertraline.[81]

CASE STUDIES

Discussion of Case Study 1: Assessment and Treatment of Cardiometabolic Obesity-Related Comorbidities

For this patient, assessment requires HBA1C screening for T2D, especially in the presence of acanthosis nigricans, along with liver enzyme testing to evaluate for NAFLD and need for further investigation including hepatic ultrasound. Her blood pressure is elevated and should be repeated within a short time frame (1 to 2 weeks) perhaps by use of a home blood pressure monitor. Mainstay of treatment is lifestyle modification with a reduced calorie diet and moderate physical activity. Important dietary plans to consider include a DASH approach (rich in fruits, vegetables, legumes, and low-fat dairy products and low in snacks, sweets, meats, and saturated and total fat) or a DPP-based low-fat diet. Lifestyle intervention may be supplemented with pharmacotherapy, such as metformin in this patient, for the additional prevention of T2D. If ambulatory blood pressures remain elevated, beginning a low-dose diuretic agent, calcium channel blocker, or angiotensin receptor blocker may be indicated. Evaluation of Janice's sleep/snoring might also assist the HCP in diagnosing an underlying sleep disorder that, through appropriate treatment, improves blood pressure control.

Discussion of Case Study 2

For this patient, discussion with psychiatry is needed to determine if mirtazapine therapy can be discontinued for his mood disorder, and instead, a less obesogenic agent be initiated. For his erectile dysfunction, lifestyle modification to promote weight loss should be initiated first to improve his symptoms; however, if no change in libido or erectile function is reported, the HCP

CASE STUDY 2:
....

ASSESSMENT AND TREATMENT OF COMORBID MOOD DISORDERS

Fred is a 42-year-old man with a history of refractory depression and class 1 obesity who presents to your office with a new complaint of erectile dysfunction. He is taking mirtazapine and is interested in testosterone replacement therapy. He has no symptoms of sleep apnea, and his wife says he does not snore. He has decreased libido and has noticed reduced frequency of needing to shave. Physical examination is notable for a BMI of 32 kg/m^2 and waist circumference of 100 cm. Genital examination is unremarkable. His prolactin and FSH levels are normal, and a pituitary MRI does not show a tumor.

should check total testosterone levels measured in the morning and repeated on two occasions, preferably 4 weeks apart. If definite biochemical hypogonadism is detected, testosterone therapy should be administered to induce and maintain secondary sex characteristics, improve his energy levels, and protect his bones from osteoporosis. Testosterone therapy will likely improve Fred's erectile dysfunction and testosterone levels.

QUIZ QUESTIONS

1. AS is a 50-year-old man who is being evaluated for complications from obesity. Known medical problems include prediabetes and HTN treated with losartan. He takes no other medications and does not smoke or drink alcohol. He has no known family history of liver disease. On physical examination, BMI is 40 kg/m^2, blood pressure 130/78, and heart rate is 84. There is no jaundice, ascites, or other signs of end-stage liver disease. On laboratory testing, AST is 95, ALT is 88, and platelet count is 100,000. His ferritin is normal, and his serological tests for hepatitis are negative. A Fibrosis 4 score is calculated as 5.1, indicating likely advanced fibrosis. Which of the following is the next best step to address his abnormal liver function tests?

   A. Reassure him that his liver will get better with weight loss
   B. Refer him to bariatric surgery
   C. Refer for an elastography scan
   D. Refer him to a gastroenterologist for a liver biopsy

   Answer: C. *NASH is a common complication of obesity that can lead to cirrhosis. Unfortunately, there are currently no highly effective pharmacotherapeutic treatments. Weight loss is beneficial. It is also important to identify those patients who are developing significant fibrosis. A liver biopsy is the best test to make a diagnosis of NASH, but it is expensive, requires expertise for interpretation, and carries with it some risk of morbidity and even mortality. The Fibrosis 4 score helps identify those patients at risk for fibrosis with a score of < 1.45 that are unlikely to have advanced fibrosis. Those with a score ≥ 3.25 are more likely to have significant fibrosis. Ultrasound elastography (Fibroscan) technology is a noninvasive test that is FDA approved for use in diagnosing significant liver fibrosis and can be used to identify those patients who are developing significant fibrosis.[71]*

2. DG is a 54-year-old male with prediabetes, dyslipidemia, and NAFLD. His NAFLD was detected incidentally on a CT scan. He takes metformin and atorvastatin. Physical examination is unremarkable except for his BMI of 39 kg/m^2 and abdominal obesity. Laboratory data show HBA1C of 5.9%, HDL 32, fasting triglycerides 178, and normal AST and ALT. The patient has been reading about obesity and elevated cancer risk and wants to know what cancer screenings he should have based on his weight. Which of the following is the most appropriate response?

   A. He should have the same cancer screening regimen as other 54-year-old men who have normal BMI
   B. He should have more frequent screening for colon cancer than other 54-year-old men since this occurs at greater frequency in people with obesity
   C. He should have more frequent screening for colon cancer than other 54-year-old men, as well as routine screening for esophageal, liver, and kidney cancer
   D. He should have more frequent screening for liver cancer than other 54-year-old men because of his diagnosis of NAFLD

   Answer: A. *There are no recommendations for increased cancer screening based on obesity alone. Thus, both answers B and C are incorrect. There is a recommendation for routine screening for hepatocellular carcinoma, but this recommendation is only for patients with NASH. This patient has NAFLD but has normal liver enzymes and thus has no evidence of NASH. Thus, he would be considered at similar risk of hepatocellular cancer compared to the general population.*

PRACTICAL RESOURCES

- DASH diet (https://dashdiet.org/sample-menu.html)
- 2019 ACC/AHA guidelines (https://www.ahajournals.org/doi/full/10.1161/CIR.0000000000000677)
- ASCVD Risk Estimator Plus from the American College of Cardiology (http://tools.acc.org/ASCVD-Risk-Estimator-Plus/#!/calculate/estimate/)
- NAFLD fibrosis score (http://gihep.com/calculators/hepatology/nafld-fibrosis-score/)
- YMCA DPP (https://www.ymca.net/diabetes-prevention/locate-participating-y)
- CDC nutrition (https://www.cdc.gov/diabetes/managing/eat-well.html)

REFERENCES

1. Johnson NB, Hayes LD, Brown K, Hoo EC, Ethier KA; Centers for Disease Control and Prevention (CDC). CDC National Health Report: Leading causes of morbidity and mortality and associated behavioral risk and protective factors–United States, 2005-2013. *MMWR Suppl.* 2014;63(4):24.
2. Dominique DS, Busetto L, Dicker D, et al. European practical and patient-centred guidelines for adult obesity management in primary care. *Obes Facts.* 2019;12(1):40-66. doi:10.1159/000496183
3. Flegal KM, Kit BK, Orpana H, Graubard BI. Association of all-cause mortality with overweight and obesity using standard body mass index categories: a systematic review and meta-analysis. *J Am Med Assoc.* 2013;309(1):71-82. doi:10.1001/jama.2012.113905
4. Rueda-Clausen CF, Ogunleye AA, Sharma AM. Health benefits of long-term weight-loss maintenance. *Annu Rev Nutr.* 2015;35:475-516. doi:10.1146/annurev-nutr-071714-034434
5. Adams TD, Davidson LE, Litwin SE, et al. Weight and metabolic outcomes 12 years after gastric bypass. *N Engl J Med.* 2017;377(12):1143-1155. doi:10.1056/NEJMoa1700459
6. Neter JE, Stam BE, Kok FJ, Grobbee DE, Geleijnse JM. Influence of weight reduction on blood pressure: a meta-analysis of randomized controlled trials. *Hypertension.* 2003;42(5):878-884. doi:10.1161/01.HYP.0000094221.86888.AE
7. Higgins M, Kannel W, Garrison R, Pinsky J, Stokes J. Hazards of obesity – The Framingham experience. *Acta Med Scand Suppl.* 1988;723:23-36. doi:10.1111/j.0954-6820.1987.tb05925.x
8. Wilson PW, D'Agostino RB, Sullivan L, Parise H, Kannel WB. Overweight and obesity as determinants of cardiovascular risk: the Framingham experience. *Arch Intern Med.* 2002;162(16):1867-1872. doi:10.1001/archinte.162.16.1867
9. Rahmouni K, Correia ML, Haynes WG, Mark AL. Obesity-associated hypertension: new insights into mechanisms. *Hypertension.* 2005;45(1):9-14. doi:10.1161/01.HYP.0000151325.83008.b4
10. U.S. Preventive Services Task Force; A and B Recommendations. *U.S. Preventive Services Task Force.* 2020.
11. Whelton PK, Carey RM, Aronow WS, et al. 2017 ACC/AHA/AAPA/ABC/ACPM/AGS/APhA/ASH/ASPC/NMA/PCNA guideline for the prevention, detection, evaluation, and management of high blood pressure in adults: a report of the American College of Cardiology/American Heart Association Task Force on clinical practice guidelines. *Hypertension.* 2018;71(6):e13-e115. doi:10.1161/HYP.0000000000000065

12. Carey RM, Whelton PK; 2017 ACC/AHA Hypertension Guideline Writing Committee. Prevention, detection, evaluation, and management of high blood pressure in adults: synopsis of the 2017 American College of Cardiology/American Heart Association Hypertension Guideline. *Ann Intern Med.* 2018;168(5):351-358. doi:10.7326/M17-3203

13. Bavikati VV, Sperling LS, Salmon RD, et al. Effect of comprehensive therapeutic lifestyle changes on prehypertension. *Am J Cardiol.* 2008;102(12):1677-1680. doi:10.1016/j.amjcard.2008.08.034

14. Appel LJ, Moore TJ, Obarzanek E, et al. A clinical trial of the effects of dietary patterns on blood pressure. DASH Collaborative Research Group. *N Engl J Med.* 1997;336(16):1117-1124. doi:10.1056/NEJM199704173361601

15. Semlitsch T, Jeitler K, Berghold A, et al. Long-term effects of weight-reducing diets in people with hypertension. *Cochrane Database Syst Rev.* 2016;3:CD008274. doi:10.1002/14651858.CD008274.pub3

16. Diabetes Prevention Program Outcomes Study; Knowler WC, Fowler SE, Hamman RF, et al. 10-year follow-up of diabetes incidence and weight loss in the Diabetes Prevention Program Outcomes Study. *Lancet.* 2009;374(9702):1677-1686. doi:10.1016/S0140-6736(09)61457-4

17. Freedman DS, Dietz WH, Srinivasan SR, Berenson GS. The relation of overweight to cardiovascular risk factors among children and adolescents: the Bogalusa Heart Study. *Pediatrics.* 1999;103(6 pt 1):1175-1182. doi:10.1542/peds.103.6.1175

18. Goldstein LB, Bushnell CD, Adams RJ, et al. Guidelines for the primary prevention of stroke: a statement for healthcare professionals from the American Heart Association/American Stroke Association. *Stroke.* 2014;45(12):3754-3832. doi:10.1161/STR.0000000000000046

19. Jensen MD, Ryan DH, Apovian CM, et al. 2013 AHA/ACC/TOS guideline for the management of overweight and obesity in adults: a report of the American College of Cardiology/American heart association Task Force on practice guidelines and the Obesity Society. *Circulation.* 2014;129(25 suppl 2):S102-S138. doi:10.1161/01.cir.0000437739.71477.ee

20. Gibbons RJ, Balady GJ, Bricker JT, et al. ACC/AHA 2002 guideline update for exercise testing: summary article. A report of the American College of Cardiology/American Heart Association Task Force on practice guidelines (committee to update the 1997 exercise testing guidelines). *J Am Coll Cardiol.* 2002;40(8):1531-1540. doi:10.1016/s0735-1097(02)02164-2

21. Estruch R, Ros E, Salas-Salvado J, et al. Retraction and republication: primary prevention of cardiovascular disease with a mediterranean diet. *N Engl J Med.* 2018;378(25):2441-2442. doi:10.1056/NEJMc1806491

22. Hu FB. Plant-based foods and prevention of cardiovascular disease: an overview. *Am J Clin Nutr.* 2003;78(3 suppl):544S-551S. doi:10.1093/ajcn/78.3.544S

23. Grundy SM, Stone NJ, Bailey AL, et al. 2018 AHA/ACC/AACVPR/AAPA/ABC/ACPM/ADA/AGS/APhA/ASPC/NLA/PCNA guideline on the management of blood cholesterol: a report of the American College of Cardiology/American Heart Association Task Force on clinical practice guidelines. *Circulation.* 2019;139(25):e1082-e1143. doi:10.1161/CIR.0000000000000625

24. Caspard H, Jabbour S, Hammar N, Fenici P, Sheehan JJ, Kosiborod M. Recent trends in the prevalence of type 2 diabetes and the association with abdominal obesity lead to growing health disparities in the USA: an analysis of the NHANES surveys from 1999 to 2014. *Diabetes Obes Metab.* 2018;20(3):667-671. doi:10.1111/dom.13143

25. *Estimates of Diabetes and its Burden in the United States, 2017.* Center of Disease Control. Accessed December, 2019. https://www.cdc.gov/diabetes/data/index.html

26. Senel E, Salmanoğlu M, Solmazgül E, Berçik İnal B. Acrochordons as a cutaneous sign of impaired carbohydrate metabolism, hyperlipidemia, liver enzyme abnormalities and hypertension: a case-control study. *J Eur Acad Dermatol Venereol.* 2011. doi:10.1111/j.1468-3083.2011.04396.x

27. Diabetes Prevention Program (DPP) Research. Group. The Diabetes Prevention Program (DPP): description of lifestyle intervention. *Diabetes Care.* 2002;25(12):2165-2171. doi:10.2337/diacare.25.12.2165

28. Salas-Salvadó J, Bulló M, Babio N, et al. Erratum. Reduction in the incidence of type 2 diabetes with the mediterranean diet: results of the PREDIMED-reus nutrition intervention randomized trial. Diabetes care 2011;34:14-19. *Diabetes Care.* 2018;41(10):2259-2260. doi:10.2337/dc18-er10

29. Ley SH, Hamdy O, Mohan V, Hu FB. Prevention and management of type 2 diabetes: dietary components and nutritional strategies. *Lancet.* 2014;383(9933):1999-2007. doi:10.1016/S0140-6736(14)60613-9

30. Sigal RJ, Alberga AS, Goldfield GS, et al. Effects of aerobic training, resistance training, or both on percentage body fat and cardiometabolic risk markers in obese adolescents: the healthy eating aerobic and resistance training in youth randomized clinical trial. *JAMA Pediatr.* 2014;168(11):1006-1014. doi:10.1001/jamapediatrics.2014.1392

31. Russo LM, Nobles C, Ertel KA, Chasan-Taber L, Whitcomb BW. Physical activity interventions in pregnancy and risk of gestational diabetes mellitus: a systematic review and meta-analysis. *Obstet Gynecol.* 2015;125(3):576-582. doi:10.1097/AOG.0000000000000691

32. Look AHEAD Research Group; Pi-Sunyer X, Blackburn G, Brancati FL, et al. Reduction in weight and cardiovascular disease risk factors in individuals with type 2 diabetes: one-year results of the look AHEAD trial. *Diabetes Care.* 2007;30(6):1374-1383. doi:10.2337/dc07-0048

33. Franz MJ, MacLeod J, Evert A, et al. Academy of nutrition and dietetics nutrition practice guideline for type 1 and type 2 diabetes in adults: systematic review of evidence for medical nutrition therapy effectiveness and recommendations for integration into the nutrition care process. *J Acad Nutr Diet.* 2017;117(10):1659-1679. doi:10.1016/j.jand.2017.03.022

34. Franz MJ, MacLeod J, Evert A, et al. Academy of nutrition and dietetics nutrition practice guideline for type 1 and type 2 diabetes in adults: nutrition intervention evidence reviews and recommendations. *J Acad Nutr Diet.* 2017;117(10):1637-1658. doi:10.1016/j.jand.2017.03.023

35. Wheeler ML, Dunbar SA, Jaacks LM, et al. Macronutrients, food groups, and eating patterns in the management of diabetes: a systematic review of the literature, 2010. *Diabetes Care.* 2012;35(2):434-445. doi:10.2337/dc11-2216

36. Boulé NG, Haddad E, Kenny GP, Wells GA, Sigal RJ. Effects of exercise on glycemic control and body mass in type 2 diabetes mellitus: a meta-analysis of controlled clinical trials. *J Am Med Assoc.* 2001;286(10):1218-1227. doi:10.1001/jama.286.10.1218

37. American Diabetes Association. 9. Pharmacologic approaches to glycemic treatment: standards of medical care in diabetes-2020. *Diabetes Care.* 2019;42(suppl 1):S90-S102. doi:10.2337/dc19-S009

38. Legro RS, Arslanian SA, Ehrmann DA, et al. Diagnosis and treatment of polycystic ovary syndrome: an Endocrine Society clinical practice guideline. *J Clin Endocrinol Metab.* 2013;98(12):4565-4592. doi:10.1210/jc.2013-2350

39. Azziz R, Woods KS, Reyna R, Key TJ, Knochenhauer ES, Yildiz BO. The prevalence and features of the polycystic ovary syndrome in an unselected population. *J Clin Endocrinol Metab.* 2004;89(6):2745-2749. doi:10.1210/jc.2003-032046

40. Sam S. Obesity and polycystic ovary syndrome. *Obes Manag.* 2007;3(2):69-73. doi:10.1089/obe.2007.0019

41. Castillo-Martínez L, López-Alvarenga JC, Villa AR, González-Barranco J. Menstrual cycle length disorders in 18- to 40-y-old obese women. *Nutrition.* 2003;19(4):317-320. doi:10.1016/s0899-9007(02)00998-x

42. Lake JK, Power C, Cole TJ. Women's reproductive health: the role of body mass index in early and adult life. *Int J Obes Relat Metab Disord.* 1997;21(6):432-438. doi:10.1038/sj.ijo.0800424

43. Practice Committee of the American Society for Reproductive Medicine. Obesity and reproduction: a committee opinion. *Fertil Steril.* 2015;104(5):1116-1126. doi:10.1016/j.fertnstert.2015.08.018

44. Fernandez CJ, Chacko EC, Pappachan JM. Male obesity-related secondary hypogonadism – pathophysiology, clinical implications and management. *Eur Endocrinol.* 2019;15(2):83-90. doi:10.17925/EE.2019.15.2.83

45. Bhasin S, Brito JP, Cunningham GR, et al. Testosterone therapy in men with hypogonadism: an endocrine society clinical practice guideline. *J Clin Endocrinol Metab.* 2018;103(5):1715-1744. doi:10.1210/jc.2018-00229

46. Ravesloot MJ, van Maanen JP, Hilgevoord AA, van Wagensveld BA, de Vries N. Obstructive sleep apnea is underrecognized and underdiagnosed in patients undergoing bariatric surgery. *Eur Arch Oto-Rhino-Laryngol.* 2012;269(7):1865-1871. doi:10.1007/s00405-012-1948-0

47. Peppard PE, Young T, Palta M, Dempsey J, Skatrud J. Longitudinal study of moderate weight change and sleep-disordered breathing. *J Am Med Assoc.* 2000;284(23):3015-3021. doi:10.1001/jama.284.23.3015

48. US Preventive Services Task Force; Bibbins-Domingo K, Grossman DC, Curry SJ, et al. Screening for obstructive sleep apnea in adults: US Preventive Services Task Force recommendation statement. *J Am Med Assoc.* 2017;317(4):407-414. doi:10.1001/jama.2016.20325

49. Netzer NC, Stoohs RA, Netzer CM, Clark K, Strohl KP. Using the Berlin questionnaire to identify patients at risk for the sleep apnea syndrome. *Ann Intern Med.* 1999;131(7):485-491. doi:10.7326/0003-4819-131-7-199910050-00002

50. Johns MW. A new method for measuring daytime sleepiness: the Epworth sleepiness scale. *Sleep.* 1991;14(6):540-545. doi:10.1093/sleep/14.6.540

51. Chung F, Abdullah HR, Liao P. STOP-bang questionnaire: a practical approach to screen for obstructive sleep apnea. *Chest.* 2016;149(3):631-638. doi:10.1378/chest.15-0903

52. Epstein LJ, Kristo D, Strollo PJ, et al. Clinical guideline for the evaluation, management and long-term care of obstructive sleep apnea in adults. *J Clin Sleep Med.* 2009;5(3):263-276.

53. Kapur VK, Auckley DH, Chowdhuri S. et al. Clinical practice guideline for diagnostic testing for adult obstructive sleep apnea: an American academy of sleep medicine clinical practice guideline. *J Clin Sleep Med.* 2017;13(3):479-504. doi:10.5664/jcsm.6506

54. Gottlieb DJ, Punjabi NM. Diagnosis and management of obstructive sleep apnea: a review. *J Am Med Assoc.* 2020;323(14):1389-1400. doi:10.1001/jama.2020.3514

55. Mokhlesi B, Masa JF, Brozek JL, et al. Evaluation and management of obesity hypoventilation syndrome. An official American thoracic society clinical practice guideline. *Am J Respir Crit Care Med.* 2019;200(3):e6-e24. doi:10.1164/rccm.201905-1071ST

56. Kaw R, Hernandez AV, Walker E, Aboussouan L, Mokhlesi B. Determinants of hypercapnia in obese patients with obstructive sleep apnea: a systematic review and meta-analysis of cohort studies. *Chest.* 2009;136(3):787-796. doi:10.1378/chest.09-0615

57. Katz PO, Gerson LB, Vela MF. Guidelines for the diagnosis and management of gastroesophageal reflux disease. *Am J Gastroenterol.* 2013;108(3):308-328; quiz 329. doi:10.1038/ajg.2012.444

58. Emerenziani S, Rescio MP, Guarino MP, Cicala M. Gastroesophageal reflux disease and obesity, where is the link? *World J Gastroenterol.* 2013;19(39):6536-6539. doi:10.3748/wjg.v19.i39.6536

59. Camilleri M, Malhi H, Acosta A. Gastrointestinal complications of obesity. *Gastroenterology.* 2017;152(7):1656-1670. doi:10.1053/j.gastro.2016.12.052

60. Chalasani N, Younossi Z, Lavine JE, et al. The diagnosis and management of nonalcoholic fatty liver disease: practice guidance from the American Association for the Study of Liver Diseases. *Hepatology.* 2018;67(1):328-357. doi:10.1002/hep.29367

61. Liu B, Balkwill A, Spencer E, Beral V; Million Women Study Collaborators. Relationship between body mass index and length of hospital stay for gallbladder disease. *J Public Health (Oxf).* 2008;30(2):161-166. doi:10.1093/pubmed/fdn011

62. Bray GA. Medical consequences of obesity. *J Clin Endocrinol Metab.* 2004;89(6):2583-2589. doi:10.1210/jc.2004-0535

63. Weinsier RL, Wilson LJ, Lee J. Medically safe rate of weight loss for the treatment of obesity: a guideline based on risk of gallstone formation. *Am J Med.* 1995;98(2):115-117. doi:10.1016/S0002-9343(99)80394-5

64. Vincent HK, Heywood K, Connelly J, Hurley RW. Obesity and weight loss in the treatment and prevention of osteoarthritis. *PM R.* 2012;4(5 suppl):S59-S67. doi:10.1016/j.pmrj.2012.01.005

65. Bartlett S. *Role of Body Weight in Osteoarthritis.* Johns Hopkins Arthritis Center. Accessed December 2019. https://www.hopkinsmedicine.org/health/conditions-and-diseases/arthritis

66. Felson DT, Chaisson CE. Understanding the relationship between body weight and osteoarthritis. *Baillieres Clin Rheumatol.* 1997;11(4):671-681. doi:10.1016/s0950-3579(97)80003-9

67. Kolasinski SL, Neogi T, Hochberg MC, et al. 2019 American College of Rheumatology/Arthritis Foundation guideline for the management of osteoarthritis of the hand, hip, and knee. *Arthritis Rheumatol.* 2020;72(2):220-233. doi:10.1002/art.41142

68. Li W, Ayers DC, Lewis CG, Bowen TR, Allison JJ, Franklin PD. Functional gain and pain relief after total joint replacement according to obesity status. *J Bone Joint Surg Am.* 2017;99(14):1183-1189. doi:10.2106/JBJS.16.00960

69. Steele B, Cheryll T, Henley J, Massetti G, Galuska D. Vital signs: trends in incidence of cancers associated with overweight and obesity – United States, 2005-2014. *MMWR Morb Mortal Wkly Rep.* 2017;66(39):1052-1058.

70. Gregor MF, Hotamisligil GS. Inflammatory mechanisms in obesity. *Annu Rev Immunol.* 2011;29:415-445. doi:10.1146/annurev-immunol-031210-101322

71. Randi G, Franceschi S, La Vecchia C. Gallbladder cancer worldwide: geographical distribution and risk factors. *Int J Canc.* 2006;118(7):1591-1602. doi:10.1002/ijc.21683

72. Heimbach JK, Kulik LM, Finn RS, et al. AASLD guidelines for the treatment of hepatocellular carcinoma. *Hepatology.* 2018;67(1):358-380. doi:10.1002/hep.29086

73. Stroud A, Dewey E, Husian FA. Association between weight loss and serum biomarkers with risk of incident cancer in the Longitudinal Assessment of Bariatric Surgery cohort. *Surg Obes Relat Dis.* 2019;16:1086-1094.

74. Keum N, Greenwood DC, Lee DH, et al. Adult weight gain and adiposity-related cancers: a dose-response meta-analysis of prospective observational studies. *J Natl Cancer Inst.* 2015;107(2):djv088. doi:10.1093/jnci/djv088

75. Griggs JJ, Mangu PB, Anderson H, et al. Appropriate chemotherapy dosing for obese adult patients with cancer: American Society of Clinical Oncology clinical practice guideline. *J Clin Oncol.* 2012;30(13):1553-1561. doi:10.1200/JCO.2011.39.9436

76. Apovian CM, Aronne LJ, Bessesen DH, et al. Pharmacological management of obesity: an Endocrine Society clinical practice guideline. *J Clin Endocrinol Metab.* 2015;100(2):342-362. doi:10.1210/jc.2014-3415

77. Maurer DM, Raymond TJ, Davis BN. Depression: screening and diagnosis. *Am Fam Physician.* 2018;98(8):508-515.

78. Igel LI, Kumar RB, Saunders KH, Aronne LJ. Practical use of pharmacotherapy for obesity. *Gastroenterology.* 2017;152(7):1765-1779. doi:10.1053/j.gastro.2016.12.049

79. Brownley KA, Berkman ND, Peat CM, Lohr KN, Bulik CM. Binge-eating disorder in adults. *Ann Intern Med.* 2017;166(3):231-232. doi:10.7326/L16-0621

80. Gallant AR, Lundgren J, Drapeau V. The night-eating syndrome and obesity. *Obes Rev.* 2012;13(6):528-536. doi:10.1111/j.1467-789X.2011.00975.x

81. O'Reardon JP, Allison KC, Martino NS, Lundgren JD, Heo M, Stunkard AJ. A randomized, placebo-controlled trial of sertraline in the treatment of night eating syndrome. *Am J Psychiatr.* 2006;163(5):893-898. doi:10.1176/ajp.2006.163.5.893

DIETARY TREATMENT

Maria L. Collazo-Clavell

CASE STUDY

You are seeing a 42-year-old woman who is concerned about her weight. She has previously lost 10 to 15 lb following various commercial and self-directed dietary interventions, but weight was always gradually regained. She is currently at her heaviest weight. She does not have an exercise program in place. The patient feels confused about dietary changes to pursue at this time. She has a history of hypertension and depression both well controlled on stable doses of losartan/hydrochlorothiazide 50 mg/12.5 mg/day and fluoxetine 20 mg/day, respectively. She has a family history of diabetes and is concerned about developing diabetes herself.

A 24-hour diet recall reveals busy days fulfilling home and work responsibilities.

- **Breakfast** is skipped, but mid-morning will have a granola bar and a flavored coffee drink.
- **Lunch** is various greens, diced chicken, sliced avocado, dried fruit, pumpkin seeds, and an olive oil–based vinaigrette.
- **Mid-afternoon**—snacks on nuts and regular soda pop.
- **Dinner** is a pasta dish with a meat- or cream-based sauce, bread with olive oil, salad with various veggies and vinaigrette dressing, and a glass of wine.
- **After dinner** may snack on sweet potato chips, sunflower seeds, nuts, or popcorn.

On physical examination, height is 5′5″ (165 cm), weight 233 lb (106 kg), blood pressure (BP) 130/88 mm Hg, heart rate (HR) 78 bmp, waist circumference 102 cm, and body mass index (BMI) 39.3 kg/m^2.

She presents as a well-developed female with upper body fat distribution without Cushingoid features. The remainder of the examination is unremarkable.

Laboratory tests:

- Complete blood count (CBC), thyroid function test, renal function, and liver function tests are normal.
- Fasting blood glucose: 115 mg/dL.
- Glycosylated hemoglobin: 5.9%.
- Total cholesterol: 198 mg/dL.
- Triglycerides: 183 mg/dL.
- High-density lipoprotein cholesterol (HDL-c): 39 mg/dL.
- Low-density lipoprotein cholesterol (LDL-c): 122 mg/dL.

CLINICAL SIGNIFICANCE

Nutrition is critical to health. Poor nutrition and a sedentary lifestyle are the main contributors to the rising prevalence of obesity and preventable chronic diseases that impact health. Over half of adults in the United States are overweight or obese and suffer from at least one diet-related chronic health condition including cardiovascular disease (CVD), type 2 diabetes mellitus (T2D), and hypertension, among others.[1] Following a healthy calorie-reduced diet that is practical, sustainable, and consistent with the patient's lifestyle and social norms is foundational to obesity care. It is also notable that despite excess caloric intake in the US population, nutrient deficiencies among adults with obesity are increasingly recognized as a result of poor food quality.[2]

DIETARY COUNSELING IN THE OFFICE SETTING

Dietary counseling in the office setting can be challenging. Time restraints and low healthcare professional (HCP) confidence in nutrition knowledge can lead to oversimplification of the recommendations provided. For many patients with obesity, dietary education is not enough to effectively promote and sustain changes in eating habits. As a result, a more deliberate and thorough approach is recommended, often implemented by other clinicians such as a registered dietitian nutritionist (RDN). Multidisciplinary teams for obesity care commonly include an HCP (physician and advanced practice providers [nurse practitioner or physician assistant]), RDNs, as well as behavioral health and exercise specialists. Collaboratively, these disciplines can help HCPs by dedicating their time and expertise to develop, implement, and support an individualized care plan for the patient.[3] When these disciplines are not readily available within a practice, a "virtual" care team can be created by identifying specialists in the community or healthcare system that can serve as valuable resources for patients. However, with proper guidance, the HCP should be able to initiate meaningful and effective dietary counseling during a dedicated office visit.

Several tools are available that can facilitate dietary counseling. The US Department of Agriculture (www.choosemyplate.gov/resources/all-resources)[4] offers online resources to develop meal plans that can be individualized to a specific calorie goal and eating pattern. There are also several smartphone apps and websites that can help with meal planning and dietary tracking (Table 5.1). Depending upon the electronic literacy of the patient, web-based technologies and mobile devices that help HCPs and patients track progress and support dietary change should be routinely considered.

TABLE 5.1 Weight Management Resources and Tracking Tools for Internet and Smartphone Apps[a]

WEIGHT MANAGEMENT RESOURCES AND TRACKING TOOLS FOR INTERNET AND SMARTPHONE APPS	SPECIAL FEATURES
Calorie King www.calorieking.com	Food nutrition database
Bitesnap www.bitesnap.com	Photo food tracker
Cooking Light www.cookinglight.com	*Cooking Light* magazine recipes
EatingWell www.eatingwell.com	Healthy recipes and meal plans
Fitday www.fitday.com	Food tracker
Fooducate www.fooducate.com	Scans barcodes of items and gives it a nutritional grade with information
Hungry Girl www.hungrygirl.com	Low-calorie recipes
Livestrong www.livestrong.com	Food tracker
Lose It! www.loseit.com	Food tracker
MyFitnessPal www.myfitnesspal.com	Food tracker
My-Food-Diary www.myfooddiary.com	Food tracker
Noom www.noom.com	Digital weight management program using cognitive behavioral therapy
Skinny Taste www.skinnytaste.com	Healthy recipes
Spark People www.sparkpeople.com	Online weight management program
USDA Foodkeeper www.choosemyplate.gov	US Department of Agriculture food tracker that uses the MyPlatefood groups and meal plans
WW (formally Weight Watchers) www.weightwatchers.com	Digital and in-person comprehensive weight management program

[a]*Selected items as of May 2020.*

CALORIE RESTRICTION FOR WEIGHT LOSS

The key principle to achieve weight loss is to create an energy deficit, i.e., to consume fewer calories than are being burned.[5] This is consistent with the first law of thermodynamics. Yet, as simple as this seems, successful implementation is limited by multiple factors including individual genetic, physiologic, psychological, environmental, and social determinants that can impact energy balance. As a result, long-term success at losing and maintaining weight with dietary intervention alone is challenging.[6] However, understanding the principles of energy balance and how they impact weight loss can establish a sound foundation on which to help patients succeed.

Individual energy requirements (i.e., calories needed to maintain or to lose weight) are determined by many factors including age (drops as we age), sex (higher for men than women), height (the taller you are, the higher your energy needs), and weight (the heavier you are, the higher your energy needs).[7] The single largest predictor of energy requirement is muscle mass. Energy expenditure (calories burned) comprises three components:

- basal metabolic rate (calories used to maintain bodily functions [60% to 70% of total daily energy expenditure])
- thermic effect of food (energy required for digestion [8% to 10% of total daily energy expenditure])
- physical activity (both purposeful exercise and non-exercise activity thermogenesis—NEAT—[20% to 30% of total daily energy expenditure])[7,8]

Both basal and total energy requirements can be measured; however, precise measurement of energy expenditure is impractical in the primary care setting. Several prediction equations, such as the Harris-Benedict equation,[9] Mifflin-St Jeor equation,[10] and WHO,[11] are available to estimate energy expenditure if a more precise estimation is desired for an individual patient. These formulas are often employed by RDNs when calculating dietary requirements. When using one of these equations, the next step is to introduce a caloric restriction for weight loss. Reducing calorie intake by 500 to 750 kcal/day (or 30% of calorie needs) can be expected to lead to weight loss. However, from a practical perspective, use of the American Heart Association/American College of Cardiology/The Obesity Society (AHA/ACC/TOS) recommendations of 1,200 to 1,500 kcal/day for women and 1,500 to 1,800 kcal/day for men is suitable for most patients with obesity as an initial treatment goal. The calorie target can then be adjusted up or down over the first 1 to 2 months of treatment, based on the patient's weight loss.

Due to biological changes that occur with weight loss, a weight reduction of just 10% of initial body weight leads to a phenomenon called "adaptive thermogenesis."[12] This term describes the observation that an individual who has lost weight burns fewer calories per 24-hour period, compared to an identical individual who is not weight reduced. For patients, this sobering reality means that, once weight loss stabilizes, the patient must maintain the same (lower) level of calorie intake in order to maintain the weight loss they have achieved. Adaptive thermogenesis appears to persist for at least 1 year after weight loss or longer.[13] Thus, regardless of which dietary intervention is selected, the patient must be prepared for the weight loss plateau that inevitably occurs after the body's energy expenditure has dropped to be equivalent with the lower calorie intake that initially led to weight loss.

DIETARY INTERVENTIONS TO INTRODUCE A CALORIE RESTRICTION

The most important dietary factor to lose weight is caloric reduction. As long as calories are reduced, the macronutrient composition of food (percent of carbohydrate, protein, and fat) can vary.[5,14] Patients and their HCPs can choose a meal plan based upon the presence of comorbid conditions, taste/food preference, family culture, access, affordability, and overall health. Often, patients will benefit from seeing an RDN for individual dietary counseling. In the section below, the composition and research behind several evidence-based healthy eating patterns are discussed, followed by several shorter-term restrictive diets that are commonly used in clinical practice (Table 5.2).

Healthy Eating Patterns

Despite the confusion that exists regarding healthy eating, the key components of a healthy diet have not changed dramatically over time. The key components include daily consumption of fruits and vegetables, whole grains, fat-free or low-fat dairy products, a variety of protein sources including lean meats and plant-based protein sources, limited intake of saturated fat, and elimination of *trans* fats. One recent change in the US dietary guidelines was the removal of recommended intake of total dietary fat. Thus, if patients can limit intake of saturated fat, they can increase intake of unsaturated fat from foods such as nuts, avocados, salmon, and other healthy high-fat foods. Several studies have shown that adherence to healthy eating patterns lower the risk for CVD, T2D, and some type of cancers.[1]

Case Study Discussion

Individualizing dietary recommendations to achieve weight loss and specific health goals can improve adherence. In our case study, there are several health goals that can guide the dietary interventions. If hypertension is the focus, the Dietary Approaches to Stop Hypertension diet (DASH diet) would be a reasonable recommendation.[15] If the goal is to improve her hyperglycemia, a Mediterranean-type eating pattern or a meal replacement program could be considered.

Dietary Approaches to Stop Hypertension Diet

The DASH diet was developed as a dietary treatment for hypertension and was then applied for weight loss by reducing overall calories. One trial evaluated the impact of three dietary interventions among 459 subjects with hypertension. The control diet was similar to the current American diet, low in fruits, vegetables, and legumes and high in high-calorie snacks, meat, and saturated fats. A second dietary intervention included high intake of fruits, vegetables, and legumes and low intake of high-calorie snacks. The DASH diet comprised high intake of fruits (4 to 5/day), vegetables (4 to 5/day), legumes, and low-fat dairy products (2 to 3/day) and limited the intake of high-calorie snacks, meats, and saturated and total fat (<25% of calories per day) (Figure 5.1).[15]

Lower blood pressure values were observed with the DASH diet when compared to the control diet. The greatest benefit with the DASH diet was observed in patients with hypertension, compared to those with normal blood pressure, with drops of 11.4/5.5 mm Hg compared to 3.5/2.1 mm Hg, respectively.[16] The DASH diet also reduced blood pressure independent of sodium intake.[16] However, for the DASH diet to produce weight loss, calorie restriction is needed. In the landmark 4-month ENCORE study, weight loss was 19 lb in the DASH-weight loss group (caloric reduction, exercise, and behavioral support) compared to < 1 lb in the DASH diet group.[17]

TABLE 5.2 Dietary Counseling in the Office Setting

DIETARY PATTERNS	CLINICAL CONSIDERATIONS	KEY NUTRITIONAL FEATURES	RESOURCES (ACCESSED MAY 2020)
DASH (dietary approaches to stop hypertension)	Hypertension	High intake of fruits (4-5 servings/day); vegetables (4-5 servings/day); legumes; low-fat dairy	https://www.nhlbi.nih.gov/files/docs/public/heart/dash_brief.pdf https://www.nhlbi.nih.gov/files/docs/public/heart/new_dash.pdf http://www.healthyinfo.com/consumers/ho/nut.dash.diet.pdf
Mediterranean	Type 2 diabetes mellitus Prediabetes Metabolic syndrome CVD	Vegetables (3-9 servings/day); fresh fruit (up to 2 servings/day); cereals: mostly whole grain (from 1 to 13 servings/day); oil (up to 8 servings of olive oil/day); fat—mostly unsaturated—up to 37% of the total calories; nuts, legumes, fish, and poultry	https://health.usnews.com/best-diet/mediterranean-diet https://oldwayspt.org/traditional-diets/mediterranean-diet https://www.medicalnewstoday.com/articles/149090
Low-fat diet	Hyperlipidemia CVD	<30% of total calories from fat <10% saturated fats	https://health.usnews.com/wellness/food/articles/what-is-a-low-fat-diet https://www.healthline.com/nutrition/healthy-low-fat-foods

CVD, cardiovascular disease.

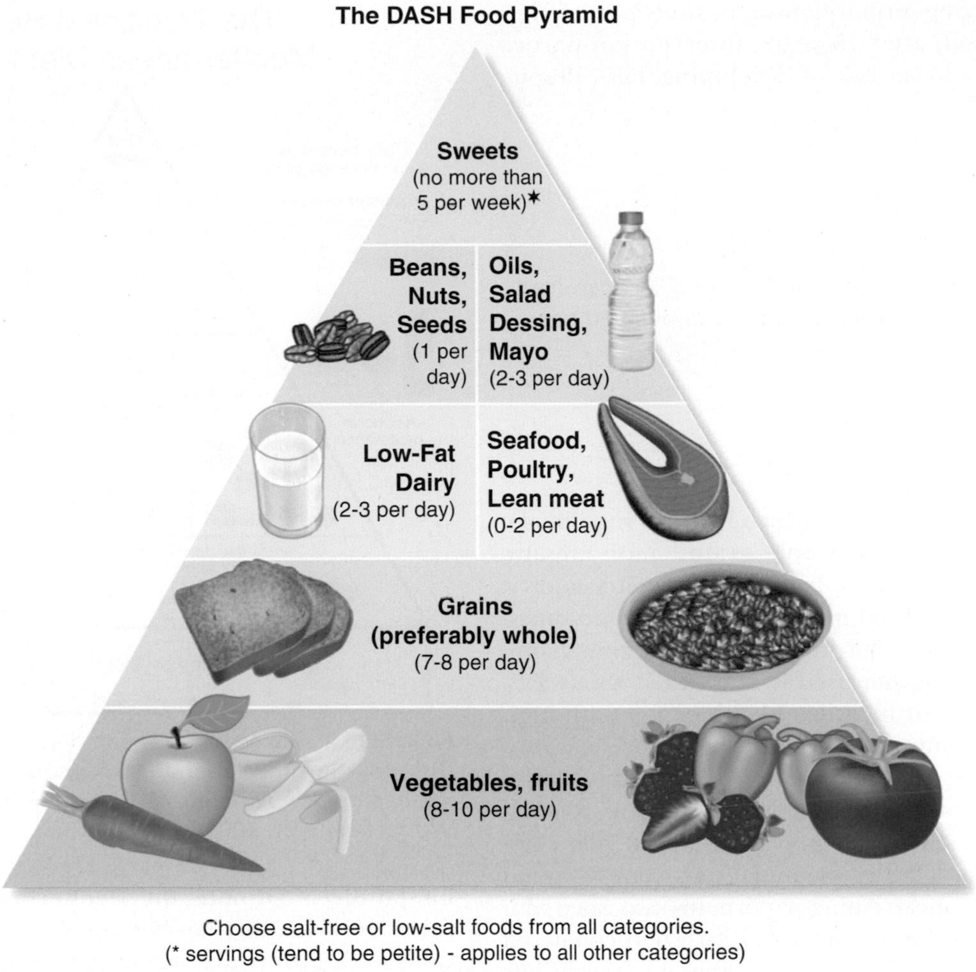

The DASH Food Pyramid

Choose salt-free or low-salt foods from all categories.
(* servings (tend to be petite) - applies to all other categories)

FIGURE 5.1 The DASH (dietary approaches to stop hypertension) food pyramid.

Take-Home Point

The DASH diet can reduce blood pressure, independent of weight loss, and, when accompanied with caloric restriction, is effective for weight loss and blood pressure reduction.

Low-Fat Diet in the Diabetes Prevention Program

The Diabetes Prevention Program (DPP) was an intensive lifestyle intervention (ILI) study in patients with impaired glucose tolerance, with the goal of avoiding progression to T2D. The dietary intervention introduced a calorie restriction to achieve a weight loss of 5% to 10% of initial body weight. The intervention diet was low in fat (<30 % of total calories), low in saturated fat (<10%), and high in fiber (≥15 grams). The intervention cohort was encouraged to participate in ≥150 minutes of exercise per week and received intensive support from coaches (16 sessions in the first 24 weeks, followed by monthly contact). The control cohort was provided oral and written recommendations on diet and exercise.[18]

After nearly 4 years of follow-up, the intervention cohort experienced a decrease in the progression to T2D of 58%, relative to controls. The intervention group lost 7% of initial body weight, and 43% experienced a weight loss >5%. However, study participants struggled with implementation of the dietary interventions, with fewer than half of the intervention group achieving the dietary goal recommendations for fat and fiber intake. The most commonly attained goal was to exercise ≥150 minutes/week, achieved by 86% and 71% of the intervention and the control cohorts, respectively.[18] Long-term follow-up of study participants has revealed that, after 15 years, intervention participants still had a lower risk of developing T2D, despite weight regain.[19]

> **Take-Home Point**
>
> A low-fat diet, as implemented in the DPP, can lead to clinically significant weight loss and delayed onset of T2D.

Mediterranean-Style Diet

The Mediterranean eating pattern features high intake of fruits and vegetables, whole grains, monounsaturated fats (olive oil), nuts, legumes, fish, and poultry. It limits the intake of red meat, high-fat dairy products, and processed foods. Fat intake can be higher (compared to the low-fat diet used in the DPP), about 35% of total calories, but includes healthier fats with high amounts of monounsaturated oils (Figure 5.2).

A randomized trial comparing three dietary interventions—a calorie-restricted Mediterranean diet, a calorie-restricted low-fat diet (<30% of calories), and a low-carbohydrate diet (<20 g/day initial restriction)—found that the Mediterranean eating pattern was associated with greater weight loss at 2 years (−9.5 lb) when compared to the low-fat diet (−6.8 lb) and comparable weight loss to a low-carbohydrate diet (−10.3 lb).[20] At 4 years, the Mediterranean diet was associated with greater weight maintenance (−6.8 lb) when compared to the low-fat diet (−1.3 lb) and the low-carbohydrate diet (−3.7 lb).[21] However, other trials have not reported superior weight loss with the Mediterranean eating pattern comparable to low-fat and low-carbohydrate diet interventions.[22]

The Mediterranean diet offered a greater benefit on hyperglycemia when compared to the other dietary interventions.[20] This metabolic benefit for patients with T2D and prediabetes has been confirmed by several other studies.[23] The PREDIMED Study was the first randomized trial to show a reduction in a combined endpoint of cardiovascular disease morbidity and mortality. Participants were randomized to three groups: (1) Mediterranean eating pattern supplemented with extra virgin olive oil; (2) Mediterranean eating pattern supplemented with mixed nuts; and (3) control diet (advice to reduce dietary fat). Despite challenges in methodology of the initial study (i.e., at least one study site did not randomize participants to an intervention group), in subsequent reanalysis, the Mediterranean eating pattern was still shown in both intervention groups (supplementation of extra virgin olive oil or nuts) to lower the risk for cardiovascular events when compared to a

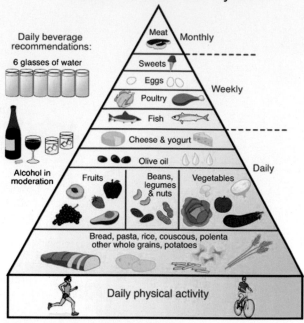

FIGURE 5.2 The Mediterranean diet food pyramid. (Reprinted from Weber JR, Kelley JH. *Health Assessment in Nursing*, 4th Edition. Philadelphia, Wolters Kluwer, 2009.)

low-fat diet.[24] Of note, the Mediterranean eating plan is the only diet that has been shown to produce reductions in cardiovascular events (with minimal weight loss in the PREDIMED Study). As with the DASH diet, a caloric restriction is needed to produce weight loss.[5,24] The greatest challenge for patients choosing to follow this eating plan may be cost (i.e., higher cost for items such as fish and extra virgin olive oil). The benefit of the diet is that the Mediterranean plan may be associated with greater satiety due to the higher fat content and, as described above, the potential benefit in reducing T2D and cardiovascular disease risk.

> **Take-Home Point**
>
> The Mediterranean eating plan has a number of potential health benefits, including weight loss and reduction in CVD, but may be more costly to follow.

Meal Replacement Products in the Look AHEAD Trial

The Look AHEAD trial (Action for Health in Diabetes) studied an ILI compared to diabetes support and education (DSE) among patients with T2D and BMI ≥ 25 kg/m². [25] Goals were to achieve a weight loss of at least 7%

of initial body weight and to report the impact on various health outcomes including the risk for cardiovascular events. The ILI used meal replacements to create a calorie restriction and recommended 175 minutes of moderate-intensity exercise per week. Meal replacement products create a calorie restriction by limiting food choice and portions. A meal replacement is defined as a bar or shake that has approximately 200 calories, 15 to 20 grams of protein, and 5 grams of fiber and provides complete nutrition (supplemented with all vitamins and minerals). Sometimes the term meal replacement is also ascribed to frozen entrees, although the calorie and sodium levels of these products exceed those typically found in bars and shakes. Meal replacement products can be purchased in any grocery store.

For the first 6 months of the dietary intervention, two meal replacements per day were recommended. This was decreased to one meal replacement per day for the latter 6 months of the year, and also, shorter weight loss "sprints" were offered later in the trial during which intervention participants could use meal replacements for two meals per day for 1 week at a time. The intervention cohort participated in weekly group/individual sessions for 6 months. The DSE group participated in three group sessions per year reviewing diet and exercise recommendations for 4 years.

The ILI group experienced greater weight loss compared to the control condition (8.6 % vs. 0.7%) at 1 year.[22,26] There was narrowing of the difference in weight loss over the course of the trial. After 12 years of follow-up, there was no significant difference between the groups in the risk for cardiovascular events. However, the intervention cohort experienced decreased need for blood pressure–lowering and glucose-lowering medications, as well as improved urinary incontinence, sleep apnea, depression, quality of life, physical functioning, sexual functioning, and mobility.[27] Of note, initial weight loss observed within the first 1 to 2 months predicted weight loss at 1 year. Furthermore, for those participants who achieved a weight loss of ≥10% at 1 year, a reduced risk was observed for cardiovascular events at 10 years.[28]

Preprepared meal replacement products (bars, shakes, or meals) that are either purchased from the internet or incorporated into the clinical practice is a useful strategy. Most meal replacement programs in this category have a calorie target of approximately 1,000 to 1,200 kcal/day when consumed either alone or with one or more self-selected meals. These products vary by calorie level, macronutrient content, and cost. Examples of prepackaged meal replacement programs that can be incorporated into clinical practice include:

* HMR (https://www.hmrprogram.com/)
* Optifast (https://www.optifast.com/)
* Medifast (https://www.medifast1.com/)
* New Directions (https://www.robard.com/programs/)

Take-Home Point

Although not a food-based meal pattern similar to DASH, low-fat or Mediterranean diet, incorporation of meal replacement products can be a safe and effective strategy of producing clinically significant weight loss. This is particularly relevant for patients who are unable to spend time preparing and cooking meals at home and/or those who eat "on the run."

Short-Term Dietary Interventions for Calorie Restriction

Variations in macronutrient composition of food intake (carbohydrate, protein, fat) have all been shown to lead to weight loss when calorie restriction is achieved.[5] Dietary interventions that limit the intake of carbohydrates to < 20 g/day for the first 3 months (i.e., very-low-carbohydrate ketogenic diet [VLCKD; Atkins or keto]) are associated with greater weight loss in the short term (3 to 6 months) when compared to other dietary interventions with different macronutrient composition. Most studies suggest that weight loss at 12 months is similar with VLCKD vs. more standard macronutrient composition.[29,30] One trial reported that among healthy premenopausal women, a low-carbohydrate diet was shown to promote greater weight loss at 12 months when compared to other dietary interventions of differing macronutrient composition (Zone, Ornish, LEARN).[31] However, when all of the participants were analyzed by level of adherence, there was no difference between diets. It has become clear that improved adherence, even when self-reported, is associated with greater weight loss regardless of macronutrient composition of the dietary intervention.[32,33] In one clinical trial that tested four different diets with varying macronutrient content, attendance at visits was a stronger predictor of weight loss, rather than treatment group.[14]

Many patients find a low-carbohydrate dietary approach attractive since it essentially eliminates an easily identifiable food group, i.e., starches such as rice, potatoes, pasta, and breads, and is associated with early rapid weight loss. Common side effects may include halitosis, constipation, and headache. Patients with diabetes treated with sulfonylureas or insulin and patients taking diuretics require special attention and adjustment of their medications to avoid complications.

Commercial Weight Loss Programs

Several commercial and proprietary weight-loss programs (WW, Jenny Craig, Nutrisystem) are a practicable option for patients. Early studies were short in duration (<12 months) with limited long-term outcomes

TABLE 5.3 Three Evidence-based National Commercial Programs

	WW (FORMALLY WEIGHT WATCHERS)	JENNY CRAIG	NUTRISYSTEM
Meal plan	Based on point system, subscribers choose one of three food-based programs	Provides preprepared low-calorie foods that are shelf-stable for three meals and two snacks per day; patients supplement with fruits, vegetables, and dairy	Provides preprepared low-calorie foods that are shelf-stable, with patients supplementing fruits and vegetables. Eat six times per day. Foods are delivered every 4 weeks
Counseling services	Begins with personal assessment, followed by options of digital, in-person, and virtual workshops and personal coaching; social community support	Weekly 1:1 meeting with a coach for weight loss guidance (in-person or telephonic), personalized feedback, and meal planning	No counseling services are offered

reported. However, the 2013 AHA/ACC/TOS guideline[5] for the management of overweight and obesity in adults, as well as an updated systematic review article, support their use as a valid alternative for a calorie-reduced diet.[34] A brief description of the three commercial programs is displayed in Table 5.3. These programs offer an alternative resource for patients depending upon their individual needs, such as desire for group support, face-to-face coaching, social support through in-person or online participation, availability of calorie-controlled meals, and low cost.

Intermittent Fasting

There has been increasing interest in "fasting" strategies to promote weight loss. However, fasting strategies differ and have not all been studied extensively. They can be divided into "intermittent fasting" or "alternate day fasting" (ADF) strategies and "time-restricted eating" (TRE) strategies. Importantly, when patients use the term fasting, they are typically describing a TRE strategy, even though there is much more published evidence to support an ADF approach. Table 5.4 lists common regimens studied.[35-39] A systematic review by Rynders et al.[40] summarized the literature in this area quite well to date. The only published randomized trials have compared ADF to daily calorie restriction (DCR) and the impact on weight loss and several metabolic parameters, including patients with T2D and prediabetes.[41,42] When compared to DCR, ADF led to similar weight loss. In one of two trials that included patients with diabetes, individuals on glucose-lowering medications were at increased risk for hypoglycemia.[42]

TRE schedules vary from 16 hours fasting:8 hours feeding (16:8) to 18 hours fasting:6 hours feeding (18:6). Early time-restricted eating (eTRE) is defined as

TABLE 5.4 Intermittent Fasting Strategies

Intermittent Fasting Strategies	Fast Day	Nonfasting Day
ADF (alternate-day fasting)	Complete fasting	Ad libitum eating
mADF (modified alternate-day fasting)	Modified fasting = 25% of daily calories	125% of daily calories
1:6	Fasting 1 day/week	6 days ad libitum eating
2:5	75% of daily requirements 2 days/week	Isocaloric diet 5 days/week
Time-Restricted Eating Strategies	Fasting Period	Eating Period
18:6[a]	18 hours fasting	6 hours eating
16:8	16 hours fasting	8 hours eating

[a]Early time-restricted eating 8 AM-3 PM (dinner meal before 3:00 PM) has been associated with greater metabolic benefit.

6 hours of eating with the latest meal consumed prior to 3:00 PM. The eTRE strategy was associated with the greatest metabolic benefit with improved insulin resistance, improved beta cell function, and lower blood pressure and oxidative stress (even in the absence of weight loss) when compared to a 12:12 fasting/feeding schedule.[38] Preliminary studies of TRE are encouraging, but intervention trials to date are limited and show modest weight loss. Intermittent fasting strategies represent another intervention to create a calorie restriction. However, long-term adherence was challenging for all fasting strategies, likely because of the social restriction in stopping all food intake by 6 to 7 PM (or by 3 PM with the eTRE strategy).

Case Study Discussion

The healthy eating patterns and short-term calorie-reduction diets reviewed above can be briefly discussed with the patient with the aim of reducing her confusion. Using shared decision-making, counseling can focus on establishing a reduced caloric goal, desired eating pattern, resources, and implementation strategies. Alternatively, a referral can be placed to see an RDN or recommend a commercial weight management program. Self-monitoring has been consistently shown to enhance weight loss which can be accomplished by asking the patient to track her diet using a commercial tracker app for the smartphone or tablet or an online website.

USING A PROGRESSIVE DIETARY COUNSELING APPROACH

As described above, patient adherence is the most important factor in predicting weight loss regardless of the diet prescribed. In turn, dietary adherence can be strengthened by recommending a diet that is personalized to the patient's lifestyle, food preferences, culture, accessibility, and affordability. Oftentimes, a progressive approach to diet is used early in treatment, where the patient's current diet is tweaked toward healthier food items and patterns of eating. Rather than recommending one of the dietary patterns or short-term interventions reviewed above, the patient's diet recall is used as a starting point for counseling. Keeping in mind that diet exists in a continuum ranging from healthy to unhealthy choices, the goal is to slowly transition food selection and preparation techniques toward healthier options. Preferably, under guidance from the HCP, the patient provides suggestions on what would be healthier meal or snack ideas based on past dietary attempts or common knowledge. In this case, the HCP would act as an "agent of change," reinforcing the patient's

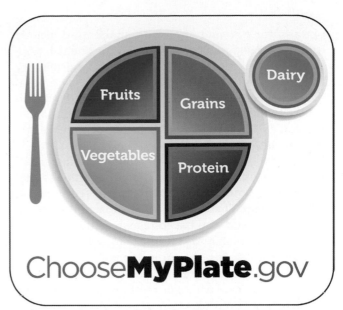

FIGURE 5.3 Plate method recommended by the United States Department of Agriculture to help simplify meal planning. (Reprinted from U.S. Department of Agriculture. MyPlate. https://www.choosemyplate.gov/.)

suggestions and providing encouragement. In the case where the patient does not have the experience or knowledge of what would be healthier options, the HCP can make specific recommendations. To initiate weight loss, the goal would be to reduce the patient's current diet by 500 to 750 kcal/day (about 30% of baseline calorie intake).

General dietary recommendations include:

- When eating, divide your plate into sections where one-half is filled with vegetables and fruits, one-quarter is lean proteins, and one-quarter is whole grains and starchy vegetables (Figure 5.3).
- Substitute lower calorie foods for higher calorie foods. For example, snack on vegetables and fruits instead of chips, nuts, and candy.
- Reduce added fats such as fried foods, butter, margarine, cream sauces, and full-fat salad dressings.
- Reduce or eliminate sugar-sweetened beverages such as soda and juice, and replace with water, flavored water, or unsweetened ice tea or coffee.
- Reduce portions sizes by using smaller plates, splitting entrees, and downsizing menu items.

Case Study Discussion

A useful counseling technique would be to review the patient's 24-hour dietary recall to identify opportunities for healthier meals and snacks. For example, instead of skipping breakfast, she can introduce a protein bar and piece of fruit. Suggested healthier options for her mid-afternoon snack may include fruit, fresh vegetables, low-fat string cheese, popcorn, and flavored water. For dinner, she may try to reduce her pasta portions and use a tomato-based sauce with 99% lean ground turkey and limit bread consumption. These changes can be implemented as a first step to increase her confidence and self-efficacy.

The second approach to strengthen dietary adherence is to utilize behavior change techniques that focus on self-monitoring, environmental control, and reinforcement. There are free and subscription smartphone apps and web-based resources (limited list in Table 5.1) available for diet tracking where patients can monitor foods consumed, caloric intake, and macronutrient composition. Attention to environmental cues to eating will also reinforce healthy eating behaviors. A full discussion of behavioral treatment for obesity is covered in Chapter 7.

CLINICAL HIGHLIGHTS

- As long as daily caloric intake is reduced by 500 to 750 kcal/day, the macronutrient composition of the diet (percent of calories from protein, carbohydrates, and protein) can vary.
- A progressive approach to dietary counseling is often the first step in obesity treatment, where the patient's current diet is tweaked toward healthier selection of foods, beverages, and preparation methods.
- Several evidence-based dietary patterns can be recommended based on the patient's medical profile and goals of treatment. These include the DASH diet, low-fat diet, Mediterranean style diet, and use of meal replacement products.
- Adherence to the dietary plan can be enhanced by self-monitoring (tracking), daily self-weighing, and incorporating cognitive behavior therapy strategies.
- Several meal replacement programs are available that include bars, shakes, and entrees that are purchased from the internet or can be incorporated into a medical practice.
- Commercial weight management programs, such as WW (formally Weight Watchers), Jenny Craig, and NutriSystem offer patients additional support for weight loss, including group support, face-to-face coaching, and social support through in-person or online participation, and availability of calorie controlled meals.

CASE STUDY

Discussion

The case study represents a common occurrence in clinical practice. She has moderately severe obesity (BMI 39 kg/m^2), hypertension, and prediabetes. Yet, despite multiple attempts at dietary change to achieve weight loss and improve her health, she has not been successful and is confused regarding dietary changes to pursue in the future.

Given the evidence for multiple eating plans, which one should she pursue? Recognizing that any dietary intervention that introduces a calorie restriction will be effective and that long-term adherence is key to success, it is beneficial to ask her where to start, inquiring about her experience and interest in following a specified meal plan, using meal replacements, tweaking her current diet, meeting with a dietitian, or knowledge about intermittent fasting strategy as treatment options.

Regardless of the dietary intervention that she chooses, there are many opportunities to support her efforts. Encouraging behaviors that are associated with greater weight loss is a good start, the most important of which is self-monitoring food intake, specifically total calories. Using resources available such as a referral to a previously defined RDN or a local commercial program will enhance results. Helping your patient become more physically active will also offer health benefits beyond weight loss. The initial goal is to achieve a weight loss of 5% to 10% after 3 to 6 months of treatment. If further weight loss is desired, then additional treatment options can to be discussed such as more deliberate and structured dietary changes, engagement in increased physical activity and exercise, and the potential use of an antiobesity medication.

WHEN TO REFER?

- Registered dietitian nutritionist—Referral to an RDN should be considered for patients who need more detailed or concrete assistance with meal planning than can be provided by online or written information, or who need more frequent feedback and support on their efforts than can be provided by the HCP. The RDN can review patient's current eating habits, identify challenges, and develop an individualized plan.
- Commercial weight management program—Considered for patients who are looking for a cost-effective approach for weight loss support, calorie-reduced meals, and options of in-person meetings or online support.
- Behavioral program—Intensive lifestyle intervention programs are offered by a trained behavioral interventionist and consist of at least 14 visits in the first 6 months to support behavior modification, as well as at least monthly contact for maintenance of weight loss. See Chapter 7 for additional details.

QUIZ QUESTIONS

1. Our case study patient decided to pursue a Mediterranean style diet. She is interested in lowering her risks for diabetes and heart disease. She has visited with an RDN and has a meal plan to create a calorie restriction of 500 cal/day.

   Which of the following is true regarding weight loss expectations?

   A. She will lose exactly one pound per week for the first 6 months
   B. She will lose less weight at 1 year than if she followed a very-low-carbohydrate diet
   C. She will lose more weight with a Mediterranean diet if she keeps a food record
   D. She will not lose additional weight by joining a behavioral program at this point

   Answer: C. *Although a common goal is an average weight loss of a pound per week, there is significant variability observed during weight loss making this an unrealistic expectation (thus, A is incorrect). Although low-carbohydrate diets may be associated with greater weight loss in the short term (3 to 6 months), weight loss would be expected to be similar at 1 year (thus, B is incorrect). Tracking eating habits has been consistently shown to lead to greater weight loss as is participation in a behavioral program (thus, C is correct). As described in the AHA/ACC/TOS guideline, intensive behavioral programs have consistently been shown to lead to 5% to 10% weight loss in the first 6 months of treatment (thus, D is incorrect).*

2. Our patient returns for follow-up 4 months into her weight loss effort. Her baseline weight was 106 kg (233 lb), her current weight is 98.5 kg (217 lb) (= 7.1% of initial body weight). She has been adhering to the meal plan created by the RDN. She has not been tracking her food intake as regularly as she did at the start. She is not doing planned exercise but is trying to be more active throughout the day and reports that her step count ranges from 5,000 to 7,000 per day. She is frustrated that she has not experienced more weight loss.

   What is the most accurate assessment of her current efforts?

   A. She is unlikely to continue to lose weight because of metabolic adaptations to weight loss
   B. She has reduced her risk for developing type 2 diabetes with the weight loss achieved so far
   C. She is currently getting all the benefits of physical activity
   D. She would not be a good candidate for weight loss medication because she has already lost more than 5% of initial body weight

   Answer: B. *The Diabetes Prevention Program reported a decrease in the risk for developing type 2 diabetes of close to 60% among subjects who lost ≥ 7% of their weight. Our patient has lost 7.5 kg (16.5 lb), or 7.1% of her baseline weight (thus, B is correct). She will likely continue to lose weight, although the rate of weight loss will drop after 6 months (thus, A is incorrect). Introducing regular physical activity will create an additional energy deficit and thus should improve weight loss. Increasing physical activity also will enhance her chances at maintaining weight after a weight loss effort (thus, C is incorrect). She is clearly motivated to pursue weight loss, it is reasonable to consider a medication to enhance the weight loss observed (thus, D is incorrect).*

PRACTICE RESOURCES

- The Practical Guide to the Identification, Evaluation, and Treatment of Overweight and Obesity in Adults (https://www.nhlbi.nih.gov/files/docs/guidelines/prct-gd_c.pdf)
- 2015-2020 Dietary Guidelines for Americans, eighth edition (https://health.gov/dietaryguidelines/2015/guidelines/)
- Nutrition Care Manual (https://www.nutritioncare-manual.org)
- ChooseMyPlate (https://choosemyplate.gov/resources/all-resources)

ACKNOWLEDGMENT

The author and editors thank Nicole Rubenstein, MS, RDN, CDE for her review and comments on this chapter.

REFERENCES

1. U.S. Department of Health and Human Services and U.S Department of Agriculture. *2015-2020 Dietary Guidelines for Americans.* 8th ed., 2015. https://health.gov/dietaryguidelines/2015/guidelines/

2. Roust LR, DiBaise JK. Nutrient deficiencies prior to bariatric surgery. *Curr Opin Clin Nutr Metab Care.* 2017;20(2):138-144.

3. Kushner RF. Providing nutritional care in the office practice: teams, tools, and techniques. *Med Clin North Am.* 2016;100:1157-1168.

4. U.S. Department of Agriculture. Accessed April 6, 2020. http://www.choosemyplate.gov/resources/all-resources

5. Jensen MD, Ryan DH, Apovian CM, et al. 2013 AHA/ACC/TOS guideline for the management of overweight and obesity in adults: a report of the American College of Cardiology/American Heart Association Task Force on Practice Guidelines and the Obesity Society. *J Am Coll Cardiol.* 2014;63(25 pt B):2985-3023.

6. Heymsfield SB, Wadden TA. Mechanisms, pathophysiology, and management of obesity. *N Engl J Med.* 2017;376(15):1492.

7. Harris JA, Benedict FG. *A Biometric Study of Basal Metabolism in Man.* Vol 279. Carnegie Institute of Washington; 1919.

8. Villablanca PA, Alegria JR, Mookadam F, Holmes DR Jr, Wright RS, Levine JA. Nonexercise activity thermogenesis in obesity management. *Mayo Clin Proc.* 2015;90(4):509-519.

9. Ravussin E, Lillioja S, Anderson TE, Christin L, Bogardus C. Determinants of 24-hour energy expenditure in man. Methods and results using a respiratory chamber. *J Clin Invest.* 1986;78(6):1568-1578.

10. Mifflin MD, St Jeor ST, Hill LA, Scott BJ, Daugherty SA, Koh YO. A new predictive equation for resting energy expenditure in healthy individuals. *Am J Clin Nutr.* 1990;51(2):241-247.

11. Joint FAO/WHO/UNU Expert Consultation on Energy and Protein Requirements. Energy and protein requirements: report of a joint FAO/WHO/UNU Expert Consultation. *World Health Organ Tech Rep Ser.* 1985;724:1-206.

12. Leibel RL, Rosenbaum M, Hirsch J. Changes in energy expenditure resulting from altered body weight. *N Engl J Med.* 1995;332(10):621-628.

13. Rosenbaum M, Hirsch J, Gallagher DA, Leibel RL. Long-term persistence of adaptive thermogenesis in subjects who have maintained a reduced body weight. *Am J Clin Nutr.* 2008;88(4):906-912.

14. Sacks FM, Bray GA, Carey VJ, et al. Comparison of weight-loss diets with different compositions of fat, protein, and carbohydrates. *N Engl J Med.* 2009;360(9):859-873.

15. Sacks FM, Svetkey LP, Vollmer WM, et al; DASH-Sodium Collaborative Research Group. Effects on blood pressure of reduced dietary sodium and the Dietary Approaches to Stop Hypertension (DASH) diet. DASH-Sodium Collaborative Research Group. *N Engl J Med.* 2001;344(1):3-10.

16. Appel LJ, Moore TJ, Obarzanek E, et al. A clinical trial of the effects of dietary patterns on blood pressure. DASH Collaborative Research Group. *N Engl J Med.* 1997;336(16):1117-1124.

17. Blumenthal JA, Babyak MA, Hinderliter A, et al. Effects of the DASH diet alone and in combination with exercise and weight loss on blood pressure and cardiovascular biomarkers in men and women with high blood pressure: the ENCORE study. *Arch Intern Med.* 2010;170(2):126-135.

18. Knowler WC, Barrett-Connor E, Fowler SE, et al; Diabetes Prevention Program Research Group. Reduction in the incidence of type 2 diabetes with lifestyle intervention or metformin. *N Engl J Med.* 2002;346(6):393-403.

19. Diabetes Prevention Program Research Group; Knowler WC, Fowler SE, Hamman RF, et al. 10-year follow-up of diabetes incidence and weight loss in the Diabetes Prevention Program Outcomes Study. *Lancet.* 2009;374(9702):1677-1686.

20. Shai I, Schwarzfuchs D, Henkin Y, et al. Weight loss with a low-carbohydrate, Mediterranean, or low-fat diet. *N Engl J Med.* 2008;359(3):229-241.

21. Schwarzfuchs D, Golan R, Shai I. Four-year follow-up after two-year dietary interventions. *N Engl J Med.* 2012;367(14):1373-1374.

22. Mancini JG, Filion KB, Atallah R, Eisenberg MJ. Systematic review of the mediterranean diet for long-term weight loss. *Am J Med.* 2016;129(4):407-415.e4.

23. Esposito K, Maiorino MI, Bellastella G, Chiodini P, Panagiotakos D, Giugliano D. A journey into a Mediterranean diet and type 2 diabetes: a systematic review with meta-analyses. *BMJ Open.* 2015;5(8):e008222.

24. Estruch R, Martinez-Gonzalez MA, Corella D, et al; PREDIMED Study Investigators. Retracted: effect of a high-fat Mediterranean diet on bodyweight and waist circumference. A prespecified secondary outcomes analysis of the PREDIMED randomised controlled trial. *Lancet Diabetes Endocrinol.* 2016;4(8):666-676.

25. Pi-Sunyer X, Blackburn G, Brancati FL, et al. Reduction in weight and cardiovascular disease risk factors in individuals with type 2 diabetes: one-year results of the Look AHEAD trial. *Diabetes Care.* 2007;30(6):1374-1383.

26. Wadden TA, West DS, Neiberg RH, et al. One-year weight losses in the Look AHEAD study: factors associated with success. *Obesity (Silver Spring).* 2009;17(4):713-722.

27. Wing RR, Bolin P, Brancati FL, et al. Cardiovascular effects of intensive lifestyle intervention in type 2 diabetes. *N Engl J Med.* 2013;369(2):145-154.

28. Gregg EW, Jakicic JM, Blackburn G, et al. Association of the magnitude of weight loss and changes in physical fitness with long-term cardiovascular disease outcomes in overweight or obese people with type 2 diabetes: a post-hoc analysis of the Look AHEAD randomised clinical trial. *Lancet Diabetes Endocrinol.* 2016;4(11):913-921.

29. Johnston BC, Kanters S, Bandayrel K, et al. Comparison of weight loss among named diet programs in overweight and obese adults: a meta-analysis. *J Am Med Assoc.* 2014;312(9):923-933.

30. Tsai AG, Wadden TA. The evolution of very-low-calorie diets: an update and meta-analysis. *Obesity (Silver Spring).* 2006;14(8):1283-1293.

31. Gardner CD, Kiazand A, Alhassan S, et al. Comparison of the Atkins, Zone, Ornish, and LEARN diets for change in weight and related risk factors among overweight premenopausal women. The A to Z weight loss study: a randomized trial. *J Am Med Assoc.* 2007;297(9):969-977.

32. Alhassan S, Kim S, Bersamin A, King AC, Gardner CD. Dietary adherence and weight loss success among overweight women: results from the A to Z weight loss study. *Int J Obes.* 2008;32(6):985-991.

33. Dansinger ML, Gleason JA, Griffith JL, Selker HP, Schaefer EJ. Comparison of the Atkins, Ornish, Weight Watchers, and Zone diets for weight loss and heart disease risk reduction: a randomized trial. *J Am Med Assoc.* 2005;293(1):43-53.

34. Gudzune KA, Doshi RS, Mehta AK, et al. Efficacy of commercial weight-loss programs: an updated systematic review. *Ann Intern Med.* 2015;162(7):501-512.

35. Trepanowski JF, Kroeger CM, Barnosky A, et al. Effect of alternate-day fasting on weight loss, weight maintenance, and cardioprotection among metabolically healthy obese adults: a randomized clinical trial. *JAMA Intern Med.* 2017;177(7):930-938.

36. Klempel MC, Kroeger CM, Varady KA. Alternate day fasting (ADF) with a high-fat diet produces similar weight loss and cardio-protection as ADF with a low-fat diet. *Metabolism.* 2013;62(1):137-143.

37. Sundfor TM, Svendsen M, Tonstad S. Effect of intermittent versus continuous energy restriction on weight loss, maintenance and cardiometabolic risk: a randomized 1-year trial. *Nutr Metabol Cardiovasc Dis.* 2018;28(7):698-706.

38. Sutton EF, Beyl R, Early KS, Cefalu WT, Ravussin E, Peterson CM. Early time-restricted feeding improves insulin sensitivity, blood pressure, and oxidative stress even without weight loss in men with prediabetes. *Cell Metab.* 2018;27(6):1212-1221.e3.

39. de Cabo R, Mattson MP. Effects of intermittent fasting on health, aging, and disease. *N Engl J Med.* 2019;381(26):2541-2551.

40. Rynders CA, Thomas EA, Zaman A, Pan Z, Catenacci VA, Melanson EL. Effectiveness of intermittent fasting and time-restricted feeding compared to continuous energy restriction for weight loss. *Nutrients.* 2019;11(10):2442. doi:10.3390/nu11102442

41. Carter S, Clifton PM, Keogh JB. The effect of intermittent compared with continuous energy restriction on glycaemic control in patients with type 2 diabetes: 24-month follow-up of a randomised noninferiority trial. *Diabetes Res Clin Pract.* 2019;151:11-19.

42. Corley BT, Carroll RW, Hall RM, Weatherall M, Parry-Strong A, Krebs JD. Intermittent fasting in Type 2 diabetes mellitus and the risk of hypoglycaemia: a randomized controlled trial. *Diabet Med.* 2018;35(5):588-594.

6

PHYSICAL ACTIVITY TREATMENT

Seth A. Creasy, Danielle Marie Ostendorf, Victoria A. Catenacci

CASE STUDY 1

A 47-year-old male nonsmoker with a body mass index (BMI) of 30 kg/m² would like to begin an exercise program to lose weight. He has no current symptoms of cardiovascular disease (CVD). He purchased a stationary bicycle for his wife for Mother's Day, which she has never used. He plans to ride the stationary bicycle for 20 minutes in the morning before work every weekday. How would you counsel him on the likelihood of him losing weight with this exercise alone?

CLINICAL SIGNIFICANCE

Increasing physical activity is recognized as a significant, modifiable risk factor for the prevention and treatment of overweight and obesity. In 2018, the US Department of Health and Human Services published the second edition of the Physical Activity Guidelines (PAG) for Americans, which provides scientific evidence of the benefits of physical activity.[1] There were four main recommendations for US adults (see Table 6.1). Importantly, the PAG recommend ≥150 to 300 minutes/week of moderate-intensity aerobic activity or ≥75 to 150 minutes/week of vigorous-intensity aerobic activity and muscle strengthening activities at least two times per week for overall health benefits. The PAG also recognize that higher levels of aerobic activity (≥300 minutes/week of moderate-intensity aerobic activity or ≥150 minutes/week of vigorous-intensity aerobic activity) are associated with additional health benefits including prevention of weight gain and regain following weight loss.[2] However, in 2018, only 54.2% (53.2% to 55.3%) of adults nationwide self-reported achieving the minimum aerobic threshold of ≥150 minutes/week of moderate-intensity physical activity or ≥75 minutes of

vigorous-intensity physical activity and even fewer adults, 37.4% (36.4% to 38.4%), reported achieving ≥300 minutes/week of moderate-intensity physical activity or ≥150 minutes/week of vigorous-intensity aerobic activity.[3] Individuals with obesity engage in even lower amounts of physical activity compared with adults without obesity. It is difficult to determine the extent to which low levels of physical activity precede the development of obesity diagnosis or whether the presence of obesity limits an individual's ability to engage in physical activity.

Health Benefits of Physical Activity

There is extensive literature outlining the benefits of regular physical activity for individuals with and without obesity. Physical activity helps to lower risk for CVD, hypertension, type 2 diabetes (T2D), and some cancers.[1] An increase from being inactive to achieving 150 minutes/week of moderate-intensity physical activity is associated with a 34% lower risk for CVD mortality, a 21% lower incidence of CVD, and a 27% lower incidence of T2D.[4] A meta-analysis of cohort studies found a 14% reduction in risk for all-cause mortality associated with engaging in 150 minutes/week of moderate-to-vigorous physical activity (MVPA) and a 26% reduction in risk for mortality associated with engaging in 300 minutes/week of MVPA.[5] In addition, there are other benefits of physical activity such as providing opportunities to have fun, be with friends and family, and enjoy the outdoors.

Consequences of Sedentary Behavior and Inactivity

Sedentary behavior is defined as any behavior during waking hours characterized by low energy expenditure, while in a sitting, reclining, or lying posture.[6] Common sedentary behaviors include watching television, playing video games, using a computer, and driving a car. On average, Americans spend ~55% (7.7 hours/day)

TABLE 6.1 Summary of Key Recommendations From the 2018 Physical Activity Guidelines for Americans

KEY RECOMMENDATIONS

1. Adults should move more and sit less throughout the day. Some physical activity is better than none. Adults who sit less and do any amount of moderate-to-vigorous physical activity gain some health benefits.

2. For substantial health benefits, adults should do at least 150 minutes (2 hours and 30 minutes) to 300 minutes (5 hours) a week of moderate-intensity aerobic physical activity, or 75 minutes (1 hour and 15 minutes) to 150 minutes (2 hours and 30 minutes) a week of vigorous-intensity aerobic physical activity, or an equivalent combination of moderate-intensity and vigorous-intensity aerobic activity. Preferably, aerobic activity should be spread throughout the week.

3. Additional health benefits are gained by engaging in physical activity beyond the equivalent of 300 minutes (5 hours) of moderate-intensity physical activity a week.

4. Adults should also do muscle strengthening activities of moderate or greater intensity and that involve all major muscle groups on 2 or more days a week, as these activities provide additional health benefits.

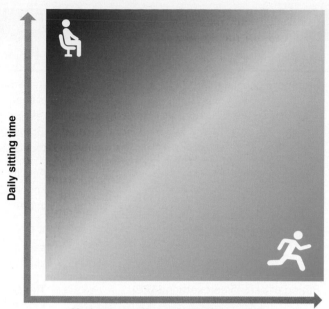

Moderate-to-vigorous physical activity
Risk of all-cause mortality decreases as one moves from red to green

FIGURE 6.1 Relationship between moderate-to-vigorous physical activity (MVPA), sitting time, and risk of all-cause mortality in adults. Having high amounts of sitting time concomitantly with low amounts of MVPA is associated with the highest risk of all-cause mortality (indicated in red in upper left corner). As one increases MVPA, the risk associated with high amounts of sitting begins to decrease (indicated by orange color). Engaging in high amounts of MVPA is associated with lower risk of all-cause mortality even when combined with high amounts of sitting (indicated by green in the upper right corner). At the lowest levels of MVPA and the lowest levels of sitting time, there is still increased risk of all-cause mortality (indicated by orange in lower left corner). Risk of mortality increases with increased sitting. The highest levels of MVPA and lowest levels of sitting time are associated with the lowest risk of all-cause mortality (indicated by green in lower right corner). (Adapted from Physical Activity Guidelines Advisory Committee. *2018 Physical Activity Guidelines Advisory Committee Scientific Report*. U.S. Department of Health and Human Services; 2018. Adapted from data from Ekelund U, Steene-Johannessen J, Brown WJ, et al. Does physical activity attenuate, or even eliminate, the detrimental association of sitting time with mortality? A harmonised meta-analysis of data from more than 1 million men and women. *Lancet*. 2016;388(10051):1302-1310.)

of their waking hours engaged in sedentary behaviors.[7] Studies have shown a link between sedentary behaviors and increased rates of obesity, independent of the overall level of physical activity.[8-10] Higher levels of sedentary behavior are also associated with greater risk for all-cause mortality, CVD, CVD mortality, T2D, and cancers of the colon, endometrium, and lung.[1] Thus, both increasing physical activity and decreasing sedentary behavior are important for overall health. As illustrated in Figure 6.1, the risk of all-cause mortality is associated with both behaviors. To summarize this figure, individuals would benefit from making efforts to increase levels of MVPA as well as decreasing sitting time.

Physical inactivity, which is distinct from sedentary behavior, is defined as a lack of any MVPA (see Table 6.2) beyond basic movement from daily activities. Physical inactivity is considered the fourth leading risk factor for death due to noncommunicable disease worldwide and contributes to >3 million preventable deaths annually. In sum, overwhelming evidence supports the benefits of regular physical activity and the negative consequences of inactivity and sedentary behavior. Current PAG (see Table 6.1) focus not only on increasing physical activity but also on making an effort to sit less. Thus, a simple message to "move more and sit less" can summarize this information succinctly for patients.

REVIEW OF EVIDENCE FOR PHYSICAL ACTIVITY IN OBESITY TREATMENT

Physical Activity and Weight Gain Prevention

Epidemiological data suggest that adults tend to gain an average of 1 to 2 pounds of body weight per

TABLE 6.2 Physical Activity and Exercise Terminology

TERMS	DEFINITION
Metabolic equivalents (METs)	A method of standardizing the intensity of an activity. This method is based on the energy cost of an activity. 1 MET is equivalent to the resting energy expenditure. 3 METs, which is considered moderate-intensity physical activity, means that the activity elicits an energy cost that is threefold resting energy expenditure.
Aerobic activity	Activities where the energy demand is met via aerobic pathways; also known as cardiovascular activities; typically associated with increases in breathing and heart rate.
Strength/resistance activity	A form of physical activity that focuses on muscular contraction and seeks to improve muscular strength and endurance. Typically done for shorter periods of time compared with aerobic activity.
Rating of perceived exertion (RPE)	The perceived intensity of an activity. Usually rated on a 0-10 scale. Moderate intensity is typically associated with an RPE of 3-5.
Sedentary behavior	Time spent awake with a low energy expenditure (<1.5 METs) in a sitting/reclining posture. Examples: watching TV, desk work, driving
Light physical activity	Activities where heart rate is not elevated much above resting (≥1.5-<3.0 METs). Examples: normal daily activity, intermittent periods of normal walking, some forms of yoga
Moderate physical activity	Activities where heart rate is moderately elevated (50%-70% of maximum heart rate); ≥3.0-<6.0 METs. Examples: brisk walking, cycling <10 miles/hour, water aerobics
Vigorous physical activity	Activities where heart is elevated (70%-85% of maximum heart rate); ≥6.0 METs. Examples: running, swimming, cycling >10 miles/hour
Moderate-to-vigorous physical activity	Any activity ≥3.0 METs. Commonly used in public health recommendations. This is a summary measure that includes both moderate and vigorous physical activity
Dose/volume	The total dose or volume of activity is usually a summary of weekly activity. For overall health benefits, the dose of physical activity should progress up to 300 minutes/week. For weight loss and weight loss maintenance, even higher amounts of physical activity may be necessary. Energy expenditure per week: Physical activity and exercise can be prescribed based on the energy expenditure of activity. This type of prescription is difficult and requires careful measurements. It is typically done in controlled research studies. MET-minutes per week: This prescription takes into account the intensity and duration of physical activity. The MET value of each activity is multiplied by the duration of the activity. Measuring physical activity as MET-min is typically done in research studies only.

year.[11] This annual weight gain places individuals at an increased risk for becoming overweight or obese with age. Physical activity has been postulated as a potential strategy for either attenuating or preventing this age-related weight gain. Several prospective, observational studies provide evidence that engaging in regular physical activity helps to prevent weight gain.[12] Randomized trials have also examined the relationship between physical activity and weight gain with most studies suggesting that engaging in moderate-intensity physical activity is sufficient to prevent weight gain.[12] In a study by Church et al., postmenopausal women who engaged in three different doses of supervised moderate-intensity aerobic activity (approximately 72, 136, and 194 minutes/week) over 6 months lost 3.0, 4.6, and 3.3 lb of body weight, respectively, compared with a 2 lb weight loss in the nonactive control group.[13] In a similar study, McTiernan et al. found that men and women who participated in a facility-based and home-based physical activity program over 1 year lost 3.0 and 4.0 lb compared with 0.2 and 1.5 lb weight gain in nonactive controls.[14] The combination of these studies and others suggest that a dose of approximately 150 to 250 minutes/week of moderate-intensity aerobic activity is effective for preventing weight gain and potentially eliciting modest weight loss.

Physical Activity Alone for Weight Loss

It has long been believed that increasing physical activity leads to increased energy expenditure and subsequent weight loss. Between 2013 and 2016, ~63% of the US adults who attempted to lose weight reported using exercise as a primary strategy.[15] Despite its frequent use as a weight loss strategy, physical activity alone typically results in only modest weight loss. Several well-designed prospective intervention trials have shown that prescribing physical activity alone (i.e., without dietary modification) typically produces weight losses of 1% to 3%.[12] Furthermore, the changes in body weight observed in these studies are on average only ~30% of predicted based upon the expected energy expenditure of the activity prescription. This is true even when exercise is supervised and adherence to physical activity is carefully monitored. Studies have also shown marked interindividual variability in weight loss in response to exercise, with some individuals losing substantial amounts of weight and others gaining weight. Recent studies suggest that a subset (~50%) of individuals may "compensate" for the increase in physical activity with increased energy intake and/or increased sedentary behavior and thereby lose less weight than expected. A recent study found that compensation to supervised physical activity was largely due to increases in energy intake rather than increases in sedentary behavior.[16] In addition, individuals who compensated had increased hunger and cravings for sweets. Thus, compensation and nonadherence mitigate the beneficial effects of physical activity on body weight in some individuals.

Despite the number of studies demonstrating relatively modest weight loss from physical activity alone, a few studies have shown that physical activity alone, when dosed in high amounts and supervised, results in clinically significant (≥5%) weight loss.[12] For example, when men and women engaged in 225 minutes of supervised physical activity per week for 16 months, men reduced body weight by 11.4 lb (~5%) more than nonactive controls and women had 5.0 lb (~3%) less weight gain compared with nonactive controls.[17] This large difference in weight change in men versus women was believed to be due to sex differences in physical activity energy expenditure. Notably, engaging in physical activity at the same intensity for the same duration would likely lead to higher energy expenditure during physical activity sessions for men compared with women due to their larger body size. Additional studies suggest that high volumes of physical activity can elicit weight loss of ≥5% in men and women when dosed based on energy expenditure rather than exercise duration. In addition, there appears to be a dose-response relationship with more physical activity energy expenditure being associated with greater weight loss.

In summary, engaging in ≥150 minutes/week of MVPA will elicit modest (1% to 3%) weight loss on average; however, higher amounts of MVPA (≥250 minutes/week) are needed to elicit clinically significant (≥5%) weight loss. Weight loss with physical activity is typically less than predicted from the energy expended in activity due to compensatory changes in eating and nonexercise activity behaviors, and there is considerable variability in weight change in response to physical activity alone. Future research is needed to understand strategies to reduce compensation and make physical activity alone a more effective weight management strategy.

Physical Activity Combined With Dietary Restriction for Weight Loss

Most behavioral weight loss interventions encourage individuals to increase physical activity in combination with an energy-reduced diet.[18] These interventions also employ behavioral support in order to maximize adherence to these recommendations. If the reduced energy diet severely restricts calories (i.e., >800 to 1,000 kcal/day deficit), similar weight losses are observed between a diet plus physical activity program and a diet-only program.[12] However, several studies have found that the combination of a more modest energy-reduced diet (i.e., 500 to 750 kcal/day deficit) and physical activity produces greater weight loss than diet alone.[12] A systematic review of studies lasting ≥12 months found that diet plus physical activity resulted in a mean weight loss of 8.8% compared with a weight loss of 6.9% from diet alone.[19]

Physical Activity and Weight Loss Maintenance

High levels of physical activity, and more specifically MVPA, are consistently and positively associated with long-term weight loss and weight loss maintenance success.[12,20,21] One study found that individuals who maintained a weight loss of >10% at 18 months engaged in an amount of physical activity equivalent to brisk walking for ~260 minutes/week[20] or approximately 10,000 steps per day.[22] Importantly, ~35% of their total steps were at a moderate-to-vigorous intensity and were taken in bouts ≥10 minutes. In a recent cross-sectional study, successful weight loss maintainers (WLMs, individuals maintaining a weight loss of >30 lb for >1 year) engaged in a total of 665 minutes/week of MVPA with 272 minutes of MVPA accumulated in bouts ≥10 minutes.[21] In addition, WLMs engaged in ≥60 minutes of MVPA on 73% of days of the week suggesting they achieve high levels of activity with consistency across the week. These and other studies[23] suggest that WLMs maintain their body weight by engaging in high amounts of physical activity, thereby allowing them to eat a similar amount of calories as they were consuming prior to weight loss.

In summary, physical activity is one of the best predictors of long-term weight loss success. The dose of physical activity necessary to achieve weight loss maintenance may vary among individuals; however, most evidence would suggest ≥200 minutes/week is necessary. Importantly, the above studies noted that MVPA was accumulated in bouts of ≥10 minutes. This suggests that sustained bouts of MVPA may be important for achieving such high levels of MVPA per week and that these sustained bouts are important for maintaining weight loss.

Physical Activity and Bariatric Surgery

Metabolic and bariatric surgery has been shown to be highly effective for reducing body weight. While metabolic and bariatric surgery is a potent treatment alone, several observational studies have found higher amounts of physical activity are associated with greater weight loss following bariatric surgery.[24-26] In addition, physical activity following surgery may improve quality of life. To date, there have been very few interventional studies that have examined the extent to which physical activity following bariatric surgery can improve long-term weight loss and health outcomes. Two randomized studies examining the effects of supervised physical activity over 3 to 6 months following bariatric surgery found that exercise resulted in no additional weight loss compared with nonactive controls.[23,27] However, adherence to the physical activity program was associated with improvements in insulin sensitivity, glucose control, and aerobic fitness.

Resistance Training and Weight Management

The 2018 PAG for Americans recommend that adults engage in muscle strengthening activities at least 2 days/week for general health benefits.[1] Within the context of weight management, it has been hypothesized that resistance training may help people retain lean mass during weight loss and/or alter eating behavior. These hypotheses would suggest that resistance training during or following weight loss may be beneficial. However, there is little evidence in support of this hypothesis.

Resistance training alone without dietary modification does not elicit weight loss or reductions in body fat.[12] Resistance training combined with aerobic training results in superior weight loss, increased fat loss, and increased lean mass compared with an aerobic physical activity program alone. When resistance training is combined with dietary modification, it does not result in increased weight loss or fat loss compared with dietary modification only; however, lean body mass is improved. In sum, the major benefit of resistance training for weight management may be the improvements in lean body mass, rather than changes in fat mass and body weight. Resistance training may become more important for weight loss maintenance and prevention of weight gain. Following weight loss, muscular efficiency is increased. This means that for the same amount of work, energy expenditure is lower.[28] This metabolic adaption is one reason why weight regain following weight loss is so common. A recent study found that resistance training following weight loss helps maintain muscle efficiency, which may in turn help to promote weight loss maintenance.[29] However, in one randomized trial, resistance training did not attenuate weight regain following 6 months of an energy-restricted diet.[30] Additional studies are needed to understand the effectiveness of resistance training for promoting long-term weight loss maintenance.

In summary, resistance training is not an effective weight loss strategy when done in isolation. In addition, resistance training does not result in greater weight loss when combined with dietary modification compared with diet alone. However, resistance training does help to retain and increase lean mass during weight loss and may help with weight loss maintenance.

Sedentary Behavior and Weight Management

Sedentary behavior is associated with overweight and obesity.[8,9] Occupational physical activity has declined over the past several decades which may be linked to the increased prevalence of overweight and obesity.

Few studies have examined how changing sedentary behavior is related to weight management. Two studies examining this question found that changes in sedentary behavior were not associated with greater weight loss.[31,32] However, it is possible that the observation period may need to be longer (>1 year) to observe an effect of changes in sedentary behavior. Although reducing sedentary behavior may not directly lead to weight loss, there are other health benefits associated with decreased sedentary behavior. In addition, decreasing sedentary behavior can be the first step toward increasing physical activity for some patients.

ASSESSMENT OF PHYSICAL ACTIVITY

Assessment of current level of physical activity can be quickly achieved using the Exercise Is Medicine (EIM) (https://exerciseismedicine.org/) Physical Activity Vital Sign (PAVS), which consists of just two questions.

The PAVS can be added to a health history intake form and provides a snapshot of whether patients are meeting the minimum PAG of 150 minutes/week of moderate-intensity activity each week. Patients not meeting these guidelines can be flagged so that the healthcare providers (HCPs) can provide targeted advice or resources. Additional follow-up questions can be asked in patients not meeting guidelines based on the brief PAVS screening tool to further evaluate level of activity and areas for potential intervention. These could include questions related to physical activity enjoyment, types of activities performed, access to exercise facility, and perceived benefits/barriers to physical activity. A more detailed set of questions designed to assess how active patients are in daily life including level of sedentary behavior, current level of exercise participation, and perceived barriers to exercise are covered in detail in Chapter 2.

EXERCISE PREPARTICIPATION HEALTH SCREENING

A strong body of evidence suggests that promoting increased physical activity in adults with overweight and obesity will result in substantial health and weight management benefits. A recommendation to engage in physical activity is generally safe with appropriate preparticipation health screening to identify individuals who may be at elevated risk for exercise-related sudden cardiac death and/or acute myocardial infarction. There is considerable evidence that exercise is safe for most people, that exercise-related cardiovascular events are often preceded by warning signs/symptoms, and that the cardiovascular risk associated with exercise lessens as individuals become more physically active/

fit.[33] The current American College of Sports Medicine (ACSM) algorithm for preparticipation screening provides an evidence-informed flowchart on the basis of three risk modulators of exercise-related cardiovascular events: (1) the individual's current level of physical activity, (2) presence of signs or symptoms and/or known cardiovascular, metabolic, or renal disease, and (3) desired exercise intensity.[33] These ACSM guidelines are shown in Figure 6.2 and provide a practical approach to determine which patients require medical clearance from an HCP prior to beginning or modifying their current exercise program. All patients with symptoms suggestive of CVD or arrhythmia should be referred for further evaluation with exercise or pharmacologic stress testing and/or consultation with a cardiologist prior to starting exercise. Inactive individuals with known cardiovascular, metabolic, or renal disease should receive medical clearance from a healthcare provider prior to beginning an exercise program. These individuals should also obtain medical clearance from a healthcare provider prior to pursuing a vigorous-intensity exercise program, even if they are already active at a moderate-intensity. Whether asymptomatic patients with known cardiovascular, metabolic, or renal disease should undergo further evaluation with stress testing and/or consultation with a cardiologist prior to beginning exercise or increasing their exercise to vigorous intensity should be decided on a case-by-case basis. Vigorous-intensity physical activity is associated with an increased risk of acute myocardial infarction and sudden cardiac death compared with less vigorous activity. Expert guidelines from the American Heart Association[34] recommend exercise stress testing before vigorous exercise in high-risk asymptomatic individuals who are classified as coronary artery disease equivalents by the National Cholesterol Education Program. This includes those with diabetes mellitus, symptomatic carotid disease, peripheral vascular disease, and a calculated Framingham 10-year risk (https://www.mdcalc.com/framingham-risk-score-hard-coronary-heart-disease) of ≥20%. However, no studies have compared outcomes from pre-exercise stress testing versus encouraging light exercise with gradual increases in exertion in these high-risk but asymptomatic individuals.

PERSONALIZING THE PHYSICAL ACTIVITY PRESCRIPTION IN ADULTS WITH OBESITY

Treating obesity should always start with a conversation with the patient about preferences and goals. If weight loss is the primary goal, overwhelming data would suggest a combination of an energy-reduced diet and increased physical activity be employed. If the patient is primarily interested in increasing physical activity, the

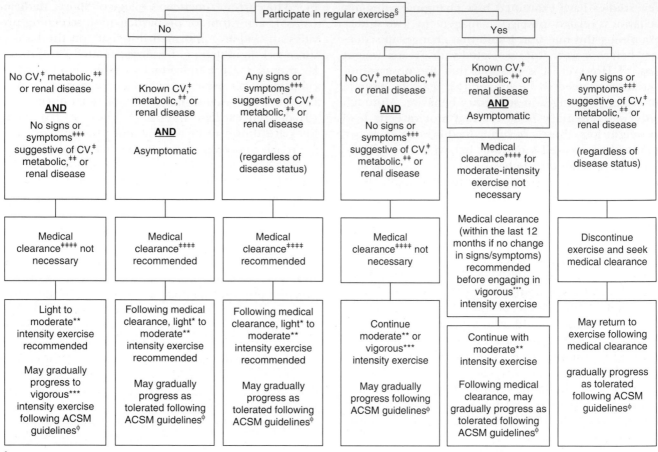

§Exercise participation, performing planned, structured physical activity at least 30 min at moderate intensity on at least 3 d.wk^{-1} for at least the last 3 months.

*Light-intensity exercise, 30% to < 40% HRR or VO$_2$R, 2 to <3 METs, 9-11 RPE, an intensity that causes slight increases in HR and breathing.

**Moderate-intensity exercise, 40% to, <60% HRR or VO$_2$R, 3 to <6 METs, 12-13 RPE, an intensity that causes noticeable increases in HR and breathing.

***Vigorous-intensity exercise ≥60% HRR or VO2R, ≥6 METs, ≥14 RPE, an intensity that causes substantial increases in HR and breathing.

‡CVD, cardiac, peripheral vascular, or cerebrovascular disease.

‡‡Metabolic disease, type1 and 2 diabetes mellitus.

‡‡‡Signs and symptoms, at rest or during activity, include pain, discomfort in the chest, neck, jaw, arms, or other areas that may result from ischemia; shortness of breath at rest or with mild exertion; dizziness or syncope; orthopnea or paroxysmal nocturnal dyspnea; ankle edema; palpitations or tachycardia; intermittent claudication; known heart murmur; or unusual fatigue or shortness of breath with usual activities.

‡‡‡‡Medical clearance, approval from a health care professional to engage in exercise.

ϕACSM Guidelines, see *ACSM's Guidelines for Exercise Testing and Prescription, 9th edition, 2014.*

FIGURE 6.2 American College of Sports Medicine preparticipation screening algorithm. (Reprinted from Riebe D, Franklin BA, Thompson PD, et al. Updating ACSM's recommendations for exercise preparticipation health screening. *Med Sci Sports Exerc.* 2015;47(11):2473-2479.)

provider should emphasize the health benefits of physical activity, regardless of weight loss. The patient should be provided with realistic expectations about the role of physical activity relative to diet modification in weight loss as the expectation that physical activity alone will produce significant weight loss may be counterproductive. In a qualitative study of adults with overweight and obesity, failure to lose weight was found to strongly affect motivation to continue or re-engage in exercise.[35] It may be best to move beyond weight loss as the primary reason for participating in physical activity, focusing on both the immediate health benefits (improved mood, sleep, cognition, physical function) and the long-term health benefits (even if weight is unchanged). Asking patients about their willingness and readiness to begin a physical activity program is particularly important if a long-term behavior change is expected. If a patient is willing and ready to begin a physical activity program, then several factors should be considered prior to initiating treatment.

The type and dose (i.e., amount, frequency, and duration) of physical activity will impact health outcomes. For example, if weight loss is the goal, then high amounts of aerobic physical activity may be necessary. If increased lean mass is the goal, then resistance training may be best. Once a patient's goal is identified, the patient's current health status and barriers to physical activity should be assessed in order to develop an individualized prescription that is safe and can enhance adherence. The provider should begin by considering the patient's current BMI, physical activity level, fitness, and preferences. In addition, barriers to physical activity should be considered including functional limitations, health restrictions, medications, time constraints, and access to resources. Overweight and obesity are associated with higher risk of musculoskeletal injury, especially in the foot, knee, and hip. Thus, special care should be taken to increase the volume and intensity of physical activity gradually to avoid injuries that can lead to cessation of physical activity. It is important to recognize that individuals with overweight and obesity can increase energy expenditure significantly with even low-intensity activities, and even low levels of physical activity provide health benefits.[1] As individuals acclimate to activity and progress in total duration, higher intensity activity may be introduced based on patient preference. If possible, recurring contact should be made to evaluate the prescription and modify as necessary. A physical activity prescription pad can serve as a helpful tool in this regard (Figure 6.3). Supervision of physical activity progression by a

Name: _____ Date: _____

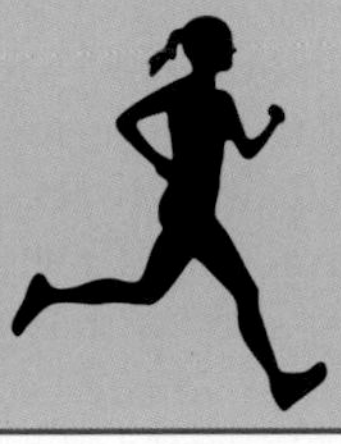

Physical Activity Prescription Pad

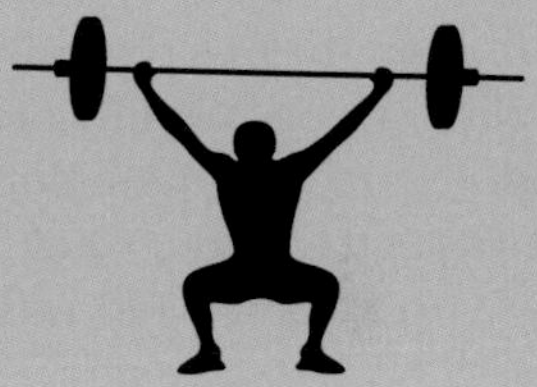

Current Physical Activity Level: _____

Patient Goals (i.e. weight loss, increase fitness level, walk up a flight of stairs, etc.):

a. _____

b. _____

c. _____

Exercise Prescription:

Frequency (days/week): ☐ 1 ☐ 2 ☐ 3 ☐ 4 ☐ 5 ☐ 6 ☐ 7

Intensity: ☐ Light (casual walk) ☐ Moderate (brisk walk) ☐ Vigorous (jogging)

Time (minutes/day): ☐ 10 ☐ 20 ☐ 30 ☐ 40 ☐ 50 ☐ 60 ☐ Other_____

Type: ☐ walk ☐ Run ☐ Bike

☐ Group Class ☐ Strength Training ☐ Swim

☐ Other _____

Details (i.e. Progressions, HR goal, follow-up in a month, etc.): _____

_____

_____

_____

Prescriber's Signature: _____

FIGURE 6.3 Physical activity prescription pad.

knowledgeable exercise professional may be helpful to enhance adherence, ensure appropriate progression, and reduce risk of injury.

When developing the physical activity prescription, aspects of the prescription that can be individualized include frequency, intensity, time, and type (FITT).

Frequency

The frequency of physical activity should be realistic, fit the patient's needs, and progress slowly. For example, an unfit patient who has engaged in no recreational physical activity should start with a frequency of 1 to 2 days/week; this prescription can progress to 3 to 5 days/week over the first few months. The frequency of physical activity prescribed may also depend on the patient's goal. Studies that have utilized physical activity alone for weight loss typically prescribe physical activity 5 to 7 days/week. Weight maintenance and prevention of weight gain may be achieved by engaging in physical activity 3 to 5 days/week. Even engaging in physical activity 1 to 2 days/week will decrease risk of all-cause mortality, CVD, and cancer mortality.[36] Any activity is better than no activity. The frequencies outlined above should serve as an initial guide.

Intensity

The intensity of the physical activity can be assessed in several different ways depending on available resources. Heart rate monitors are one way to measure activity intensity. In general, 50% to 70% of the maximum heart rate (HR_{max} = 220 bpm– person's age) is equivalent to moderate activity and 70% to 85% HR_{max} is equivalent to vigorous-intensity activity. Another intensity guide is ratings of perceived exertion (RPE), a simple 1 to 10 scale (1 = minimal exertion, 10 = maximal exertion). An RPE rating of 3 to 5 is considered moderate with higher levels being associated with vigorous activity. If neither of those resources is available, participants can use the talk test. While engaging in activity, if a person can sing, then it is light activity; if the person cannot sing but can talk, then it is moderate activity; and if the person can only say a few words between breaths, then it is likely vigorous activity. High-intensity interval training (HIIT) is a novel training method that may be of interest for some patients. HIIT involves alternating short bursts (up to 4 minutes) of high-intensity exercise with recovery periods. The definition of high-intensity exercise may vary by participant. It could vary from uphill walking to sprinting. Small, short-term studies suggest HIIT elicits similar enjoyment and adherence levels compared with continuous moderate-intensity physical activity in adults with overweight and obesity.[37] HITT offers the advantage of taking 40% less total training time compared with moderate-intensity physical activity; thus, individuals who report time as a barrier to physical activity may adhere better to this type of training. However, no studies have determined long-term adherence to HITT or the long-term efficacy of this type of training in adults with obesity.

Duration

The time or duration of physical activity that is being prescribed should also depend on the patient's current activity level, barriers to physical activity, and their goals. A good starting point is to recommend engaging in physical activity in a single bout of ~10 minutes. Jakicic and colleagues found that individuals who were prescribed the same dose of physical activity in multiple 10-minute bouts versus one prolonged bout engaged in higher amounts of physical activity and had similar increases in cardiorespiratory fitness compared with the long bout group.[38] Participants in both groups lost similar amounts of weight. For individuals who report time as a barrier, short bouts may be a practical alternative. In addition, shorter bouts of physical activity may be an effective strategy for increasing physical activity in inactive patients. As physical activity and physical activity self-efficacy increase, the bout duration can be lengthened.

Type of Activity

Finally, the type of physical activity should be considered. All forms of physical activity are beneficial for overall health and should be encouraged. Recommendations on the type of physical activity should be guided by the patient's preferences, goals, and environmental factors such as family income, access, and safety of neighborhood. In addition, the patient's health status, current activity level, and personal barriers to physical activity are additional considerations. For patients who are currently inactive, activities in which the body weight is supported may be preferred to higher impact activities, especially for those with higher BMI or musculoskeletal conditions.[39] Options for low-impact activities include walking, stationary or recumbent cycle, water aerobics, or water walking (which supports body weight and reduces impact on joints). The type of activity may also be influenced by community resources. Local community recreation centers may provide lower cost alternatives (exercise equipment and group-based activity programs) to traditional fitness center memberships.

Aerobic physical activity generally burns more calories than resistance training and thus works best for weight loss. However, resistance training can lead to favorable changes in body composition, physical function, metabolic health, and muscle efficiency in adults with overweight and obesity. Furthermore, resistance training may be easier and more enjoyable for some individuals with overweight and obesity.[40] In a patient who prefers resistance training over aerobic exercise or who struggles with motivation or adherence to aerobic training, resistance training should be encouraged as an acceptable alternative that will provide health benefits (albeit perhaps less weight loss than aerobic physical activity). In addition, enjoyment of the activity should be a major consideration.

BEHAVIORAL SUPPORT FOR INCREASING PHYSICAL ACTIVITY

Although high levels of physical activity are needed for long-term weight loss, producing substantial, long-term changes in physical activity is difficult. Additional support may be needed, especially for individuals who are using physical activity as a strategy for weight management. Referral to an exercise physiologist, personal trainer, or a supported exercise program can be considered based on the patient's goals and preferences. Developing referral relationships with local fitness facilities and exercise professionals who can provide educated support and guidance may help patients increase physical activity levels. Certifications that are accredited by the National Commission for Certifying Agencies (NCCA) are recommended including the following:

- The American College of Sports Medicine (ACSM)
- American Council on Exercise (ACE)
- The Cooper Clinic
- National Strength and Conditioning Association (NSCA)
- National Academy of Sports Medicine (NASM)

Inquiring about accredited fitness certifications and specific experience in working with patients with overweight and obesity may help identify the best exercise professionals. The ACSM EIM program also offers a credential to ensure that exercise professionals are properly prepared to work with referred patients, and the ACSM EIM Action Guide (https://www.exerciseismedicine.org/) can help identify certified professionals. In addition to providing a network of exercise professionals, the ACSM EIM Health Care Providers Action Guide provides specific guidance for increasing physical activity, regardless of an individual's level of readiness to make a change. The EIM Action Guide includes tips for starting conversations about physical activity with patients, safety screening tools and instructions, a PAVS questionnaire, and a downloadable EIM Physical Activity Prescription form. The EIM Rx for Health Series also provides guidelines on physical activity for individuals with various chronic diseases and medical conditions, including overweight and obesity. These downloadable patient handouts provide specific recommendations, strategies, and motivational tips to support patient efforts to increase physical activity and are developed by ACSM subject matter experts. Some patients may have limited access to reimbursed exercise programs. Thus, it is important for physicians to be aware of community-based solutions that provide opportunities for people to be active. Local resources, such as the YMCA (https://www.ymca.net/healthy-living/), offer memberships (including financial assistance programs), group fitness classes, and a range of exercise classes for different chronic disease conditions. Developed by the Arthritis Foundation, the Arthritis Foundation Exercise Program (AFEP, formerly called PACE) is a community-based program that offers group physical activity classes and is offered in some YMCAs (and in other community organizations) that may be suitable for some patients with overweight and obesity (https://www.cdc.gov/arthritis/interventions/programs/afep.htm).

Barriers and Facilitators for Physical Activity

What are the major reasons why people choose not to exercise?

Some of the most common reported barriers to maintaining an exercise program include illness, injury, work commitments, poor weather (e.g., snow storm, heat and humidity), time, vacation, boredom, and family commitments (Table 6.3).[41] Women with overweight or obesity report additional barriers compared with women with normal weight, including feeling too overweight, feeling self-conscious, minor aches and pains, and a lack of self-discipline. Furthermore, women who reported not meeting 120 minutes/week of exercise or who were not physically active more than three times per week typically had very narrow definitions of what counts as physical activity.[42] For example, these participants felt that physical activity only counted if they were exerting themselves in high-intensity exercise and for the "right" amount of time (e.g., 30 minutes). Lastly, these participants acknowledged some degree of anticipated negative affect (e.g., negative emotions such as anger, contempt, disgust, guilt) about being physically active. For example, some participants mentioned that even just thinking about exercise was stressful, and some mentioned feelings of "dreading" exercise or experiencing soreness and pain during exercise. In general, people tend to approach what feels good and avoid what feels bad.[43] How an individual feels during physical activity (i.e., their affective response) is predictive of their future involvement with physical activity.[44] Thus, it is important for HCPs to encourage patients to choose activities that make them feel good and avoid activities that make them feel bad.

Use of Mobile Applications and Wearable Technologies for Enhancing Physical Activity Adherence

HCPs have a limited amount of time to provide counseling for patients on weight loss and physical activity

TABLE 6.3 Strategies to Overcome Common Barriers to Physical Activity

COMMON BARRIERS TO PHYSICAL ACTIVITY	SUGGESTED STRATEGIES TO OVERCOME BARRIERS
Time	Is it true that you do not have time for one more step? Or, is it that you do not have a full 30 minutes to spare, so you think it's not worth doing anything at all? Most people find it's the latter. You can almost always choose to modify your plans and just move—even if it's only a few more steps.
Family commitments	1. Communicate with your family about your self-care needs. Bring your partner and children on board with your plans and let them know things that you may need help with in order to be more active. Examples include asking your partner to make dinner two nights a week, telling your child that during their soccer practice, you will be walking at an area nearby but that you will be back in time to pick them up, etc. 2. Incorporate your family into your physical activities. You can go for a family walk, bike ride, or hike. You can play with the kids at the playground, instead of sitting and watching them play.
Work commitments	Physical activity and your work commitments do not have to conflict. In fact, physical activity can help you be more productive at work, reduce anxiety/stress, and improve your memory and cognition. 1. Communicate with your boss and/or coworkers about your self-care needs. Some language you could use include, "I know that you are used to me working at the office past 5:00 PM, but I wanted to communicate with you that I am trying to take better care of myself. I'd like to plan to be out of the office by 5:00 PM on Mondays and Wednesdays so that I can get to a Zumba class. On these days, I'll be sure to be in by 8:00 AM." 2. Working walk/walking meeting: Many people find that they have better ideas and feel freed up for creativity when they walk and work outside of the office environment. 3. Standing work station: Instead of sitting at your desk, try standing up and working.
Weather	Think creatively about things you can do when the weather is poor. 1. Walk around an indoor mall. 2. Wear proper gear so you can be active outside. For the winter, activities like snow shoeing or cross-country skiing can be quite enjoyable. 3. Try out your local gym. Most gyms offer a complimentary day pass. 4. Search YouTube for exercise videos to do at home.
Illness/injury	1. For any serious illness/injury, seek a healthcare professional. 2. Ease back into being physically active and take it slow. 3. Modify the activity. For lower body injuries, try the arm ergometer. For overuse injuries, try swimming or water aerobics—these can help take pressure off your joints.
Boring	1. Focus on enjoyment. What are movements that you actually enjoy doing? Try those instead! 2. Try moving while spending time with a friend or family member. Go for a hike, call someone just to catch up while walking around a park. 3. Try a sport. For example, pickleball is easy to learn and easy on your body.

COMMON BARRIERS TO PHYSICAL ACTIVITY	SUGGESTED STRATEGIES TO OVERCOME BARRIERS
	TABLE 6.3 Strategies to Overcome Common Barriers to Physical Activity (Continued)
Travel/vacation	1. Walk the airport. You are going to be sitting on the plane for hours, right? Instead of sitting and working while waiting to board the plan, walk around with your wheeled luggage. 2. Try booking a hotel that has a fitness room. 3. Walking can be a great way to explore a new city, as long as you feel safe.
Feeling self-conscious when exercising	Remind yourself that at one point and time, everyone was where you were, and they just took the time to learn how to do it. 1. Practice acceptance of your weaknesses, strengths, and yourself. 2. Focus on comfort. Wear comfortable clothes (such as a loose T-shirt and shorts). Choose a place that you are familiar with such as a nearby park, your neighborhood, or inside your home. 3. Find an exercise buddy. Having a workout partner can help you feel less shy and more confident when trying new things. 4. Find a coach or personal trainer. Once you take the time to learn more about how to use different equipment in a fitness center, you will be more confident in your movements.
Money/resources	You do not need a membership to a fitness center to be active. There are lots of other ways to incorporate activities that do not hurt the budget. Ideas include the following: 1. Walking: As long as you have a good pair of shoes and a safe place, walking can be one of the best ways to increase your physical activity. 2. YouTube exercise video: There are several YouTube videos for workouts that are freely available, including yoga, high-intensity interval training, Zumba, and many more. 3. Go to a local park: Some parks offer courts for basketball, tennis, pickleball, playgrounds for kids, sidewalks for walking/biking/or roller skating, and grassy areas for kickball, softball, volleyball, yard games, etc.
Negative perception of exercise	1. Move in ways that make you feel good and stop moving in ways that make you feel bad. 2. Choose your own pace. Try light-intensity or moderate-intensity movements and avoid vigorous-intensity movements. 3. Try a new activity that you have not done before. It is never too late to create new, positive perceptions of exercise.

Taken from No Sweat *by Michelle Segar. Copyright © 2015 by Michelle Segar. Used by permission of HarperCollins Leadership. www.harpercollinsleadership.com*

and they may benefit from resources or referrals that can help their patients lose weight and keep the weight off. Mobile technologies are attractive as one of these resources. However, a review of 30 mobile apps for weight loss indicated that the majority of these apps made only limited use of evidence-based behavioral strategies.[45] In fact, the apps on average only included 3 to 4 of 20 evidenced-based strategies. Recent studies have shown mixed evidence for the efficacy of mobile apps that target weight management. In a systematic review on mobile health applications in weight management, results suggested that overall app use for weight management was found to be widely accepted and considered as useful by study participants.

There is mixed evidence about the use of wearable devices for increasing physical activity and facilitating weight loss. Observational studies have found that participants who use pedometers on average increase their steps per day by ~2000 from baseline levels. Pedometer users who set a goal of achieving 10,000 steps per day were also more likely to increase their physical activity.[46] These results confirm the importance of goal setting and indicate that pedometers may be a useful tool to help patients increase their physical activity levels in the short term. However, studies examining the long-term effectiveness of pedometers and wearable devices are lacking. One study examined the long-term effectiveness of wearable technology within the context of a behavioral weight loss intervention. This study compared a standard behavioral weight loss intervention to a technology-enhanced weight loss intervention which included a wearable device (SenseWear) as well as a web interface (FIT Core; BodyMedia) to monitor diet and physical activity.[47] In this study, the standard behavioral weight loss intervention resulted in similar changes in physical activity and weight loss compared to the group that received the wearable device. However, the device (worn on the upper arm) used in this study did not provide immediate physical activity feedback to participants. Whether the provision of more current wrist-worn devices that provide immediate feedback enhances physical activity adherence as well as short-term and long-term weight loss over a standard intervention remains to be determined.

CASE STUDIES

Discussion of Case Study 1

The patient should be encouraged and provided positive reinforcement for purchasing the bike and preparing to exercise. Physical activity alone typically produces modest weight loss (1% to 3%). This is an important consideration because often weight loss is a primary motivator for beginning an exercise program, and lack of weight loss can lead to disappointment and discontinuation of exercise. Thus, it would be important to emphasize the substantial health benefits (including immediate benefits such as improved sleep, less stress, etc.) of exercise that will accrue regardless of whether he achieves any weight loss. Furthermore, the amount of exercise required to produce clinically significant weight loss is relatively high. For example, men who exercised at 80% maximum heart rate for approximately 155 and 210 minutes/week for 10 months lost 8.4 lb (4%) and 13 lb (6%), respectively, from exercise alone. However, there was substantial individual variability with weight loss of up to 22% to weight gain of 4% despite high (>90%) adherence to the intervention. Current evidence suggests that diet and physical activity combined typically produce substantially greater weight loss than physical activity alone, so it is likely that his weight loss would be greater if he added dietary modification to his physical activity program.

CASE STUDY 2
....

A 30-year-old female nonsmoker with a previous BMI of 33 kg/m² and no medical problems lost 40 pounds over the past 6 months by following a low-calorie diet (current BMI: 26 kg/m²). She is finding it more challenging to stick to her daily calorie goal and has started to regain some of the weight that she has lost. She works full time and has three school-aged children who are busy with soccer and lacrosse practices. She has a fitness center membership but has trouble finding time to go to the gym and staying motivated to exercise. Currently, she is only exercising for 45 minutes 1 to 2 times a week. She was a swimmer in high school and met her husband salsa dancing but has not engaged in these activities in years. What is your recommendation?

Discussion of Case Study 2

Congratulate her for continuing to exercise 1 to 2 days/week and help her feel good about the activity she is doing. Have her revisit her reasons for wanting to lose weight in the first place and have her consider setting new physical activity goals such as completing a 5K run. Having a goal of "maintaining weight loss" may not be very motivating, so helping her shift her focus to other goals such as "enjoying time with my family while doing something active" may be a better start. Let her know that in order for her activity to "count," it does not have to be done at the fitness center. Encourage her to incorporate her family into increasing physical activity. Ideas include walking around the fields while her kids are at their respective sports practices or going for a family walk in the evenings. To increase the likelihood of sustaining activity long term, she could be encouraged to get other parents to walk with her, since we know that social support is highly predictive of physical activity adherence. In addition, have her consider getting back into salsa dancing with her husband. She could search for local places that offer salsa dancing or try dancing at home (if there is space and appropriate flooring). Starting off small (approximately one night per month of salsa dancing) can be very approachable. If salsa dancing is out of the question, you could ask her whether her fitness center offers Zumba group exercise classes. She may find that she really enjoys the class and it could bring back positive memories from salsa dancing with her husband.

CLINICAL HIGHLIGHTS

- Engaging in ≥150 minutes/week of MVPA will elicit modest (1% to 3%) weight loss on average; however, higher amounts of MVPA (≥250 minutes/week) are needed to elicit more clinically significant (≥5%) weight loss.
- Physical activity is one of the best predictors of long-term weight loss success. The dose of physical activity necessary to achieve weight loss maintenance may vary among individuals; however, most evidence would suggest ≥200 minutes/week is necessary.
- Resistance training is not an effective weight loss strategy when done in isolation. However, resistance training does help to retain and increase lean mass during weight loss and may help with weight loss maintenance.
- An individualized physical activity prescription should include all elements of the FITT acronym: frequency, intensity, time, and type.

WHEN TO REFER?

- Patient has symptoms suggestive of CVD or arrhythmia and needs further evaluation with exercise or pharmacologic stress testing and/or consultation with a cardiologist.
- Patient would benefit from more guidance and accountability by an accredited personal trainer.
- Patient has physical disabilities that would benefit from seeing physical therapist.

QUIZ QUESTIONS

1. Mrs. S is a 47-year-old woman with a body mass index of 32 kg/m², prediabetes, and mild degenerative joint disease of her knees who comes to see you with concerns about her weight. She is now at her peak lifetime weight and wants to do everything she can to lose weight. Although she was a cheerleader in high school and enjoyed being active, she has engaged in no planned physical activity for the last 10 years due to family responsibilities. She is self-conscious about her appearance and this has made her avoid exercising. Which of the following would be the best first suggestion to make to her today?

    A. Reduce her time watching television from 2 to 1 hour/day.
    B. Begin walking for 10 minutes two times per week.
    C. Begin walking at a moderate intensity for 30 minutes 5 days a week.
    D. Over the next month increase her activity to 60 minutes of walking 6 days/week.

    Answer: B. *While a longer duration of activity at a higher intensity will be more likely to produce more weight loss, she is currently inactive. She has arthritis and this may increase her risk of pain and injury with starting an exercise program which will lead to a perceived sense of failure. Starting at a modest level of activity even two times per week has been shown to have health benefits and will increase self-efficacy. While reducing sedentary time may have health benefits, the evidence for this is not as strong as the evidence for the benefits of increasing physical activity.*

2. Mr. J is a 39-year-old man with a body mass index of 35 kg/m² who has been seeing you for help managing his weight. He has been on a moderate 1,500 kcal/day restricted diet and began a walking program 6 months ago. He has increased his activity from 15 minutes twice a week to his current level of 40 minutes 5 days a week. He is enjoying walking but is finding it hard to make time for these walks. He is interested in increasing his intensity of activity. Which of the following could he use during exercise to know he is exercising at a vigorous level?

    A. He is able to say a few words between breaths.
    B. His perceived exertion level is 5 out of 10.
    C. His heart rate of 118 bpm.
    D. His walking pace is > 3.5 miles/hour.

    Answer: A. *Vigorous activity is defined by a perceived exertion on a 10-point scale that is 6 or greater. A target heart rate associated with vigorous activity is 70% to 85% of the predicted maximum heart rate (220 − age x 0.7-0.85 which for this man would be 127 to 154 bpm). There is no particular speed of walking or running that would be predictive.*

REFERENCES

1. US Department of Health and Human Services. *Physical Activity Guidelines for Americans.* 2nd ed. U.S. Department of Health and Human Services; 2018.

2. Centers for Disease Control and Prevention. Adult participation in aerobic and muscle-strengthening physical activities–United States, 2011. *MMWR Morb Mortal Wkly Rep.* 2013;62(17):326-330. PubMed PMID: 23636025; PMCID: PMC4604926.

3. National Center for Chronic Disease Prevention and Health Promotion Division of Nutrition. *Physical Activity, and Obesity. Data, Trend and Maps* [online]. Centers for Disease Control and Prevention; 2018. Accessed April 29, 2020. https://www.cdc.gov/physicalactivity/downloads/trends-in-the-prevalence-of-physical-activity-508.pdf

4. Wahid A, Manek N, Nichols M, et al. Quantifying the association between physical activity and cardiovascular disease and diabetes: a systematic review and meta-analysis. *J Am Heart Assoc.* 2016;5(9):e002495. doi:10.1161/JAHA.115.002495. PubMed PMID: 27628572; PMCID: PMC5079002.

5. Samitz G, Egger M, Zwahlen M. Domains of physical activity and all-cause mortality: systematic review and dose-response meta-analysis of cohort studies. *Int J Epidemiol.* 2011;40(5):1382-1400. doi:10.1093/ije/dyr112. PubMed PMID: 22039197.

6. Owen N, Healy GN, Matthews CE, Dunstan DW. Too much sitting: the population health science of sedentary behavior. *Exerc Sport Sci Rev.* 2010;38(3):105-113. doi:10.1097/JES.0b013e3181e373a2. PubMed PMID: 20577058; PMCID: PMC3404815.

7. Matthews CE, Chen KY, Freedson PS, et al. Amount of time spent in sedentary behaviors in the United States, 2003-2004. *Am J Epidemiol.* 2008;167(7):875-881. doi:10.1093/aje/kwm390. PubMed PMID: 18303006; PMCID: PMC3527832.

8. Banks E, Jorm L, Rogers K, Clements M, Bauman A. Screen-time, obesity, ageing and disability: findings from 91 266 participants in the 45 and up study. *Public Health Nutr.* 2011;14(1):34-43. doi:10.1017/S1368980010000674. PubMed PMID: 20409356.

9. Duncan MJ, Vandelanotte C, Caperchione C, Hanley C, Mummery WK. Temporal trends in and relationships between screen time, physical activity, overweight and obesity. *BMC Public Health.* 2012;12:1060. doi:10.1186/1471-2458-12-1060. PubMed PMID: 23216917; PMCID: PMC3541208.

10. Xie YJ, Stewart SM, Lam TH, Viswanath K, Chan SS. Television viewing time in Hong Kong adult population: associations with body mass index and obesity. *PLoS One.* 2014;9(1):e85440. doi:10.1371/journal.pone.0085440. PubMed PMID: 24427309; PMCID: PMC3888420.

11. Dutton GR, Kim Y, Jacobs DR Jr, et al. 25-year weight gain in a racially balanced sample of U.S. adults: the CARDIA study. *Obesity.* 2016;24(9):1962-1968. doi:10.1002/oby.21573. PubMed PMID: 27569121; PMCID: PMC5004783.

12. Donnelly JE, Blair SN, Jakicic JM, Manore MM, Rankin JW, Smith BK. American College of Sports Medicine Position Stand. Appropriate physical activity intervention strategies for weight loss and prevention of weight regain for adults. *Med Sci Sports Exerc.* 2009;41(2):459-471.

13. Church TS, Martin CK, Thompson AM, Earnest CP, Mikus CR, Blair SN. Changes in weight, waist circumference and compensatory responses with different doses of exercise among sedentary, overweight postmenopausal women. *PLoS One.* 2009;4(2):e4515. doi:10.1371/journal.pone.0004515. PubMed PMID: 19223984; PMCID: PMC2639700.

14. McTiernan A, Sorensen B, Irwin ML, et al. Exercise effect on weight and body fat in men and women. *Obesity.* 2007;15(6):1496-1512. doi:10.1038/oby.2007.178. PubMed PMID: 17557987.

15. Martin CB, Herrick KA, Sarafrazi N, Ogden CL. Attempts to lose weight Among adults in the United States, 2013-2016. *NCHS Data Brief.* 2018;313:1-8. PubMed PMID: 30044214.

16. Martin CK, Johnson WD, Myers CA, et al. Effect of different doses of supervised exercise on food intake, metabolism, and non-exercise physical activity: the E-MECHANIC randomized controlled trial. *Am J Clin Nutr.* 2019;110(3):383-592. doi: 10.1093/ajcn/nqz054. PubMed PMID: 31172175.

17. Donnelly JE, Hill JO, Jacobsen DJ, et al. Effects of a 16-month randomized controlled exercise trial on body weight and composition in young, overweight men and women: the Midwest Exercise Trial. *Arch Intern Med.* 2003;163(11):1343-1350.

18. Jensen MD, Ryan DH, Apovian CM, et al. 2013 AHA/ACC/TOS guideline for the management of overweight and obesity in adults: a report of the American College of Cardiology/American Heart Association Task Force on Practice Guidelines and The Obesity Society. *J Am Coll Cardiol.* 2014;63(25 pt B):2985-3023. doi:10.1016/j.jacc.2013.11.004. PubMed PMID: 24239920.

19. Washburn RA, Szabo AN, Lambourne K, et al. Does the method of weight loss effect long-term changes in weight, body composition or chronic disease risk factors in overweight or obese adults? A systematic review. *PLoS One.* 2014;9(10):e109849. doi:10.1371/journal.pone.0109849. PubMed PMID: 25333384; PMCID: PMC4198137.

20. Jakicic JM, Tate DF, Lang W, et al. Objective physical activity and weight loss in adults: the step-up randomized clinical trial. *Obesity.* 2014;22(11):2284-2292.

21. Ostendorf DM, Lyden K, Pan Z, et al. Objectively measured physical activity and sedentary behavior in successful weight loss maintainers. *Obesity (Silver Spring).* 2018;26(1):53-60. doi:10.1002/oby.22052. PubMed PMID: 29090513; PMCID: PMC5739988.

22. Creasy SA, Lang W, Tate DF, Davis KK, Jakicic JM. Pattern of daily steps is associated with weight loss: secondary analysis from the step-up randomized trial. *Obesity (Silver Spring).* 2018;26(6):977-984. doi:10.1002/oby.22171. PubMed PMID: 29633583; PMCID: PMC5970037.

23. Coen PM, Tanner CJ, Helbling NL, et al. Clinical trial demonstrates exercise following bariatric surgery improves insulin sensitivity. *J Clin Invest.* 2015;125(1):248-257. doi:10.1172/jci78016. PubMed PMID: 25437877; PMCID: PMC4382227.

24. Bond DS, Phelan S, Wolfe LG, et al. Becoming physically active after bariatric surgery is associated with improved weight loss and health-related quality of life. *Obesity (Silver Spring).* 2009;17(1):78-83. doi:10.1038/oby.2008.501. PubMed PMID: 18997679.

25. Evans RK, Bond DS, Wolfe LG, et al. Participation in 150 min/wk of moderate or higher intensity physical activity yields greater weight loss after gastric bypass surgery. *Surg Obes Relat Dis.* 2007;3(5):526-530. doi:10.1016/j.soard.2007.06.002. PubMed PMID: 17903772.

26. Josbeno DA, Kalarchian M, Sparto PJ, Otto AD, Jakicic JM. Physical activity and physical function in individuals post-bariatric surgery. *Obes Surg.* 2011;21(8):1243-1249. doi:10.1007/s11695-010-0327-4. PubMed PMID: 21153567; PMCID: PMC4887858.

27. Shah M, Snell PG, Rao S, et al. High-volume exercise program in obese bariatric surgery patients: a randomized, controlled trial. *Obesity (Silver Spring).* 2011;19(9):1826-1834. doi:10.1038/oby.2011.172. PubMed PMID: 21681226.

28. Rosenbaum M, Hirsch J, Gallagher DA, Leibel RL. Long-term persistence of adaptive thermogenesis in subjects who have maintained a reduced body weight. *Am J Clin Nutr.* 2008;88(4):906-912. doi:10.1093/ajcn/88.4.906. PubMed PMID: 18842775.

29. Rosenbaum M, Heaner M, Goldsmith RL, et al. Resistance training reduces skeletal muscle work efficiency in weight-reduced and non-weight-reduced subjects. *Obesity (Silver Spring).* 2018;26(10):1576-1583. doi:10.1002/oby.22274. PubMed PMID: 30260099.

30. Kukkonen-Harjula KT, Borg PT, Nenonen AM, Fogelholm MG. Effects of a weight maintenance program with or without exercise on the metabolic syndrome: a randomized trial in obese men. *Prev Med.* 2005;41(3-4):784-790. doi:10.1016/j.ypmed.2005.07.008. PubMed PMID: 16125218.

31. Jakicic JM, King WC, Marcus MD, et al. Short-term weight loss with diet and physical activity in young adults: the IDEA study. *Obesity (Silver Spring).* 2015;23(12):2385-2397.

32. Kerrigan SG, Call C, Schaumberg K, Forman E, Butryn ML. Associations between change in sedentary behavior and outcome in standard behavioral weight loss treatment. *Transl Behav Med.* 2018;8(2):299-304. doi:10.1093/tbm/ibx038. PubMed PMID: 29425373; PMCID: PMC6257008.

33. Riebe D, Franklin BA, Thompson PD, et al. Updating ACSM's recommendations for exercise preparticipation health screening. *Med Sci Sports Exerc.* 2015;47(11):2473-2479. doi:10.1249/mss.0000000000000664. PubMed PMID: 26473759.

34. Fletcher GF, Ades PA, Kligfield P, et al. Exercise standards for testing and training: a scientific statement from the American Heart Association. *Circulation.* 2013;128(8):873-934. doi:10.1161/CIR.0b013e31829b5b44. PubMed PMID: 23877260.

35. Guess N. A qualitative investigation of attitudes towards aerobic and resistance exercise amongst overweight and obese individuals. *BMC Res Notes.* 2012;5:191. doi:10.1186/1756-0500-5-191. PubMed PMID: 22533863; PMCID: PMC3490848.

36. O'Donovan G, Lee IM, Hamer M, Stamatakis E. Association of "weekend warrior" and other leisure time physical activity patterns with risks for all-cause, cardiovascular disease, and cancer mortality. *JAMA Intern Med.* 2017;177(3):335-342. doi:10.1001/jamainternmed.2016.8014. PubMed PMID: 28097313.

37. Vella CA, Taylor K, Drummer D. High-intensity interval and moderate-intensity continuous training elicit similar enjoyment and adherence levels in overweight and obese adults. *Eur J Sport Sci.* 2017;17(9):1203-1211. doi:10.1080/17461391.2017.1359679. PubMed PMID: 28792851; PMCID: PMC6104631.

38. Jakicic JM, Wing RR, Butler BA, Robertson RJ. Prescribing exercise in multiple short bouts versus one continuous bout: effects on adherence, cardiorespiratory fitness, and weight loss in overweight women. *Int J Obes Relat Metab Disord.* 1995;19(12):893-901. PubMed PMID: 8963358.

39. Nantel J, Mathieu ME, Prince F. Physical activity and obesity: biomechanical and physiological key concepts. *J Obes.* 2011;2011:650230. doi:10.1155/2011/650230. PubMed PMID: 21113311; PMCID: PMC2990021.

40. Ten Hoor GA, Plasqui G, Schols A, Kok G. A benefit of being heavier is being strong: a cross-sectional study in young adults. *Sports Med Open.* 2018;4(1):12. doi:10.1186/s40798-018-0125-4. PubMed PMID: 29492711; PMCID: PMC5833324.

41. Tulloch H, Sweet SN, Fortier M, Capstick G, Kenny GP, Sigal RJ. Exercise facilitators and barriers from adoption to maintenance in the diabetes aerobic and resistance exercise trial. *Can J Diabetes.* 2013;37(6):367-374. doi:10.1016/j.jcjd.2013.09.002. PubMed PMID: 24321716.

42. Segar M, Taber JM, Patrick H, Thai CL, Oh A. Rethinking physical activity communication: using focus groups to understand women's goals, values, and beliefs to improve public health. *BMC Public Health.* 2017;17(1):462. doi:10.1186/s12889-017-4361-1. PubMed PMID: 28521756; PMCID: PMC5437577.

43. Petruzzello SJ. Doing What Feels Good (and Avoiding What Feels Bad)-a Growing Recognition of the Influence of Affect on Exercise Behavior: a Comment on Williams et al. *Ann Behav Med.* 2012;44(1):7-9. doi:10.1007/s12160-012-9374-5. PubMed PMID: WOS:000308822700004.

44. Williams DM, Dunsiger S, Jennings EG, Marcus BH. Does affective valence during and immediately following a 10-min walk predict concurrent and future physical activity? *Ann Behav Med.* 2012;44(1):43-51. doi:10.1007/s12160-012-9362-9. PubMed PMID: WOS:000308822700008.

45. Pagoto S, Schneider K, Jojic M, DeBiasse M, Mann D. Evidence-based strategies in weight-loss mobile apps. *Am J Prev Med.* 2013;45(5):576-582. doi:10.1016/j.amepre.2013.04.025. PubMed PMID: 24139770.

46. Bravata DM, Smith-Spangler C, Sundaram V, et al. Using pedometers to increase physical activity and improve health: a systematic review. *J Am Med Assoc.* 2007;298(19):2296-2304. doi:10.1001/jama.298.19.2296. PubMed PMID: 18029834.

47. Jakicic JM, Davis KK, Rogers RJ, et al. Effect of wearable technology combined with a lifestyle intervention on long-term weight loss: the IDEA randomized clinical trial. *J Am Med Assoc.* 2016;316(11):1161-1171. doi:10.1001/jama.2016.12858. PubMed PMID: 27654602; PMCID: PMC5480209.

7

BEHAVIORAL TREATMENT

Ariana M. Chao, Kerry M. Quigley, Thomas A. Wadden

CASE STUDY 1

A 60-year-old female patient with a history of osteo-arthritis presents to your office complaining of bilateral knee pain. She states that 6 months ago she lost 20 lb by following a ketogenic diet, which helped relieve her knee pain. However, she has since gained back almost all the weight, and her knee pain is returning. She is taking naproxen prn over the counter. The patient comments that she does not understand why she is gaining weight. You ask her to tell you about her eating habits. She states they vary a lot day to day. She says that yesterday she had a yogurt and fruit for breakfast, turkey sandwich for lunch, a few cookies for a snack, and chicken for dinner but she cannot remember all the details. Two days ago, she was very busy with work and did not eat anything until dinner, which was a burger, milkshake, and fries from a fast-food restaurant. She wants to lose weight but feels like no matter what she does, she cannot keep the weight off. On examination, weight is 185 lb, height 5'4", blood pressure (BP) 132/84, heart rate (HR) 88, and body mass index (BMI) 31.8 kg/m². The remainder of examination and laboratory tests are unremarkable.

CLINICAL SIGNIFICANCE

Behavioral modification is a core component of obesity treatment. Behavioral weight control consists of a package of principles and techniques that aims to help patients make long-term changes in their eating behaviors and physical activity.[1] It is goal directed and process oriented and emphasizes that new habits can be learned.

Numerous expert panels have recommended that adults with a BMI ≥30 kg/m² be offered intensive, multicomponent, behavioral interventions for weight loss.

These include the US Preventive Services Task Force[2]; the American Association of Clinical Endocrinologists the American College of Endocrinology[3]; the American Heart Association, the American College of Cardiology and The Obesity Society.[4] The Centers for Medicare and Medicaid Services (CMS) has approved reimbursement for intensive behavioral weight loss counseling provided to Medicare beneficiaries in primary care settings by physicians, nurse practitioners, clinical nurse specialists, and physician assistants, as well as other auxiliary personnel (e.g., registered dietitian nutritionists) who bill "incident to" one of the aforementioned health professionals. Coverage is provided for brief (15 minute) weekly counseling visits for the first month, followed by biweekly visits for the following 5 months. Patients who lose >3 kg (6.6 lb) in the first 6 months are eligible for six additional monthly visits.

The purpose of this chapter is to discuss strategies to deliver efficient and effective behavioral treatment for obesity within the context of primary care. First, this chapter will provide an overview of the basic theoretical principles and core components of behavioral treatment for obesity, followed by a description of the efficacy of this approach. It then will describe the 5 *A's* framework for obesity counseling, as well as a treatment protocol that can be used by providers to deliver treatment in primary care settings.

BEHAVIORAL TREATMENT OF OBESITY

Theoretical Basis

Behavioral treatment of obesity incorporates a number of different theories of behavior change. These include the transtheoretical model, behavioral and cognitive-behavioral theories, and social cognitive theory.[5] The transtheoretical model describes behavior change as a series of six stages: *precontemplation, contemplation, preparation, action, maintenance,* and *termination.* This model supports matching behavioral counseling strategies to different stages of change.[6] For example, patients who are not interested in actively working on their weight would be identified in the *precontemplation* stage of change. For these patients, simply mentioning that weight loss may help them achieve improved health and that you are there to assist when they are ready is sufficient. In contrast, some patients present in the *preparation* stage, having already downloaded a smart phone app to track their diet and joined a health club. These patients are ready and interested in receiving further guidance on how to take action to lose weight.

Behavioral and cognitive-behavioral theories posit that individuals have learned maladaptive patterns of eating and exercise which contribute to weight gain and/or maintenance of their weight status.[7-9] These patterns may be influenced by external or internal factors. Behaviors can be unlearned and modified to induce weight loss. Social cognitive theory is based on the premise that behavior is the result of interactions between personal, behavioral, and environment factors.[10] People learn from watching and modeling the behaviors, attitudes, and emotional reactions of others. Learning can also occur through the observation of rewards and punishments. Social cognitive theory also emphasizes the importance of self-efficacy, an individual's confidence in their ability to take a specific action or to overcome barriers to engage in a specific behavior, as a major motivator for behavior change. For example, patients who previously lost weight by attending a commercial weight loss program may have gained self-efficacy that they can lose weight if they are provided a structured program with accountability.

Behavior Change Components

The following components of behavioral weight loss provide the foundation for what to discuss and emphasize during a focused obesity encounter. Not all components need to be included in every encounter. By using active listening, the provider can pick and choose which elements are most pertinent to assist the patient at that time. With experience, the flow of using the components becomes easier and more time efficient.

Self-monitoring

Self-monitoring of dietary intake, physical activity, and weight is a cornerstone of behavioral weight management and is the first behavioral change that should be recommended. It involves the use of food logs, activity records, and self-weighing and is a crucial element to successful weight loss and maintenance.[11-15] Self-monitoring helps patients become more aware of their behaviors, increase accountability, monitor progress, and enhance motivation. In addition, self-monitoring

can help patients and providers identify patterns and modifiable stimuli that might contribute to overeating and sedentary behaviors.

Dietary Intake and Calories

Self-monitoring of food intake is perhaps the most important behavioral strategy for weight control. Patients can be given paper copies of food journals or encouraged to use an internet program or smart phone app (e.g., MyFitnessPal). Patients are instructed to record everything they eat and drink, portion size, method of preparation, and the time of consumption. Ultimately, they should also record the calorie value for each food and drink item. They should be told that successful self-monitoring requires accuracy, consistency, and timeliness in relation to the performance of the behavior.[16] Patients should be advised that the process of self-monitoring diet is a learning process that takes time to develop. It is important to keep in mind that patients may get frustrated by the challenge of not finding the exact food item they are consuming in the electronic tracking database or the difficulty of tracking when eating out or consuming recipes with multiple ingredients. It is important to remind them that they do not need to be perfect and the very act of tracking will increase mindfulness about their dietary intake—a key therapeutic objective of self-monitoring.

It is crucial to discuss a plan for record keeping including when and where patients will record their food intake and how they will remember to record. At subsequent visits the healthcare professional (HCP) reviews the number of meals eaten per day, type of foods eaten, and calories consumed and provides brief comments about the patient's eating plan. Calorie counting is introduced early in treatment. Following methods used in the Diabetes Prevention Program[15] and the Look AHEAD study,[17-19] patients who weigh <250 lb are prescribed a diet of 1,200 to 1,499 kcal/day, with approximately 15% to 20% kcal from protein, 20% to 35% from fat, and the remainder from carbohydrate. Patients who weigh >250 lb are prescribed 1,500 to 1,800 kcal/day. These calorie goals may be reached by recommending conventional foods or meal replacements (i.e., a protein shake or protein bar that provides 15 to 20 g of protein, vitamins and minerals, and at least 5 g of fiber). Patients are shown how to determine calories using a book such as *CalorieKing* or by looking up calories online. Patients are encouraged to keep a running calorie total throughout the day. Later in treatment, patients can be encouraged to record the situations and contextual factors in which they are eating to help identify and target cues. Education on how to read food labels and measure food to increase accuracy is an important skill. It is also useful if patients are provided with meal plans which offer breakfast, lunch, and dinner options for the week. A link to examples of meal plans is available in the Practical Resources section of this chapter. In summary, the HCP should recommend that the patient monitor diet as a first step to weight loss ("Ms. Jones, I recommend that you start recording all food and liquid intake and aim for 1,200 cal/day.") For the clinician, it is important to keep in mind that patients often underestimate their calorie intake. Thus, the patient who is struggling with calorie intake despite a low-calorie count can be encouraged to lower their target by 200 to 300 kcal/day.

Physical Activity

Although individual prescriptions will vary, most patients can be instructed to engage in low- to moderate-intensity physical activity (principally walking or similar aerobic activity) 5 days/week, gradually building to ≥180 minutes/week at approximately month 6 of treatment.[19,20] The goal is increased to >225 minutes/week starting after the first 6 months of treatment, which is around the time that weight loss typically hits a plateau and is consistent with targets required for the maintenance of lost weight.[21] Patients are instructed to record the duration and type of physical activity including any bouts of physical activity of 10 minutes or more. This recommendation is based on findings that four 10-minute bouts, spread across the day, result in similar improvements in fitness as one continuous 40-minute bout.[20] Just as patients self-monitor their calorie intake through recording, they can self-monitor energy expenditure through the use of devices (e.g., Fitbit, Apple watch).

Weight

Patients should be weighed in the office regularly and also be encouraged to weigh themselves weekly or daily at home. The weight should be recorded in their food journal or on a weight tracking sheet or graph. This helps to track progress, establish relationships with their weight control behaviors, and catch small weight gains and make behavioral changes as necessary.[14,22] For patients who are sensitive about their weight and hesitant to self-weigh at home, this recommendation can be put aside until the patient gains more comfort and confidence in the process.

Goal Setting

Setting goals related to weight control behaviors and weight loss can help to focus treatment and provide structure for visits.[23] Patients are encouraged to set goals regarding weight, as well as specific weight control behaviors. We also encourage patients to set "SMART" goals that are **S**pecific, **M**easurable, **A**chievable, **R**ealistic, and **T**imely for weight loss and weight control behaviors.

There is often a mismatch between HCPs and patients in terms of weight loss goals. Many obesity treatments recommend weight loss goals of 5% to 10% of initial body weight, as these goals are achievable and also are clinically valuable.[17,24] On the other hand, patients often select goals that are two to three times larger than the average weight change outcomes and may be unrealistic.[25,26] High weight loss goals, also called stretch goals, generally do not undermine weight loss efforts in the short or long term.[27,28] Thus, they do not focus on the discrepancy between the patient's ideal goals and what is realistic and instead focus on factors that predict successful outcomes such as consistent self-monitoring. Inform patients that you seek to help them reach their goals by making gradual, healthy, and reasonable changes in their eating and activity. However, it is useful to break larger weight loss goals into smaller goals such as 0.5 to 1 kg (1.1 to 2.2 lb) loss per week or 5% to 10% of baseline weight within 6 months.[4] You can also say to patients, "Let's work toward this goal first. When you reach this goal, we'll discuss going further. You can definitely aim for higher goals if you'd like. I am here to help support you." Occasionally you may have patients who want to lose less weight than the 5% and would benefit from greater weight loss. You can respond by saying, "You can decide what goals are best for you. Tell me why you would want to aim for a lower weight loss goal."

Antecedents-Behaviors-Consequences Model

HCPs should individually tailor their treatment approach. This can be done using an analysis of the antecedents, behaviors, and consequences ("ABCs") related to the patient's weight-related behaviors. Antecedents are cues—either external or internal—that prompt a behavior, such as the sight of a high-calorie food or favorite restaurant, food cravings, hunger, or stress from work. Consequences are negative or positive actions or responses that come after the behavior, such as feeling guilty for overeating, receiving positive social reinforcement related to weight change, or having more energy. ABCs, which can be identified from self-monitoring records, form a behavior chain which can then be intervened upon to promote healthy eating and physical activity and to develop specific behavioral plans.

An example of a behavioral chain—and ways to break the chain—is provided in Figure 7.1. As shown, the patient stayed up late working on a presentation and was subsequently late for work, leaving her with no time to make breakfast or pack lunch (Links 1-3). This led to the patient eating two doughnuts in a meeting (4). This chain could be broken by making a plan to pack lunch the night before, or by calorie counting the doughnuts and planning the next meal accordingly. The patient

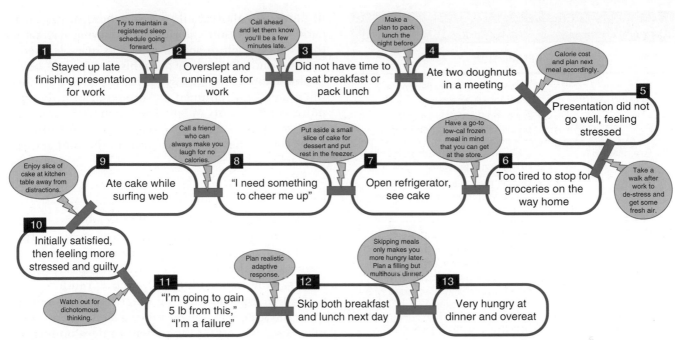

FIGURE 7.1 Example of a behavioral chain. Each chain represents a process that can lead to unhealthy eating behaviors. Examples of interventions are in yellow bubbles.

heads home after a long day and decides not to stop for groceries, even though she does not know what she will make for dinner (6). She opens the refrigerator and sees a few slices of leftover cake (7). Very hungry, she eats the cake while surfing the web, telling herself that she needs something delicious to make herself feel better (8, 9). The patient could have broken the chain by eating a go-to frozen meal option that she knows fits within her calorie goal, calling a friend instead of turning to the cake for comfort, or saving a slice of cake for after dinner and putting the rest in the freezer so it requires defrosting. The patient eating the cake might lead to negative self-talk or drastic recovery measures like skipping meals the next day to make up for calories, ultimately leading to feeling very hungry at dinner and overeating (10-13). Breaking chain links here could occur through meal planning for the following day, as skipping meals would only make one hungrier later. Ideally, an intervention should occur as early as possible in the chain. However, providing multiple strategies to break the link in several places is beneficial as patients can get an idea of what would be the "weakest link" for them to break.

While the above example is fairly extensive and detailed, it can also be effective to discuss ABCs in a more general way or to focus on a particular part of the chain with patients as a way to target intervention strategies. For example, Ms. Jones may remark that she frequently overeats cookies after dinner. The provider could ask Ms. Jones, "what events, situations, thoughts, feelings, or behaviors may contribute to overeating episodes?" One trigger that Ms. Jones may identify is that

she has a hard time resisting the cookies because she sees them on the counter. Ms. Jones and the provider could then discuss ways to decrease this behavior, such as keeping the cookies in the cabinet or by not keeping cookies in the house.

Stimulus Control

Stimulus control focuses on modifying external, environmental factors to make them more conducive to weight control goals. These strategies can be used to increase or decrease cues that foster healthy eating and exercise habits. Examples of stimulus control strategies include removing high-calorie foods from the home (or keeping them out of sight), asking work colleagues to keep high-calorie foods out of sight at work, keeping lower calorie foods (fruits and vegetables) on the counter or easily accessible, and putting gym shoes by the door (as a reminder to go for a walk). While these principles of behavior modification may seem intuitive, it is often the case that patients have not considered them. Thus, it is often helpful to check with patients that they are aware of the behavior patterns linked with excess food intake or minimal physical activity.

Problem-solving

Problem-solving is aimed at assisting individuals to develop adaptive solutions to cope effectively when faced with challenges encountered in everyday life. As outlined in Table 7.1, this approach uses a five-step problem-solving technique: (1) identify a problem; (2)

TABLE 7.1 Problem-Solving Steps

STEP	DESCRIPTION
1. Problem identification	• Establish that the patient agrees that there is a problem • Agree on the definition of the problem/target for intervention
2. Brainstorming	• Develop a list of potential solutions to the target problem • Use behavioral analysis to facilitate the development of a wide variety of potential solutions
3. Pro/con analysis	• Help patient select a strategy that will be acceptable and also likely to effectively resolve the problem • Discuss the patients' perceived benefits and costs associated with each possible solution
4. Selection of a plan	• Select and write down a plan of action including a target behavior/problem, well-defined goal, detailed plan of action tailored to the individual, specified period during which the effectiveness will be evaluated, and specified target goal defined in objective terms
5. Evaluation of effectiveness	• After a specified period of time, evaluate strategy to determine if it achieved predetermined goal • If successful, continue solution • If unsuccessful, discuss process of behavior change, problems with implementation, examine new intervention options, and repeat steps

brainstorm potential solutions; (3) consider the pros and cons of each option; (4) choose a solution and develop plans for implementing it; and (5) test the efficacy of the strategy for a specific period of time. The process can be repeated if the problem was not successfully solved.

Cognitive Restructuring

Maladaptive thought patterns can be antecedents to consumption of high-calorie food, underexercising, and reductions in weight control efforts (Figure 7.2). Thoughts such as, "I've had a tough day, so I deserve a treat," or "I gained weight again; I knew I would never be able to lose weight" may be triggers to overeating or inactivity. Cognitive restructuring involves challenging problematic thoughts, emotions, and ideas that undermine efforts and hinder treatment adherence. These strategies help patients adopt positive rather than negative self-talk (e.g., if you eat a bowl of ice cream, choose to eat fewer calories the following day, rather than feeling guilt or shame). Patients may be asked to monitor and record their thoughts and feelings before or after eating. Any negative thinking patterns are identified and then reframed or countered with thoughts more conducive to weight loss, such as "I deserve a treat, so I think I'll listen to some music," or "Although I overate this time, I can learn from this and get back on track."

Reinforcement

There are many rewards related to weight loss that can be reinforcing, especially in the early stages of treatment such as wearing smaller size clothes, observing decreased health risks, and receiving compliments from others. However, additional positive reinforcement is needed, especially during weight loss maintenance when the scale is no longer moving. Self-reinforcement incorporates assisting the patient to develop forms of self-reward. The type of reinforcement most effective for motivating behavior change differs for each person. Extrinsic motivators or incentives such as money or a new outfit are common; however, intrinsic motivation (self-enjoyment or satisfaction from achieving a goal) can also be powerful. For example, a patient who is struggling with logging her food may reward herself at the end of each day she meets the goal with 15 minutes of reading a new book or watching a new series. Patients should be encouraged to develop and keep their own reward system.

Social Support

Enhancing social support also may improve weight loss. Including family members or friends is one way to accomplish this. Patients should be asked about people who may be supportive of their weight control behaviors and what these individuals might do to further encourage the patients' success. Patients may also need to develop strategies for dealing with weight loss "saboteurs" or "enablers" such as family members, coworkers, or friends who encourage overeating (whether consciously or unconsciously).

Relapse Prevention

Setbacks in patients' weight control efforts are inevitable, and "slips" or less than perfect eating episodes are normal parts of the weight loss and maintenance process. Relapse prevention strategies have been adapted from substance abuse treatment for weight management to handle these setbacks.[18,29] Patients should also be taught the difference between a lapse versus a relapse. Lapses are expected, temporary slips. For example, overeating snack foods for a day or two,

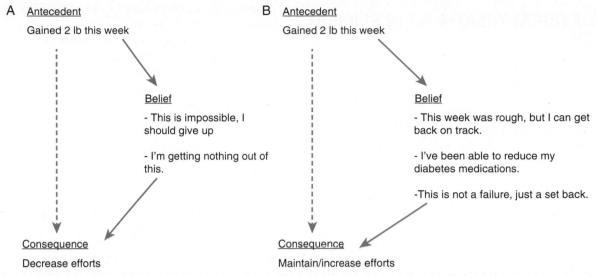

FIGURE 7.2 Example of cognitive restructuring. According to cognitive models, the link between an antecedent and the emotional or behavioral consequence is influenced by the belief about the antecedent. When the belief contains cognitive bias (e.g., dichotomous thinking), as in panel A, the consequence tends to be unfavorable. However, if the beliefs about that antecedent have been adequately challenged and replaced with more functional thoughts, the consequences are more favorable as in panel B.

or skipping exercise for a week. A relapse is a return to frequent problematic weight control behaviors and is associated with weight regain. It is essential that patients learn to reverse small weight gains or lapses as they occur. These instances can be viewed as opportunities to learn and get back on track. Using relapse prevention techniques, HCPs teach patients to identify and describe potentially risky situations in which overeating or underexercising may occur. Patients and providers discuss strategies and step-by-step plans to flexibly manage these situations. For example, a patient may identify a high-risk situation as going out for lunch with coworkers. The HCP and patient may discuss several strategies such as bringing lunch, suggesting a healthier restaurant, or making sure to look at the menu beforehand to pick a lower calorie lunch option and then sticking with that choice. Discussions should also include scenarios in which the patient does have a lapse, say by going to lunch but consuming more calories than anticipated. Patients should be encouraged to spot the problem early and to restart self-monitoring (if they have stopped) and other weight control behaviors, to ask for social support, and to identify and address the trigger of the setback.

Other Weight Control Behaviors

It is also helpful to identify and reduce other triggers that may contribute to unhealthy dietary or physical activity behaviors. These include factors such as stress, fatigue, inadequate sleep, and time constraints.

Efficacy of Behavioral Treatment

Behavioral-based treatment of obesity can help patients achieve and maintain clinically meaningful weight losses.[2,19] A meta-analysis of 89 randomized controlled trials and two observational studies compared behavior-based weight loss interventions with comparison groups that received usual care.[21] At 12 to 18 months, participants who received multicomponent, behavioral-based interventions lost an average of 5.3 lb more than those in control conditions (mean absolute weight changes ranged from −1.1 to −20.5 lb among intervention participants and 3 to −12.3 lb among control participants). Participants in the intervention groups also were more likely than controls to lose 5% or more of baseline weight (risk ratio 1.94, 95% confidence interval [CI] 1.7 to 2.2).

Maintaining weight loss is challenging. Data from a meta-analysis of long-term weight loss studies showed that after cessation of an intervention, participants typically regain more than half of lost weight within 2 years.[30] Weight regain is likely related to biological adaptations,[31,32] as well as declines in behaviors that are associated with maintenance of lost weight such as physical activity, monitoring weight, reducing calorie and fat intake, and use of meal replacements.[33,34] Primary care providers play an important role in helping patients with both weight loss and weight loss maintenance. Monthly or more frequent contacts with providers during weight loss maintenance helps to prevent weight regain.

BEHAVIORAL TREATMENT IN PRIMARY CARE

HCPs and their staff are uniquely positioned to assess weight and related health risks and give personalized recommendations for weight loss. Providers can help patients learn behavioral strategies for weight loss, support patients with weight management, and refer them to other providers who can help patients attain weight management goals. However, providing behavioral weight loss counseling can be difficult. HCPs rarely diagnose, document, or discuss overweight or obesity.[35,36] Approximately 70% of patients with obesity do not have a documented obesity diagnosis.[37] Only 21% of primary care visits include weight-related education.[37] Busy practitioners may miss the opportunity for providing behavioral weight loss counseling because of a lack of training, limited time, competing health priorities, and lack of confidence.[38] Yet, most primary care providers feel that they have a responsibility to contribute to patients' weight loss efforts.[39] Weight loss discussions with primary care providers are associated with patients having greater attempts at losing weight and achieving clinically significant weight losses.[40-42] Thus, even a brief mention of weight loss, if provided as a personalized recommendation, makes a difference in patient outcomes.

5 *A*'S FRAMEWORK

The 5 *A*'s Framework is recommended by the CMS to establish initial contacts with patients who are interested in beginning the process of weight management. The 5 *A*'s have been adapted to work for different aspects of behavioral change, but the CMS recommends "assess," "advise," "agree," "assist," and "arrange" for weight management. A description of the 5 *A*'s and sample language that providers can use is provided in Table 7.2.[43] Providers may also choose to employ the briefer "assess-advise-refer" model of care, where patients are referred

TABLE 7.2 The 5 *A*'s for Obesity Treatment in Primary Care

CMS'S 5 *A*'S	DEFINITION	EXAMPLES
Assess	Ask whether the patient feels comfortable having a discussion regarding their weight. Assess patient readiness to manage weight through behavioral changes. Assess BMI, waist circumference, "root causes" of obesity, and effects of weight on psychosocial factors.	"Would it be alright if we talked about your weight?" "Can you tell me about your diet and exercise habits?" "How confident are you that you will be able to change your eating and exercise habits?"
Advise	Encourage patient that there are benefits to healthier lifestyles regardless of their weight. Provide specific and personalized behavior change recommendations.	"You might want to try self-monitoring with a food journal and activity log." "Since it sounds like you travel a lot for work, let's brainstorm some on-the-go meals that would fit your calorie goals."
Agree	Collaborate with patient to come up with realistic behavioral changes and goals with the patient's personal interests in mind. Place emphasis on changing behavior rather than pounds lost.	"How many days a week do you think you could realistically go to the gym after work?" "How would you feel about trying to food log on just the weekdays to start?"
Assist	Help patient to identify and address any barriers or obstacles that might challenge their goals. Recommend weight-management resources or refer patient to IBT programs that could provide more specialized care.	"How do you think your friends and family could support you in your diet changes?" "Would you be interested in making an appointment with a dietitian?
Arrange	Schedule follow-up contacts with patient to check in with patient and adjust the treatment plan as needed.	"I will give you a call in 2 weeks to see how our plan is going."

BMI, body mass index; CMS, Centers for Medicare and Medicaid Services; IBT, intensive behavioral treatment.

to registered dietitian nutritionists, behavioral psychologists, self-help or commercial weight loss programs, or other obesity-treatment specialists (e.g., providers certified in obesity medicine, bariatric surgeons) instead of providing counseling themselves.

Assess

Before assessing the patient's circumstances regarding their weight, providers should first ask permission to discuss body weight. By asking patients whether they feel comfortable having a discussion, the provider verbalizes respect for the patient's autonomy, and the precedent is set for a collaborative conversation regarding a sensitive issue. If patients are unwilling to talk about their weight, the HCP can respond that they can revisit the conversation when weight becomes a concern. If the patient consents, the HCP can move forward with asking the patient about their motivation, lifestyle, and behavioral health risks to explore complications and underlying factors that might affect weight. In this discussion, it is important for HCPs to use patients' preferred terms for discussing body weight, such as "weight" or "BMI," rather than offensive terms such as "fatness" or "obesity."[44] Further information on broaching the subject of obesity with patients is covered in Chapter 2.

Advise

Once the patient's overall health practices, motivation, and BMI have been assessed, HCPs can discuss treatment options and develop a clinical management plan. They should tailor their advice based on the severity of the patient's weight and comorbid conditions. For example, antiobesity pharmacotherapy, as an adjunct to behavioral weight management, is an option for patients with BMIs > 30 kg/m^2 or > 27 kg/m^2 in the presence of one or more obesity-related comorbidities. Practitioners should acknowledge that weight management (both behavioral and pharmacologic) usually requires a long-term approach.

Agree

The "agree" step of the 5 *A*'s is crucial for establishing HCP and patient buy-in to the treatment plan. This step can also help the patient recognize realistic weight loss expectations. In addition, the patient and provider can set and sequence goals to facilitate long-term weight-management strategies.[45]

Assist

Once treatment goals are agreed upon, HCPs should help patients to anticipate obstacles or barriers that could obstruct their behavioral plans. Providers might ask about support systems, economic barriers, or other factors that could affect weight-management strategies.

Arrange

Studies show that this step in the 5 *A*'s is the most well-received among patients, as they like knowing that they will receive ongoing support and assistance to adjust treatment plans as needed.[43] HCPs have multiple options for offering behavioral weight loss treatment. They may provide treatment to patients in their practice during office visits. They may also choose to use the "assess-advise-refer" model of care. There are several formats in which behavioral weight loss counseling has been successfully administered, including group, individual, phone, internet, commercial, and mobile-based. When referring patients to other practitioners for weight management, HCPs can play a critical role in continuing to monitor changes in patients' weight and health status, supporting their weight loss and behavior change goals, and reminding them of the need for long-term behavior change. Patients should select a treatment program that best fits their needs and preferences since adherence to a behavioral weight loss program is one of the most important factors related to successful weight loss.[46] In the next section, we focus on describing a protocol for delivering individual behavioral counseling in primary care. This protocol is best delivered by a trained member in the office, such as an Advanced Practice Provider (APP), registered nurse, registered dietitian nutritionist, or medical assistant.

DELIVERING STRUCTURED BEHAVIORAL COUNSELING IN PRIMARY CARE

Until recently, HCPs had few ready-to-use protocols or curricula to follow to provide behavioral treatment for obesity in primary care. Our research team has developed a protocol that provides a structured, 21-session approach that can be delivered in 15-minute sessions. The protocol is adapted from several large clinical trials including the Diabetes Prevention Program,[47] the Lifestyle, Exercise, Attitudes, Relationships, Nutrition (LEARN) program,[48] and the Look AHEAD (Action for Health in Diabetes) intensive lifestyle intervention.[49] In a recent randomized controlled trial, 150 participants with obesity were assigned to a protocol for intensive behavioral treatment (IBT) for obesity, delivered on the visit schedule recommended by CMS.[50,51] At week 52, participants who received the IBT protocol lost a mean of 6.1% of their initial weight, and 44% of participants lost ≥5% of baseline weight. This protocol has also been used in a larger study conducted by Novo Nordisk in the

Satiety and Clinical Adiposity—Liraglutide Evidence (SCALE) IBT trial, in which 282 patients with obesity were recruited at 17 largely primary care sites across the United States.[52] At week 56, the estimated mean weight loss was 4.0% for patients who received IBT (combined with placebo), and 38.8% of participants lost ≥5% of baseline weight. The detailed protocol is posted online and available for individual practitioners to use (please see Practical Resources section).[50] The following section will review how to deliver IBT in the office setting.

With proper training and familiarity with the treatment protocol, behavioral weight loss counseling can be provided by the physician, APP (nurse practitioner, physician assistant), registered nurse, or medical assistant. Educational materials should be available at the time of the patient visit and adequate time should be allowed to deliver counseling. With practice and experience, the behavioral counseling will become more efficient and effective.

Visit Flow

Greeting and Check-in

IBT visits begin by greeting patients and asking how they have been since their last visit. If you have previously met the patient, weigh the patient in a private area at the beginning of the session. If you have not met the patient previously, you can obtain a weight at the end of the visit as part of the physical examination. It should be explained early in the program that each visit will begin with a structured check-in during which several activities are reviewed: weight change since last visit; number of days the patient self-monitored food intake; and average calories consumed for the week, minutes of physical activity, and other behaviors.

Patients should begin to associate specific weekly behaviors with weight loss (e.g., self-monitoring food intake), which can help to facilitate behavior changes. The check-in provides a good opportunity to educate patients about their body weight and to provide support to patients in the behavioral change process. Steps of the behavioral change process are (1) identifying behavior change goals; (2) reviewing when, where, and how the behaviors will be performed; (3) having the patient keep a record of the behavior change; (4) reviewing their progress at the next treatment visit; (5) congratulating the patient on successes and not criticizing shortcomings; and (6) reviewing the patient's successes and barriers. Figure 7.3 shows an example of these steps.

Curriculum Content

The next steps of the visit are to (1) review self-monitoring records (described below); (2) cover curriculum content; and (3) assign skill builders (i.e.,

homework). At each session, patients receive a short handout to focus and guide the discussion. The handout introduces one or two new topics on behavioral weight control. The curriculum helps patients learn essential behavior change techniques that are summarized above. Each handout also has an accompanying skill-building assignment to be completed daily before the next visit, including recording daily food intake and physical activity and other behavior change goals relevant to the curriculum content and/or the patient's personal goals.[17,51]

Responding to Weight Changes

Patients may have a variety of responses to their weight change ranging from joy to frustration and discouragement. After patients are told their weight change, let them respond first. It is important that providers respond in a way that is respectful and nonjudgmental. If, for example, the participant exclaims, "That's wonderful, 2 pounds!" the provider could respond, "I can see how delighted you are. Congratulations." If the patient has been working hard to record dietary intake, the provider could add, "It looks like recording your food intake has really paid off this week. Congratulations!" This acknowledges the participant's satisfaction, while making a connection between behavior change and weight change.

If the patient has not lost weight or has gained weight, ask about any challenges patients had, whether with their eating and physical activity or with social stressors. In such cases, acknowledge their frustration and also assess whether the weight gain makes sense to the participant. The provider can ask, "Is the weight gain consistent with your eating and activity habits since our last visit?" Some participants will acknowledge that they overate and that the weight gain was anticipated. Problem solve with these individuals, making a plan for handling overeating in the future.

Some patients will report that they adhered to their diet and activity plan but still maintained or gained weight. It is important to empathize with their disappointment and not to criticize patients. For example, the provider could confront and criticize the patient by saying that she must not have recorded accurately if she claims to have consumed only 1,000 kcal/day, all 7 days of the week, but gained 3 lb. Instead of being confrontational, the provider could say, "That must be confusing to you, to have eaten so little and to have gained weight. Let's review your records to make sure they are as accurate as possible." This response raises the possibility that her records are imprecise but does so in an effort to help, not criticize the participant. The discussion should include efforts to reestablish the patients' self-efficacy and positive expectations (i.e., that they can continue with their self-monitoring and that their

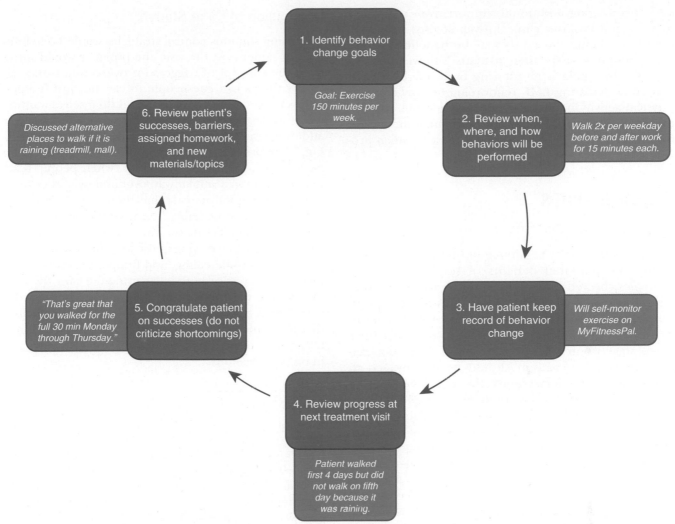

FIGURE 7.3 Behavioral change techniques. The steps of behavioral change are in blue, and an example is provided in green.

weight will eventually reflect their efforts). The above steps (greeting/check-in, curriculum content, responding to weight changes) could potentially consume more than 15 minutes, and thus, the clinician should prioritize items at each visit depending upon the patient's needs.

Weight Loss Maintenance Strategies

Obesity is a chronic disease, characterized by behavioral and biological forces that tend to drive patients' weight toward a higher set point. Although many individuals succeed in losing weight with behavioral treatment, weight regain is common, especially after 6 months when weight loss starts to plateau. Behaviors associated with weight loss maintenance that should be encouraged include eating a low-calorie diet, moving food intake to earlier in the day, developing a daily planned meal pattern, self-monitoring of food intake and physical activity, consuming low- or no-calorie beverages,

self-weighing at least once a week, limiting television viewing time (<10 hours a week), and increasing physical activity.[33,34,53]

Another factor identified with long-term weight loss maintenance is continued follow-up visits.[54] Providing patients with every-other-week weight loss maintenance counseling, following initial weight loss, can help prevent this weight regain.[55] Long-term counseling is necessary since once maintenance sessions end, patients gain weight, suggesting that this counseling only delays, rather than prevents, weight regain.[4,56-58]

Over half of the general patient population sees healthcare providers two or fewer times a year.[59] While this creates some opportunity for ongoing support and motivation for weight management, most studies testing extended care models for weight loss maintenance include at least monthly, if not more frequent, follow-up visits. This frequency of weight loss maintenance visits is ideal but may not be possible for primary care providers. Thus, using a multidisciplinary team and encouraging additional support from registered dietitian nutritionists, clinical psychologists, and other obesity medicine specialists may be beneficial. HCPs can continue to assist their patients with weight management by regularly monitoring body weight at each visit and calculating BMI, reinforcing healthy diet and physical activity habits, and addressing other risk factors for weight gain. In addition, sustaining motivation for behavior change is another key area in which providers can provide support.

CASE STUDIES

Discussion of Case Study 1

The case study at the beginning of the chapter demonstrates the potential benefits of several behavioral strategies covered in this chapter. The first behavioral weight loss strategy to discuss with this patient is self-monitoring of her food intake. As demonstrated, it can be difficult for patients to accurately remember their food intake when asked to recall this information retrospectively. The patient should be encouraged to self-monitor her dietary intake by first discussing the benefits of keeping food journals. For example, the provider would explain that "recording everything you eat and drink in your food journal will help you recognize your eating patterns and make healthy changes in your diet." Next, explain how to use a food journal or online app, such as MyFitnessPal by saying, "Here is a journal for recording your food intake or, if you prefer, you can use an electronic tracking program." It is also important to make a plan for record keeping including when and where she will journal her food intake and how she will remember. Also encourage her to start recording her food intake at the visit, starting with what she had to eat so far today. Explain that she should record how much food she ate and how it was prepared (including desserts, snacks, and caloric drinks), and to carry the food journal with her and record immediately after she eats something.

CASE STUDY 2

For the past month you have been seeing a 35-year-old male patient for behavioral weight loss counseling who has a BMI of 33 kg/m². He has lost 5 lb, but his weight loss is slowing and he has not lost any weight in the past week. He is self-monitoring his food intake using a smartphone app and has noticed a pattern where he frequently overeats while driving to and from work. What behavioral technique would you suggest for this patient?

Discussion of Case Study 2

Discussing stimulus control strategies would be helpful for this patient. At the visit, the provider would introduce the concept of triggers for overeating by saying, "many things can cue people to eat, not just hunger. For example, some people will find themselves wanting to eat while they are driving because they do this over and over again and start to associate driving with snacking." The provider would then discuss how habits can be formed or changed by saying, "when people react to a food cue in a similar way, over and over, they form a habit. The good news is that there are strategies to help you alter those habits." Some strategies to suggest would be to limit the places where he eats (e.g., discouraging eating while driving in the car), limiting the activities he does while eating, and finding positive ways to respond to stress or boredom during the car ride, such as listening to a podcast or audiobook. The provider would then ask him to identify cue control strategies that he would like to use in the next week to address triggers for overeating and evaluate their effectiveness in ongoing sessions.

CASE STUDY 3

A 66-year-old female patient who now weighs 200 lb has been coming to your office for behavioral weight loss counseling for the past year. She has lost 12% of her body weight over the year and is interested in maintaining the weight she lost. She has a history of weight-cycling and is nervous about regaining the weight, especially since she is going on a cruise with her family next month. How do you help to manage this patient? What counseling approaches would you use to help maintain her weight loss?

Discussion of Case Study 3

Weight regain after weight loss is common. The provider would first acknowledge her apprehension about weight regain and then discuss changes she has made and areas she plans to work on, such as making weight loss maintenance a priority; limiting her calorie intake to 1,200 to 1,500 kcal/day (i.e., the same calorie target that produced initial weight loss); weighing herself at least once a week or daily; exercising about 1 hour a day (including resistance training 2×/week); eating three meals and two snacks a day; going to fast-food restaurants less than once a week; and watching less than 10 hours of television per week. The provider would encourage her to keep herself accountable by performing her own check-ins. A plan for these behaviors is crucial and would discuss any challenges that might make these behaviors difficult and solutions to those challenges.

The provider would also introduce the concept of a lapse and a relapse to this patient. Weight regain usually starts with a lapse, a temporary or small slip in weight loss efforts such as overeating for a day or two. Lapses are common and happen to everyone at some point. If not addressed, a lapse can become a relapse, a return to earlier eating and activity habits that are associated with significant weight regain. The best way to prevent a lapse from becoming a relapse is to identify lapses early and deal with them before they turn into a relapse. She may have identified the upcoming cruise as a high-risk situation, and the provider would help her develop a plan of response by developing concrete goals for her vacation. The provider would suggest writing these on an index card before she leaves and bringing the card with her. Goals may include self-monitoring food intake, meal planning, or how often, when, where, and how she will exercise.

If she does have a lapse, she should start using the behaviors that initially helped her lose weight such as attending counseling sessions, recording food intake, continuing to use a calorie goal, weighing herself daily, exercising starting that day or the next with a goal of 225 minutes/week, and planning what she will eat at the next meal, and not waiting until tomorrow for healthier eating. Lastly, it can also be useful to help the patient identify resources in the community that she can use to help them maintain her weight loss.

- Cognitive restructuring
- Reinforcement
- Social support
- Relapse prevention

SMART Goals
- Broad goal: I want to walk more.
- SMART goal: I will walk for 10 minutes, three times a day (morning, afternoon, and evening) on every weekday this week.

Key Strategies for Weight Loss Maintenance
- Eating a low-calorie diet
- Moving food intake to earlier in the day
- Self-monitoring of food intake and physical activity
- Consuming low- or no-calorie beverages
- Self-weighing at least once a week
- Limiting television viewing time
- Increasing physical activity
- Attending follow-up visits

WHEN TO REFER?

- Patient is having difficulty making and sustaining behavioral change
- Patient has excessive stress or a mood disorder such as depression or anxiety that interferes with self-care
- Patient requires additional accountability for behavioral change

CLINICAL HIGHLIGHTS

Key Components of Behavioral Weight Loss
- Self-monitoring of dietary intake, physical activity, and weight
- Goal setting
- Antecedents-behaviors-consequences
- Stimulus control
- Problem-solving

Practice Pointers

Behavioral modification is the cornerstone of obesity treatment. Behavioral weight loss counseling can help patients achieve clinically significant reductions in weight. Healthcare providers can use a number of different strategies and techniques to help their patients achieve their goals related to weight, nutrition, and physical activity.

QUIZ QUESTIONS

1. A 48-year-old male patient makes an appointment to discuss his body weight. He has gained 10 lb over the past 6 months and is concerned about his most recent glycohemoglobin blood test of 6.1%. His BMI is 29 kg/m². You begin to counsel him about the benefit of modest weight loss and paying more attention to diet. At that time, the patient responds, "I know what you are going to say. I talked to my wife last night about this. She suggested that I download an app to my phone so that I can track all of the foods that I eat. I happened

to look at it this morning. It's pretty cool but not sure I know how to use it." The patient is determined to be in which stage of change regarding reducing his dietary calorie consumption?

A. Precontemplation
B. Contemplation
C. Preparation
D. Action

> **Answer: C.** *By downloading the app, the patient comes to the visit in the preparation stage of change. Your response is to congratulate him for being proactive and provide guidance on how to track his diet.*

2. You have been working with a 38-year-old female patient with obesity (BMI 32 kg/m²) and hypertension (BP 138/90) to reduce her caloric and sodium intake over the past 4 months. She is tracking her diet using a smartphone app with the goal of consuming 1,300 kcal and 2,300 mg sodium per day. During today's visit, she mentions that her husband continues to bring fatty and salty snacks into the house which makes it hard for her to meet her dietary goals, especially when she is stressed. You counsel her to talk to her husband about not bringing these foods into the house, and instead have healthier snacks available. This suggestion an example of which behavioral weight loss technique?

A. Self-monitoring
B. Stimulus control
C. Cognitive restructuring
D. Stress reduction
E. Contingency management

> **Answer: B.** *Stimulus control focuses on modifying environmental factors to make them more conducive to weight control goals. By removing problem foods from the home, the patient is less likely to consume these products.*

PRACTICAL RESOURCES

- Lifestyle intervention materials and meal plans from the University of Pennsylvania (med.upenn.edu/weight/wadden.html); these materials provide a structured protocol for offering 21 brief (15-minute) sessions of IBT.
- Lifestyle intervention materials from Look AHEAD (https://www.lookaheadtrial.org/)
- National Weight Control Registry (http://www.nwcr.ws/)
- MyFitnessPal (https://www.myfitnesspal.com/)
- The Learn Program for Weight Management

REFERENCES

1. Foster GD, Makris AP, Bailer BA. Behavioral treatment of obesity. *Am J Clin Nutr.* 2005;82:230S-235S.
2. Curry SJ, Krist AH, Owens DK, et al. Behavioral weight loss interventions to prevent obesity-related morbidity and mortality in adults: US preventive services task force recommendation statement. *J Am Med Assoc.* 2018;320:1163-1171.
3. Garvey W, Garber A, Mechanick J, et al. American Association of Clinical Endocrinologists and American College of Endocrinology position statement on the 2014 advanced framework for a new diagnosis of obesity as a chronic disease. *Endoc Pract.* 2014;20:977-989.
4. Jensen MD, Ryan DH, Apovian CM, et al. 2013 AHA/ACC/TOS guideline for the management of overweight and obesity in adults: a report of the American College of Cardiology/American Heart Association Task Force on Practice Guidelines and The Obesity Society. *Circulation.* 2014;129:S102-S138.
5. Spahn JM, Reeves RS, Keim KS, et al. State of the evidence regarding behavior change theories and strategies in nutrition counseling to facilitate health and food behavior change. *J Am Diet Assoc.* 2010;110:879-891.
6. Prochaska JO, Velicer WF. The transtheoretical model of health behavior change. *Am J Health Promot.* 1997;12:38-48.
7. Skinner BF. *Contingencies of Reinforcement: A Theoretical Analysis.* B.F. Skinner Foundation; 2013.
8. Beck AT. *Cognitive Therapy and the Emotional Disorders.* Penguin; 1979.
9. Skinner BF. *The Behavior of Organisms: An Experimental Analysis.* B.F. Skinner Foundation; 1991.
10. Bandura A. *Social Foundations of Thought and Action.* Prentice-Hall; 1986.
11. Teixeira PJ, Carraça EV, Marques MM, et al. Successful behavior change in obesity interventions in adults: a systematic review of self-regulation mediators. *BMC Med.* 2015;13:84.
12. Peterson ND, Middleton KR, Nackers LM, Medina KE, Milsom VA, Perri MG. Dietary self-monitoring and long-term success with weight management. *Obesity (Silver Spring).* 2014;22:1962-1967.
13. Wing RR, Phelan S. Long-term weight loss maintenance. *Am J Clin Nutr.* 2005;82:222S-225S.

14. Burke LE, Wang J, Sevick MA. Self-monitoring in weight loss: a systematic review of the literature. *J Am Diet Assoc.* 2011;111:92-102.

15. Michie S, Abraham C, Whittington C, McAteer J, Gupta S. Effective techniques in healthy eating and physical activity interventions: a meta-regression. *Health Psychol.* 2009;28:690-701.

16. Bandura A. Health promotion from the perspective of social cognitive theory. *Psychol Health.* 1998;13:623-649.

17. Look Ahead Research Group. Cardiovascular effects of intensive lifestyle intervention in type 2 diabetes. *N Engl J Med.* 2013;369:145-154.

18. Burgess E, Hassmén P, Welvaert M, Pumpa K. Behavioural treatment strategies improve adherence to lifestyle intervention programmes in adults with obesity: a systematic review and meta-analysis. *Clin Obes.* 2017;7:105-114.

19. Johns DJ, Hartmann-Boyce J, Jebb SA, Aveyard P, Group BWMR. Diet or exercise interventions vs combined behavioral weight management programs: a systematic review and meta-analysis of direct comparisons. *J Acad Nutr Diet.* 2014;114:1557-1568.

20. Jakicic JM, Wing R, Butler B, Robertson R. Prescribing exercise in multiple short bouts versus one continuous bout: effects on adherence, cardiorespiratory fitness, and weight loss in overweight women. *Int J Obes Relat Metab Disord.* 1995;19:893-901.

21. LeBlanc ES, Patnode CD, Webber EM, Redmond N, Rushkin M, O'Connor EA. Behavioral and pharmacotherapy weight loss interventions to prevent obesity-related morbidity and mortality in adults: updated evidence report and systematic review for the US Preventive Services Task Force. *J Am Med Assoc.* 2018;320:1172-1191.

22. Butryn ML, Phelan S, Hill JO, Wing RR. Consistent self-monitoring of weight: a key component of successful weight loss maintenance. *Obesity (Silver Spring).* 2007;15:3091-3096.

23. Locke EA, Latham GP. Building a practically useful theory of goal setting and task motivation: a 35-year odyssey. *Am Psychol.* 2002;57:705-717.

24. Diabetes Prevention Program Research Group. Reduction in the incidence of Type 2 diabetes with lifestyle intervention or metformin. *N Engl J Med.* 2002;346:393-403.

25. Foster GD, Wadden TA, Vogt RA, Brewer G. What is a reasonable weight loss? Patients' expectations and evaluations of obesity treatment outcomes. *J Consult Clin Psychol.* 1997;65:79-85.

26. Jeffrey RW, Wing RR, Mayer RR. Are smaller weight losses or more achievable weight loss goals better in the long term for obese patients? *J Consult Clin Psychol.* 1998;66:641-646.

27. Linde JA, Jeffery RW, Levy R, Pronk N, Boyle R. Weight loss goals and treatment outcomes among overweight men and women enrolled in a weight loss trial. *Int J Obes (Lond).* 2005;29:1002-1005.

28. Linde JA, Jeffery RW, Finch EA, Ng DM, Rothman AJ. Are unrealistic weight loss goals associated with outcomes for overweight women? *Obes Res.* 2004;12:569-576.

29. Perri MG, Nezu AM, McKelvey WF, Shermer RL, Renjilian DA, Viegener BJ. Relapse prevention training and problem-solving therapy in the long-term management of obesity. *J Consult Clin Psychol.* 2001;69:722-726.

30. Anderson JW, Konz EC, Frederich RC, Wood CL. Long-term weight-loss maintenance: a meta-analysis of US studies. *Am J Clin Nutr.* 2001;74:579-584.

31. Sumithran P, Prendergast LA, Delbridge E, et al. Long-term persistence of hormonal adaptations to weight loss. *N Engl J Med.* 2011;365:1597-1604.

32. Hall KD, Kahan S. Maintenance of lost weight and long-term management of obesity. *Med Clin North Am.* 2018;102:183-197.

33. Thomas JG, Bond DS, Phelan S, Hill JO, Wing RR. Weight-loss maintenance for 10 years in the National Weight Control Registry. *Am J Prev Med.* 2014;46:17-23.

34. Look AHEAD Research Group. Eight-year weight losses with an intensive lifestyle intervention: the Look AHEAD study. *Obesity (Silver Spring).* 2014;22:5-13.

35. Waring ME, Roberts MB, Parker DR, Eaton CB. Documentation and management of overweight and obesity in primary care. *J Am Board Fam Med.* 2009;22:544-552.

36. Mattar A, Carlston D, Sariol G, et al. The prevalence of obesity documentation in primary care electronic medical records. *Appl Clin Inform.* 2017;26:67-79.

37. Fitzpatrick SL, Stevens VJ. Adult obesity management in primary care, 2008–2013. *Prev Med.* 2017;99:128-133.

38. Petrin C, Kahan S, Turner M, Gallagher C, Dietz WH. Current attitudes and practices of obesity counselling by health care providers. *Obes Res Clin Pract.* 2017;11:352-359.

39. Kaplan LM, Golden A, Jinnett K, et al. Perceptions of barriers to effective obesity care: results from the national ACTION study. *Obesity (Silver Spring).* 2018;26:61-69.

40. Gudzune KA, Bennett WL, Cooper LA, Bleich SN. Perceived judgment about weight can negatively influence weight loss: a cross-sectional study of overweight and obese patients. *Prev Med.* 2014;62:103-107.

41. Post RE, Mainous AG, Gregorie SH, Knoll ME, Diaz VA, Saxena SK. The influence of physician acknowledgment of patients' weight status on patient perceptions of overweight and obesity in the United States. *Arch Intern Med.* 2011;171:316-321.

42. Rose S, Poynter P, Anderson J, Noar S, Conigliaro J. Physician weight loss advice and patient weight loss behavior change: a literature review and meta-analysis of survey data. *Int J Obes (Lond).* 2013;37:118-128.

43. Sherson EA, Yakes Jimenez E, Katalanos N. A review of the use of the 5 A's model for weight loss counselling: differences between physician practice and patient demand. *Fam Pract.* 2014;31:389-398.

44. Volger S, Vetter ML, Dougherty M, et al. Patients' preferred terms for describing their excess weight: discussing obesity in clinical practice. *Obesity (Silver Spring).* 2012;20:147-150.

45. Vallis M, Piccinini–Vallis H, Sharma AM, Freedhoff Y. Modified 5 As: minimal intervention for obesity counseling in primary care. *Can Fam Physician.* 2013;59:27-31.

46. Alhassan S, Kim S, Bersamin A, King A, Gardner C. Dietary adherence and weight loss success among overweight women: results from the A TO Z weight loss study. *Int J Obes (Lond).* 2008;32:985-991.

47. Diabetes Prevention Program Research Group. The Diabetes Prevention Program (DPP): description of lifestyle intervention. *Diabetes Care.* 2002;25:2165-2171.

48. Brownell KD. *The LEARN Program for Weight Management 2000.* American Health Publishing Company; 2000.

49. Look AHEAD Research Group. The Look AHEAD study: a description of the lifestyle intervention and the evidence supporting it. *Obesity (Silver Spring).* 2006;14:737-752.

50. Wadden TA, Tsai AG, Tronieri JS. A protocol to deliver intensive behavioral therapy (IBT) for obesity in primary care settings: the MODEL-IBT program. *Obesity.* 2019;27:1562-1566.

51. Wadden TA, Walsh OA, Berkowitz RI, et al. Intensive behavioral therapy for obesity combined with liraglutide 3.0 mg: a randomized controlled trial. *Obesity (Silver Spring).* 2019;27:75-86.

52. Wadden TA, Tronieri JS, Sugimoto D, et al. Liraglutide 3.0 mg and intensive behavioral therapy (IBT) for obesity in primary care: The SCALE IBT randomized controlled trial. *Obesity.* 2020;28(3):529-536.

53. Wing RR, Hill JO. Successful weight loss maintenance. *Annu Rev Nutr.* 2001;21:323-341.

54. Svetkey LP, Stevens VJ, Brantley PJ, et al. Comparison of strategies for sustaining weight loss: the weight loss maintenance randomized controlled trial. *J Am Med Assoc.* 2008;299:1139-1148.

55. Perri MG, Limacher MC, Durning PE, et al. Extended-care programs for weight management in rural communities: the treatment of obesity in underserved rural settings (TOURS) randomized trial. *Arch Intern Med.* 2008;168:2347-2354.

56. Perri MG, McAdoo WG, Spevak PA, Newlin DB. Effect of a multicomponent maintenance program on long-term weight loss. *J Consult Clin Psychol.* 1984;52:480-481.

57. Perri MG, McAdoo WG, McAllister DA, Lauer JB, Yancey DZ. Enhancing the efficacy of behavior therapy for obesity: effects of aerobic exercise and a multicomponent maintenance program. *J Consult Clin Psychol.* 1986;54:670-675.

58. Perri MG, McAllister DA, Gange JJ, Jordan RC, McAdoo WG, Nezu AM. Effects of four maintenance programs on the long-term management of obesity. *J Consult Clin Psychol.* 1988;56:529-534.

59. Jackson H. *Health Status and Medical Services Utilization.* U.S. Census Bureau; 2013.

OBESITY PHARMACOTHERAPY

Donna H. Ryan, Rekha Kumar

CASE STUDY 1

A 44-year-old woman presents to her healthcare professional (HCP) for an annual wellness visit. She denies any new complaints, but her provider notes a 15 lb weight gain since the prior visit. She has a past medical history of depression, irritable bowel syndrome with diarrhea (IBS-D), and migraine headaches. Her medications are a low-dose combination oral contraceptive pill, sertraline 150 mg daily, and sumatriptan 50 mg as needed for migraines. Weight history is notable for successfully losing weight several times in the past through self-directed diet and exercise; however, she always regains the weight. She is very frustrated and does not understand why she is unable to maintain the weight loss. On examination, weight is 198 lb, height 5′6″, blood pressure (BP) 118/72, heart rate (HR) 86, body mass index (BMI) 32 kg/m², and waist circumference 99 cm. The remainder of her physical examination is unremarkable. Her laboratory data are notable for blood glucose 92 mg/dL, high-density lipoprotein (HDL) 35 mg/dL, low-density lipoprotein (LDL) 180 mg/dL, triglycerides 210 mg/dL, and thyroid-stimulating hormone (TSH) 1.2 µIL/mL.

Using Shared Decision-Making

Here is a sample conversation about introducing medications in the weight management conversation. The topics to be covered are mechanisms of action, potential efficacy, cost and reimbursement issues, and need for long-term therapy.

HCP: "You have been successful in losing weight in the past but like many patients, weight regain seems to be an issue."

Patient: "Losing weight is the easy part! The hard part is keeping it off. I am frustrated and don't want to live the rest of my life on a diet. I eat healthy food, but the weight comes back anyway."

HCP: "You haven't tried medications. Some of our newer medications have been extensively studied and are safe. Taking one can make it more likely that you will lose significant weight—5% or 10%, but importantly, as long as you take the medication, the more likely you are to sustain that hard-won weight loss. What is your initial reaction to taking a medication?"

Patient: "Aren't medications cheating? I guess I want to hear more…."

HCP: "These medications don't work on their own. They reinforce your body's biology and help with hunger and fullness. There is one that doesn't affect appetite, but helps you stay on a low-fat diet. If you are not making an effort with diet and increased physical activity, you will not get optimal results. I am going to give you a handout that describes the medications (See additional resources, below, for a handout, 'Medications for Weight Loss') and I want you to go home and do some internet research. The meds all have slightly different profiles. And you will need to check with your insurance company to see which ones you have coverage for. I will see you back, answer your questions and we can decide on the one that is right for you. When we choose one, we will need to monitor you monthly over the first 3 months to make sure it is working and to deal with side effects. How does this sound?"

Patient: "I have a friend at work who lost 40 pounds when her diabetes medications were changed, so I know medications can make a difference in weight. It sounds like a good plan to me. Can we meet in a month?"

The patient returned to the office in a month and expressed a preference for phentermine/topiramate because of her history of migraine headaches. She is started on phentermine/topiramate ER 3.75/23 mg daily and instructed to increase to 7.5/46 mg daily after 2 weeks. She schedules appointments with a registered dietitian nutritionist every 4 weeks between visits with her HCP. At the visit at 12 weeks, she is found to have lost 14 lb (7% of her total body weight).

CLINICAL SIGNIFICANCE

With nearly 40% of US adults having a BMI ≥30 kg/m², and unsuccessful following lifestyle modification changes alone, many of these individuals would benefit from intensifying therapy with an antiobesity medication (AOM)[1] to help them adhere to lifestyle changes in order to lose enough weight to achieve health benefits and to sustain weight loss. On the other hand, some medications promote unintentional weight gain and providers also need to avoid prescribing certain drugs which would worsen obesity.

Since 2012, four new medications have been approved by the US Food and Drug Administration (US FDA) with an indication for chronic weight management, although one was voluntarily withdrawn in February 2020. In addition, one capsule that is considered a device was marketed in 2020. Moreover, there are several companies with active obesity drug discovery programs and promising compounds in development that appear to produce twice the amount of weight loss achievable with current medications. Thus, we are entering a period where prescribers have access to safe and increasingly effective tools to help patients with complications of excess abnormal body fat to regularly achieve enough weight loss to prevent and control obesity-driven chronic diseases. This chapter will review current best practices and context regarding using medications for patients with obesity (including avoiding medications that promote weight gain), the safety and efficacy of currently available medications (both with a weight management indication and those commonly used "off-label" to aid weight management), and the most promising AOMs on the horizon.

INDICATIONS, RATIONALE, AND CONTEXT FOR OBESITY PHARMACOTHERAPY

In the National Institutes of Health (NIH)–supported Obesity Guidelines released in 2014,[2] obesity pharmacotherapy was allowed for individuals who are unresponsive to lifestyle interventions after 6 months of treatment, have a BMI of ≥30 kg/m², or a BMI of ≥27 kg/m² with a weight-induced comorbidity where weight-loss medication may be added to the treatment plan. At the time those recommendations were drafted, orlistat was the only medication available for obesity management. In 2015, the US Endocrine Society produced the first guidelines[3] that recommended pharmacologic treatment of obesity. These evidence statements and recommendations were based on a systematic evidence review encompassing all available approved AOMs. This guidance was also notable for including recommendations for management of drug-induced weight gain.[3] The Endocrine Society guidelines review the existing evidence for the FDA-approved medicines for weight management, and the recommendations contained in them are not just permissive of medication use (as in earlier guidelines), but also directive of medication use to help patients achieve weight loss in order to attain health benefits.[3] Taking this a step further, the AACE/ACE Guidelines[4] from 2016 indicate that initial pharmacotherapy added to lifestyle intervention is appropriate if patients present with one or more severe comorbidities and would benefit from weight loss of 10% or more.[4,5]

CLINICAL HIGHLIGHTS

- The 2013 American Heart Association/American College of Cardiology/The Obesity Society (AHA/ACC/TOS) Guidelines for the Management of Overweight and Obesity in Adults[2] recommends that patients with obesity or overweight with cardiovascular risk factors should be counseled on diet, physical activity, and other lifestyle modifications. Unfortunately, behavioral interventions alone do not lead to sustained weight loss for many patients because adaptive physiologic responses reduce energy expenditure and increase appetite. Patients have measurable changes in resting metabolic rate, burn fewer calories with the same exercise, and have more hunger and cravings and reduced satiety at a lower weight. These phenomena, known as metabolic adaptation or adaptive thermogenesis, counteract weight loss and lead to weight regain.
- Healthcare professionals should consider prescribing AOMs along with diet and physical activity to help patients achieve health goals through weight loss, especially when comorbidities are compromising health.[3-5]
- The Endocrine Society's systematic evidence review of common medications that promote weight gain and use of alternative approaches is a valuable resource; this knowledge base should be a standard of care for adult HCPs. Wherever possible, for patients with overweight and obesity, using medications that are weight neutral or associated with weight loss is advisable. See Table 8.1.

- The rationale for using AOMs is to help achieve and sustain more weight loss that can be achieved with lifestyle intervention alone, thus benefitting the health of patients who need to lose weight for health reasons.
- Prescribers need to be knowledgeable about ALL medications, because there is no one medication that works in every patient. If patients do not respond in the first 12 to 16 weeks with at least 4% to 5% weight loss, the drug should be discontinued, and another medication tried.
- Obesity is a chronic disease. AOMs should be used long term, just like antihypertensive and lipid-lowering agents.

As shown in Table 8.1, there are currently four medications approved for chronic weight management by the US FDA in addition to phentermine and a few related compounds which are approved for short-term use. Although their abuse potential is low, some of these medications are scheduled by the US Drug Enforcement Agency and regulated by the states. Of note is the fact that three medications have been approved since 2012 and are approved for long-term use (reinforcing the concept that obesity is a chronic disease). The mechanism of action of FDA-approved AOMs is also shown in Table 8.1. These medications (except orlistat) work biologically to suppress appetite, affecting hunger, satiety, and response to highly rewarding foods, thus making it easier for patients to follow their dietary intentions to restrict caloric intake. The rationale for using medications to aid in weight loss and weight loss maintenance is based on an advanced understanding of the biologic regulation of body weight and food intake. Knowledge has emerged regarding the biologic basis of eating, e.g., the gut-brain

axis of the homeostatic regulation of hunger and satiety, and of the reward circuitry that governs the response to foods of high hedonic value.[6] Patients who struggle losing weight with lifestyle alone do not have weak "will power." Rather, the biologic forces opposing weight loss are very powerful. Furthermore, once weight loss occurs, metabolic adaptations reduce metabolism, adding to the forces opposing weight loss and driving regain.

Three Reasons to Use AOMs

AOMs are indicated for adults with BMI ≥30 or ≥27 kg/m² and at least one comorbidity as an adjunct to reduced calorie diet and increased physical activity when the patients

1. are unsuccessful in losing weight with lifestyle changes alone, or
2. need to lose 10% or more body weight to achieve health benefits, or
3. need to maintain weight loss (regardless of the methods used to achieve initial weight loss).

Even with our most intensive lifestyle interventions, some patients are unsuccessful at achieving adequate weight loss. In the "gold standard" Look AHEAD intensive lifestyle intervention, despite a minimum of 24 counseling sessions in the first year and the use of meal replacements, 30% of patients did not achieve 5% weight loss from baseline.[7] Furthermore, weight regain occurred even though intervention continued through year 4. At that time, there was only 3.6% difference in weight between the intensive lifestyle intervention group and control.[8] Clearly, HCPs cannot duplicate this degree of intensity of effort at the intervention deployed in Look

TABLE 8.1 Current Antiobesity Medications Approved in the United States and How They Work[a]

AGENT	ACTION	APPROVAL	SCHEDULED DRUG
Phentermine	• Sympathomimetic amine; norepinephrine release and to lesser extent releases other monoamines	Approved 1959	• Yes
Orlistat	• Pancreatic lipase inhibitor; blocks absorption of 30% of ingested dietary fat	Approved 1999 OTC Approved 2007	• No
Phentermine/ Topiramate ER	• Sympathomimetic • Anticonvulsant (GABA receptor modulator carbonic anhydrase inhibitor, glutamate antagonist)	Approved 2012	• Yes
Naltrexone SR/ Bupropion SR	• Opioid receptor antagonist • Dopamine/norepinephrine reuptake inhibitor	Approved 2014	• No
Liraglutide 3.0 mg	• GLP-1 receptor agonist	Approved 2014	• No

GABA, gamma aminobutyric acid.
[a]*Information from product labels of prescribing information, except where noted.*

AHEAD. In primary care efforts at lifestyle intervention, average weight loss is on the order of 0.9 to 2.0 kg in 6 months.[9] For the many patients who are unable to achieve and sustain weight loss with lifestyle intervention alone, AOMs are needed to help achieve enough weight loss to produce improved health benefits. Additionally, for patients with more severe complications of obesity, such as type 2 diabetes (T2D) or obstructive sleep apnea, weight loss of >10% is needed to maximize health benefits. Despite the limitations of lifestyle intervention for weight loss, high-intensity behavioral treatment of obesity (≥14 visits in the first 6 months, followed by at least monthly contact for maintenance of weight loss) is recommended as a standard of care for treatment of obesity and should produce a 5% to 10% weight loss during the first 6 months of treatment. Several randomized trials using different medications have reported that the combination of intensive behavioral treatment and pharmacotherapy is additive in terms of weight loss.

How much weight does a patient need to lose? Health benefits can be achieved without normalizing body weight or achieving a BMI <25 or <30 kg/m². One begins to see improvement in glycemic measures, triglycerides, and HDL-cholesterol with small amounts of weight loss (3% to 5%), but there appears to be a further dose response benefit with greater levels of weight loss.[2] Modest weight loss (5% to 10%) is also associated with improvement in systolic and diastolic blood pressure.[2] There are graded improvements in measures of quality of life, depression, mobility, sexual dysfunction, and urinary stress incontinence that are demonstrable with modest weight loss (5% to 10%) and continue to improve with further weight loss.[10] Additionally, for patients with higher BMI levels (≥40 kg/m²), the ability to lose the same proportion of weight with lifestyle intervention is equal to that of those with lower BMI levels, and there is equal benefit in terms of risk factor improvement with modest weight loss.[10] For some comorbid conditions, more weight loss is needed, i.e., 10% to 15%, to translate into clinical improvement. This is observed for obstructive sleep apnea and nonalcoholic steatohepatitis.[10]

Lifestyle Counseling

All patients who have obesity or overweight and abnormal cardiovascular risk factors should be counseled on diet, physical activity, and other lifestyle modifications. Specifically, patients should be advised to pursue high-intensity lifestyle modification, as defined in the 2013 AHA/ACC/TOS guideline on management of obesity. The HCP should counsel patients that the combination of pharmacotherapy and intensive lifestyle modification nearly doubles weight loss, compared to either therapy alone.

Table 8.2 shows the proportion of patients who achieved 5% or 10% weight loss at 1 year in the clinical studies which were performed for FDA approval. All medications are included except phentermine. There are no long-term studies with phentermine, and its efficacy is discussed below. It should be noted that in all cases there is a greater proportion of medication-treated subjects who achieve the 5% and 10% benchmark, compared to placebo. Also noteworthy is the wide range of success that is achieved with placebo alone. This is because the components, delivery, and intensity of the lifestyle intervention varied between the studies.

In terms of context, the studies that led to the approval of AOMs were all conducted along with a lifestyle intervention of diet and physical activity counseling. In any study where the medication was stopped, weight regain was demonstrated. Therefore, the labels state they are "indicated as an adjunct to reduced calorie diet and increased physical activity for chronic weight management in adults." As discussed later, the medication could be given after patients lose weight on a strict diet to produce more weight loss and advance maintenance. Furthermore, this chapter will later discuss the use of medications in the setting of bariatric procedures, where AOMs are used as an adjunct to the surgical procedure to treat insufficient weight loss or weight regain or to improve weight-related comorbidities.

BEST PRACTICES IN PRESCRIBING MEDICATIONS APPROVED FOR WEIGHT MANAGEMENT

Qualifications for Prescription

The FDA labels for AOMs provide the indications of BMI ≥30 kg/m² or BMI ≥27 kg/m² with a weight-related comorbidity. It is not necessary for patients to fail a weight loss attempt while under the care of an HCP for the patient to be prescribed a medication; the history of failure to maintain successful weight loss is enough. For patients with more severe complications (T2D, hypertension, and sleep apnea), practitioners should be more proactive about using medications and follow the AACE recommendations.[4,5] Those patients would benefit from 10% or more loss and should be prescribed medications to augment the weight loss effort.

Choosing an Individual Medication

The Endocrine Society guideline[3] indicates that contraindications and warnings should be the first step to match the patient to the medication profile, excluding medications from consideration if they are contraindicated or associated with serious warnings. See Table 8.3

TABLE 8.2 Antiobesity Medications Approved in the United States: Dosing and Route of Administration; Efficacy (Proportion of Treated Individuals Who Achieve >5% and >10% During Phase 3 Clinical Trials)[a]

DRUG, GENERIC NAME	DOSE AND ROUTE OF ADMINISTRATION	PROPORTION ACHIEVING >5% WEIGHT LOSS AT ONE YEAR[A]	PROPORTION ACHIEVING >10% WEIGHT LOSS AT ONE YEAR[A]
Phentermine	• 8 mg up to tid, before meals Or • 15 mg, 30 mg, or 37.5 mg once daily	In a 6-month study[11] Phentermine 7 mg = 43.3% Phentermine 15 mg = 46.2% Placebo = 15.5%	Not described
Orlistat	• 120 mg tid, before meals Or • 60 mg tid before meals • Oral	In five studies, Orlistat = 35.5%-54.8% *vs.* Placebo = 16%-27.4%	In five studies, Orlistat = 16.4%-25.8% *vs.* Placebo = 3.8%-9.9%
Phentermine/ Topiramate ER (Phen/TPM)	• 7.5 mg/46 mg qid • 15 mg/92 mg qid, indicated as rescue • Oral, once daily dosing (requires titration)	In two studies, Phen/TPM (3 doses) = 45% – 70%; *vs.* Placebo = 17% – 21% Difference from placebo = 27.6% – 49.4%	In two studies, Phen/TPM (3 doses) = 19% – 48%; *vs.* Placebo = 7% Difference from placebo = 11.4% – 40.3%
Naltrexone SR/ Bupropion SR (NB)	• 32 mg/360 mg • Oral; bid dosing (requires titration)	In three studies, NB = 44.2% – 62.3%; *vs.* Placebo = 17% – 43% Difference from placebo = 14% – 25%	In three studies, NB = 15% – 35%; *vs.* Placebo = 5% – 21% Difference from placebo – 10% – 14%
Liraglutide	• 3.0 mg • Injection; once daily dosing (requires titration)	In two studies, Liraglutide = 62%[12] and 49%[13]; *vs.* Placebo = 34.4%[12] and 16.4%[13] Difference from placebo = 32.6%[14] and 22.6%[12]	In two studies, Liraglutide = 22.4%[13] and 33.9%[12]; *vs.* Placebo = 5.5%[13] and 15.4%[12] Difference from placebo = 16.9%[12] and 18.5%[14]

[a]Information from product labels of prescribing information, except where noted.

for a description of contraindications and safety issues with AOMs. Choosing a medication requires matching the patient profile to the medication profile. If patients describe difficulty controlling their appetite, then common sense dictates that one of the medications that affect appetite should be chosen, rather than orlistat. Also, one should consider dual benefits: orlistat can enforce a low-fat diet and lower plasma LDL cholesterol.[15] Liraglutide 3.0 mg can lower glycemic measures and, at a dose of 1.8 mg in patients with T2D, is associated with reduction in cardiovascular events in addition to affecting appetite and body weight.[16] See Table 8.4 for a description of dual benefits of AOMs.

Ask Two Questions Before Selecting the Prescription AOM

Before starting pharmacotherapy for obesity, it is important to consider two questions:

1. Are there contraindications, drug-drug interactions, or undesirable adverse effects associated with this medication that could be problematic for the patient?
2. Can this medication improve other existing symptoms or conditions?

TABLE 8.3 Medications Approved in the United States: Common Side Effects and Safety Issues[a]

DRUG, GENERIC NAME	COMMON SIDE EFFECTS	CONTRAINDICATIONS AND SAFETY ISSUES
Phentermine	• Headache, elevated BP, elevated HR • Insomnia, dry mouth, constipation, anxiety • Cardiovascular: palpitation, tachycardia, elevated BP, ischemic events • Central nervous system: overstimulation, restlessness, dizziness, insomnia, euphoria, dysphoria, tremor, headache, psychosis • Gastrointestinal: dryness of the mouth, unpleasant taste, diarrhea, constipation, other gastrointestinal disturbances • Allergic: urticaria • Endocrine: impotence, changes in libido	• Anxiety disorders (agitated states), history of heart disease, uncontrolled hypertension, • Seizure • MAO inhibitors • Pregnancy and breastfeeding, • Hyperthyroidism • Glaucoma • History of drug abuse • Sympathomimetic amines
Orlistat	• Steatorrhea • Oily spotting • Flatulence with discharge • Fecal urgency • Oily evacuation • Increased defecation • Fecal incontinence	• Contraindicated in pregnancy • Warning: ↑cyclosporine exposure • Liver failure (rare) • Requires coadministration of multi-vitamin • Increased risk of gall bladder disease • Increased urine oxalate; monitor renal function
Phentermine/Topiramate ER	• Insomnia • Dry mouth • Constipation • Paresthesias • Dizziness • Dysgeusia (altered taste)	• Contraindicated in pregnancy • Fetal toxicity; monthly pregnancy test suggested • Contraindicated with hyperthyroidism, glaucoma • Do not use with MAOIs or sympathomimetic amines • Metabolic acidosis and kidney stones • Acute myopia—angle closure glaucoma (rare)
Naltrexone SR/Bupropion SR	• Nausea • Constipation • Headache • Vomiting • Dizziness	• Boxed warning: suicide risk in depression • Contraindicated in pregnancy • Contraindicated in seizure disorders, uncontrolled hypertension • Do not use with opioids, MAOIs • Hepatotoxicity (rare) • Warning: angle closure glaucoma
Liraglutide 3.0 mg	• Nausea • Vomiting • Diarrhea • Constipation • Headache • Dyspepsia • Fatigue • Dizziness • Abdominal pain	• Boxed warning: thyroid C-cell tumors in rodents • Contraindicated with personal or family history of medullary thyroid cancer or multiple endocrine neoplasia • Pancreatitis • Hypoglycemia in diabetes • Increased risk of gall bladder disease

BP, blood pressure; HR, heart rate; MAOI, monoamine oxidase inhibitor.
[a]Information from product labels of prescribing information, except where noted.

Cost and Prescribing

Financial considerations are always part of the decision about which drug to prescribe. It is unfortunate that Medicare Part D does not cover AOMs. However, more than 50% of employer-based plans will allow coverage for these medications, albeit with co-pays. Furthermore, these medications commonly require prior authorization.

TABLE 8.4 Dual Benefits to Guide Obesity Medication Selection

IF PATIENT HAS OBESITY AND	CONSIDER THIS MEDICATION (BUT NOT EXPLICITLY APPROVED)
Smoking	Naltrexone/Bupropion
Depression	Naltrexone/Bupropion
Migraines	Phentermine/topiramate
Diabetes	Liraglutide 3.0 mg
Chronic constipation	Orlistat
Elevated LDL	Orlistat

LDL, low-density lipoprotein.

Determining Response and "Stopping Rules"

The best predictor of long-term weight loss is initial weight loss. If patients lose ≥4% to 5% of their body weight in 12 to 16 weeks at the recommended dose of a drug, the patient is considered responsive with an increased likelihood of a clinically meaningful weight loss at 1 year. In contrast, if the patient loses <5% weight, the patient is considered nonresponsive and the medication should be stopped. Every medication approved for chronic weight management comes with label recommendations for stopping the medication if 4% to 5% weight loss is not achieved by 12 to 16 weeks, depending upon the specific medication. By using these label recommendations, HCPs are guided to discontinue ineffective medications as early as possible and consider use of another medication if indicated.

Timing of Follow-Up and Duration of Therapy

According to the Endocrine Guidelines,[3] after prescription, providers should follow patients monthly for the first 3 months and then every 3 months thereafter. Long-term use of medications is recommended to promote weight loss maintenance, but they may be used intermittently.[3]

Treating Obesity as a Chronic Disease

- Just as in other chronic diseases, there is no one medication that works in every patient. If patients do not respond with at least 4% to 5% weight loss in 12 to 16 weeks, try another medication.
- If patients do respond, these medications are approved for long-term use. When an AOM is discontinued, weight regain should be anticipated.

MEDICATIONS WITH AN INDICATION FOR WEIGHT LOSS OR CHRONIC WEIGHT MANAGEMENT

The characteristics of medications with a weight management indication are described below. This information is supplemented by Tables 8.1 to 8.4 and is primarily sourced from product labels.

Phentermine[17-20]

Phentermine, a sympathomimetic amine first approved in 1959, has long had the distinction of being the most prescribed agent for obesity treatment in the United States, primarily because it is the least expensive of the available agents. Other sympathomimetic agents in this class include diethylpropion and phendimetrazine. Phentermine is available in 8 mg tablets,[17] which may be given three times daily, or as 15 and 30 mg capsules, or 37.5 mg tablet, given once daily. The efficacy of phentermine is on a par with other AOMs currently available. Phentermine is a sympathomimetic agent which increases blood pressure and pulse, although it does not affect resting metabolic rate in humans.[11] The Endocrine pharmacotherapy guideline[3] recommends that phentermine NOT be prescribed in patients with preexisting cardiovascular disease. It is contraindicated in uncontrolled hypertension, hyperthyroidism, glaucoma, or within 14 days of use of a monoamine oxidase inhibitor. Phentermine is a controlled substance (Schedule IV and sometimes Schedule II) and some state licensing boards track phentermine prescribers and limit its duration of use. The Endocrine pharmacotherapy guideline endorses long-term prescribing in certain patients.[3]

CASE STUDY 2

A 37-year-old female experiences a weight gain of 17 lb after undergoing a total thyroidectomy for papillary thyroid cancer 6 months ago. She was prescribed levothyroxine for hormone replacement. She reports following a 1,200-kcal diet, exercises three times/week but cannot lose weight since the thyroidectomy. She feels very frustrated and is concerned since obesity runs in her family.

The patient initiates a food log and 8 mg tablet of phentermine, taken once or twice daily for appetite control and continues her lifestyle modification. She loses 12 pounds in 3 months and reduces the phentermine to every other day or only in situations that she believes she might overeat.

Key points: low cardiac risk, optimized on lifestyle, able to use low doses of medicines to maintain weight loss.

Phentermine/Topiramate[11,19,20]

Low-dose, controlled-release phentermine plus topiramate (as one capsule) was approved by the FDA in 2012 as a long-term treatment for obesity. Phentermine is described above and has been long used for weight management. Topiramate has also been widely used for migraine prophylaxis (approved in 2005) and epilepsy (approved in 1996), and it was observed in these settings to produce modest weight loss. The combination has been shown to have additive weight loss efficacy.[19] Phentermine/topiramate is available in four doses: 3.75/23 mg (starting dose), 7.5/46 mg (lowest treatment dose), 11.25/69 mg, or 15/92 mg. All patients start on 3.75/23 mg and most progress to 7.5/46 mg, with higher doses used if the medication is well-tolerated and maximal efficacy is required; the highest dose is 15/92 mg.

All prescribers need to be aware of the potential for development of orofacial clefts in infants exposed to topiramate during the first trimester of pregnancy. Therefore, all women of childbearing potential should have a negative pregnancy test before the drug is prescribed and should use contraception and have a monthly home test thereafter. The drug is contraindicated in patients with glaucoma, metabolic acidosis, and history of oxalate kidney stones. The most common adverse effects (AEs) with phentermine/topiramate ER include paresthesia, dizziness, dysgeusia (a distortion of the sense of taste), insomnia, constipation, and dry mouth. Medication interactions include an increased risk of malignant hypertension with monoamine oxidase (MAO) inhibitors and increased probability of elevated heart rate and blood pressure if used with other sympathomimetic amines.

Of the currently available AOMs, phentermine/topiramate is generally considered to have the greatest weight loss efficacy. As shown in Table 8.2, the odds of 5% or 10% weight loss while on this medication are generally superior to other agents. Providers must be knowledgeable about the teratogenic risk of topiramate in causing cleft palate during pregnancy. For this reason, a Risk Evaluation and Management Strategy program was authorized by the FDA to education prescribers on the importance of using active birth control among women of childbearing age (https://www.qsymiarems.com/). In addition to anxiety or history of nephrolithiasis, other contraindications including active or unstable coronary disease, hyperthyroidism, glaucoma, insomnia, or history of drug abuse or recent MAO inhibitor use. The most common AEs reported in phase III trials were paresthesia, dry mouth, and constipation.

Lorcaserin[14,21-24]

Lorcaserin was approved by the FDA for chronic weight management in 2012 and taken off the market in 2020. Lorcaserin was developed for selective agonism of the serotonin 2C receptor. This drug was generally regarded as having a favorable tolerability and safety profile, with a positive effect in dysglycemia. A cardiovascular outcome trial conducted in 12,000 volunteers over 5 years showed no meaningful difference between lorcaserin and placebo in the risk of major adverse cardiovascular events, demonstrating noninferiority.[22] The one-sided upper bound of the 95% confidence interval (CI) of the hazard ratio (HR) was less than 1.4 (the noninferiority margin). The HR (95% CI) was 1.005 (0.842, 1.198) for lorcaserin versus placebo.[22] Additionally, echocardiograms conducted during the trial did not raise the issue of valvulopathy.[22] Furthermore, this study demonstrated not only safety, but health benefits. Another publication of the same population demonstrated that lorcaserin decreased risk for incident T2D, induced remission of hyperglycemia, and reduced the risk of microvascular complications.[23]

However, on January 14, 2020, the FDA sent a Drug Safety Communication (DSC)[21] "alerting the public that results from a clinical trial assessing safety show a possible increased risk of cancer with the weight management medicine Belviq, Belviq XR (lorcaserin)."

In the initial report from lorcaserin's cardiovascular outcome trial, cancer numbers in patients taking lorcaserin were reported as 215 (3.59%) and in placebo as 210 (3.50%) with 95% CI of −0.58 to 0.75.[22] The FDA subsequently reported that there were 990 cancers diagnosed in 885 patients. Overall, 7.7% of participants in the lorcaserin group and 7.1% in the placebo group were diagnosed with cancer. In the lorcaserin group, the proportion of participants who died from cancer were 0.9% and while on placebo this was 0.6%. The trial was conducted in 12,000 patients over 5 years. A range of cancer types was reported, with several different types of cancers occurring more frequently in the lorcaserin group, including pancreatic, colorectal, and lung. Lorcaserin is no longer available in the United States. Cancer screening of patients who took lorcaserin should follow standard age and sex recommendations.

Naltrexone SR/Bupropion SR[12]

Bupropion has long been approved in the United States for treatment of depression (approved in 1985) and smoking cessation (approved in 1997). As discussed below, bupropion as a single agent can produce some weight loss on its own. In contrast, naltrexone does not cause weight loss when used alone. The FDA approved the combination with each drug in sustained release form for chronic weight management in 2014. It is thought that the combination also modulates the "reward pathway" and may reduce food cravings.

The most common side effects of naltrexone SR/bupropion SR are nausea, vomiting, constipation, headache, dizziness, insomnia, and dry mouth. In order to improve tolerability, a specified dose titration is used over the first 4 weeks beginning with one tablet per day for the first week and increased by one tablet weekly until a dose of two tablets twice daily is reached.

The chief safety issues of naltrexone SR/bupropion SR are related to the components. Bupropion lowers the seizure threshold and should therefore not be prescribed in patients with a history of seizures. Similarly, caution should be used in other instances that provoke seizures and the drug should not be given when there is abrupt discontinuation of alcohol, sedatives, antiepileptic drugs, or opioids or in patients with bulimia or anorexia nervosa. The drug is contraindicated in patients taking opioids since naltrexone will block opioid action. The medication should not be used within 14 days of MAO inhibitors. Increased blood pressure with bupropion can occur. Naltrexone SR/bupropion SR should be avoided in patients with uncontrolled hypertension.

CASE STUDY 3

A 47-year-old male presents with class III obesity (BMI 40 kg/m^2), prediabetes, and hyperlipidemia. He has lost 10 lb with diet/exercise several times but is unable to sustain the weight loss. He also reports a history of heavy alcohol use and wants to cut back on his drinking. The patient reports cravings and episodes of overeating his favorite food, ice cream, when he is on a diet. This patient is a good candidate for bupropion/naltrexone due to his cravings and desire to also lower his alcohol intake.

Liraglutide 3.0 mg[13,25-27]

Liraglutide is a GLP-1 receptor agonist that has 97% homology with native GLP-1. The GLP-1 molecule has been modified to extend the circulating half-life from 1 to 2 minutes to 13 hours. Liraglutide is approved in 2010 for treatment of T2D at a dose of up to 1.8 mg. In humans, liraglutide reduces food intake by its action on GLP-1 receptors in various regions of the brain. Liraglutide also causes weight loss through effects on

the GI tract by increasing satiety due to slowing of gastric emptying. There is no effect on energy expenditure. The chief tolerability issues with liraglutide 3.0 mg are gastrointestinal side effects, chiefly nausea and vomiting. Liraglutide is given once daily by injection. A dose escalation is required to minimize side effects, beginning at 0.6 mg subcutaneously daily for the first week and increasing by 0.6 mg weekly to the recommended dose of 3.0 mg daily.[13]

As with other drugs in the GLP-1 receptor agonist class, liraglutide carries a black box warning on the association with medullary thyroid cancer in rodents although the relevance to humans has not been determined. It is contraindicated in people with a personal or family history of medullary thyroid carcinoma or multiple endocrine neoplasia syndrome type 2 (MEN2), a hereditary condition associated with three primary types of tumors: medullary thyroid cancer, parathyroid tumors, and pheochromocytoma. As with all medications for weight management, it is contraindicated in pregnancy. Liraglutide has not been studied in patients with a history of pancreatitis and should be discontinued if acute pancreatitis develops, a rare event associated with drugs in this class. Increased rates of cholecystitis and cholelithiasis were also observed in the phase III studies, but it is unclear whether the cases were related to the medication or to weight loss, which is also associated with gall bladder disease. Although liraglutide is associated with improvements in blood pressure and blood lipids, it produces an average increase heart rate by 2.0 beats/minute.

One of the advantages of liraglutide is that it also influences glycemia. In a study of patients with prediabetes,[25] patients were followed for 3 years on liraglutide or placebo. Only 2% of individuals on liraglutide progressed to diabetes, compared to 6% of those on placebo. Although there was not a dedicated cardiovascular outcome trial with liraglutide 3.0 mg, a cardiovascular outcome trial[26] at the lower dose of 1.8 mg in patients with T2D showed reduced events which is reassuring in terms of safety for this compound. The efficacy of liraglutide in maintaining weight loss was examined in the SCALE Maintenance[27] study. In that study, 422 subjects with overweight and obesity who lost ≥5% of their initial body weight on a low-calorie diet were randomly assigned to liraglutide 3.0 mg daily or placebo for 56 weeks. Mean weight loss on the initial diet was 6.0%. By the end of the study, participants in the liraglutide group lost an additional 6.2% compared with 0.2% with placebo ($P < .0001$), for a total weight loss of >12% in the liraglutide 3.0 mg group. This trial demonstrates the benefit of sequencing the use of AOMs after an initial weight loss on lifestyle management alone.

A 32-year-old female would like to lose weight prior to pregnancy. She has a history of PCOS (polycystic ovarian syndrome) and obesity since she was a teenager and reports eating a high-carbohydrate diet. She is currently on oral contraceptive pill (OCP) but reports a history of oligomenorrhea. She has been on metformin since the age of 16 years but does not feel that it affects her appetite. She is started on liraglutide 0.6 mg daily for the first week and is titrated up to 3.0 mg daily over 4 weeks. She is seen in follow-up 3 months later and has lost 20 lb and reports regular menses off her OCP.

Key point: Liraglutide 3.0 mg is a good choice in patients with insulin resistance syndromes like PCOS.

Orlistat[28]

Prior to 2012, the only weight-loss medicine for long-term use was orlistat, which was FDA approved in 1999. The recommended dose is 120 mg taken orally three times daily before meals. It is also available over-the-counter as 60 mg capsules (alli), approved in 2007. Orlistat is not absorbed from the GI tract to any significant degree, and its side effects relate to blockade of triglyceride digestion in the intestine. If orlistat is taken with a high-fat meal or snack, then the effects of unabsorbed fat—steatorrhea—are likely to occur. Therefore, counseling patients about gastrointestinal side effects that may occur from consuming excess fat intake is important. It may also be helpful to take psyllium along with orlistat to minimize gastrointestinal side effects.[29] Because orlistat can cause small but significant decreases in fat-soluble vitamins, some patients may need vitamin supplementation given at bedtime, particularly if it is continued long term. Orlistat does not seem to affect the absorption of other drugs, except cyclosporine, where exposure is increased. Orlistat enhances the effect of Coumadin, and Coumadin doses may need to be adjusted according to the international normalized ratio (INR) level. Rare cases of severe liver injury have been reported with patients taking orlistat; however, a causal relationship has not been established.[28] Orlistat has also been associated with calcium oxalate renal stones. Despite these rare occurrences, orlistat is remarkable for its safety, as evidenced by achieving over-the-counter status for the 60 mg dose.

Orlistat is the only medication currently approved for weight management for adolescents with obesity. In 539 adolescents who received 120 mg three times per day of orlistat, on average, BMI decreased by 0.55 kg/m^2 in the drug-treated group compared to an increase of +0.31 kg/m^2 in the placebo-treated group.[30]

A 60-year-old attorney has been taking orlistat 120 mg three times daily before meals for 15 years, since an initial weight loss of 40 pounds. He reports that he believes orlistat helps him maintain the lost weight, especially during times of stress, such as a jury trial. He says, "Orlistat helps me stay on a healthier diet and I can avoid comfort foods because I know they will upset my system."

Key point: Orlistat reinforces the intention to follow a low-fat dietary approach.

Comparison of Weight Loss Efficacy of Available Medications

There are no head-to-head comparisons of these medications. However, there is an analysis[31] of 28 randomized clinical trials of weight loss medications including trials with orlistat ($N = 17$), lorcaserin ($N = 3$), liraglutide ($N = 3$), naltrexone-bupropion ($N = 4$), and phentermine-topiramate ($N = 2$). The inclusion criteria and background lifestyle interventions differed across studies, so results must be interpreted with caution. Attrition rates were 30% to 45% across these trials. All five agents were associated with significantly greater weight loss at 1 year than placebo. Across all studies, an average weight loss of ≥5% was seen in 23% of the patients treated with placebo compared to 44% of those treated with orlistat, 49% with lorcaserin, 55% with naltrexone/bupropion, 63% with liraglutide, and 75% of those treated with phentermine/topiramate. The highest odds ratios for treatment-related discontinuation of the trial were seen with liraglutide and naltrexone/bupropion.

MEDICATIONS WHICH PROMOTE WEIGHT GAIN

Table 8.5 describes the medications which were identified in the 2015 Endocrine Society systematic evidence review as promoting weight gain.[3] For patients who have overweight and obesity and who have already demonstrated susceptibility for weight gain, HCPs should inform them of the potential for further weight gain with these medications before prescribing. Not all patients will experience weight gain with the medications identified in Table 8.5, but alternative medications should be considered if possible.

TABLE 8.5 Medications Which Promote Weight Gain and Alternative Approaches

WEIGHT GAIN ASSOCIATED WITH USE	ALTERNATIVES (WEIGHT REDUCING IN PARENTHESES)
Medications for diabetes • Insulin • Sulfonylureas • Thiazolidinediones • Meglitinide	• (Metformin) • Alpha-glucosidase inhibitors • DPP-4 inhibitors • (Pramlintide) • (GLP-1 receptor agonists) • (SGLT 2 inhibitors)
Antidepressants/mood stabilizers: Tricyclic antidepressants • Amitriptyline • Doxepin • Imipramine • Nortriptyline • Trimipramine • Mirtazapine	• (Bupropion) • Nefazodone • Fluoxetine, short term • Sertraline, given <1 year
Antidepressants/mood stabilizers: Selective Serotonin Reuptake Inhibitors • Paroxetine • Fluvoxamine	
Antidepressants/mood stabilizers: Monoamine Oxidase Inhibitors • Phenelzine • Tranylcypromine	
Mood stabilizers • Lithium	
Antipsychotic medications • Clozapine • Risperidone • Olanzapine • Quetiapine • Haloperidol • Perphenazine	• Ziprasidone • Aripiprazole
Anticonvulsants • Carbamazepine • Gabapentin • Valproate	• Lamotrigine • (Topiramate) • (Zonisamide)

TABLE 8.5 Medications Which Promote Weight Gain and Alternative Approaches (Continued)

WEIGHT GAIN ASSOCIATED WITH USE	ALTERNATIVES (WEIGHT REDUCING IN PARENTHESES)
Hypertension medications • α-blocker • β-blocker, i.e., atenolol, metoprolol, nadolol, propranolol	• ACE inhibitors • Calcium channel blockers • Angiotensin-2 receptor antagonists
Contraceptives • Injectable progesterone • Oral progesterone	• Barrier methods • IUDs • Oral contraceptives preferable to injectable
Endometriosis treatment • Depot leuprolide acetate	• Surgical treatment
Chronic inflammatory diseases • Glucocorticoids	• Nonsteroidal anti-inflammatory drugs • Disease-modifying antirheumatic drugs
AIDS treatment • Antiretroviral therapies may adversely affect body fat distribution	• No therapeutic alternatives but monitoring and counseling are appropriate

ACE, angiotensin-converting enzyme; AIDS, acquired immunodeficiency syndrome; IUD, intrauterine device.
Adapted from Apovian CM, Aronne LJ, Bessesen DH, et al. Pharmacological management of obesity: An Endocrine Society clinical practice guideline. J Clin Endocrinol Metab. 2015;100(2):342-362. Erratum in: J Clin Endocrinol Metab. 2015;100(5):2135-2136.

MEDICATIONS USED OFF-LABEL FOR WEIGHT MANAGEMENT

Because of the variable coverage for AOMs, providers have prescribed certain medications off-label for weight management. Whenever possible, it is preferable to prescribe FDA-approved drugs because there are more available data on their long-term use. However, for patients without coverage, these agents may be a safe and affordable option to aid weight management.

• Metformin. This is probably the most often prescribed medication in patients with obesity. It is commonly prescribed in patients who have insulin resistance, and metformin also produces modest weight loss. In the DPP (Diabetes Prevention Program) study, metformin was associated with about 2% weight loss. In prescribing metformin to assist in weight management, it is advisable to use

500 mg ER tablets at a dose of 2,000 mg/day. The ER tablets produce less diarrhea.

- Bupropion. This agent is approved for smoking cessation and depression. It was evaluated as a potential single agent for weight loss, but the efficacy did not support pursuing approval. Still, some patients do well with weight loss on a dose of 360 mg bupropion given in extended-release form, and bupropion may be a good option for individuals with obesity who need an antidepressant medication. See the section above for other comments.
- GLP-1 receptor agonists. These medications are approved for T2D, and they are used frequently in patients with obesity to aid weight loss. Liraglutide 1.8 mg, exenatide, dulaglutide, and others are associated with weight loss. Semaglutide, recently approved for diabetes, produces the most weight loss on average of these options. See section above for other comments.
- Topiramate. This medication is used for migraine prophylaxis and for epilepsy. At higher doses, it can depress brain function and memory, particularly affecting word-finding. If used off-label for weight management, careful dose titration is needed and caution with its use in women of childbearing potential, as described above.
- SGLT 2 inhibitors. These medications are approved for T2D and are frequently used in patients with obesity and T2D, although occasionally they are used in patients who do not have T2D to aid in weight loss. In patients who are not restricting their diet, the calorie deficit with glycosuria is usually compensated for by increasing food intake. Therefore, to achieve maximal weight loss, patients must be counseled to restrict food intake while on SGLT 2 inhibitors. While these compounds have positive effects on glycemia, body weight, blood pressure, and serum uric acid, they also have been shown to increase risk for yeast infections, urinary tract infections, diabetic ketoacidosis, fracture, and foot amputation.
- Pramlintide. This drug is a human amylin analogue approved for use in conjunction with insulin therapy in patients with type 1 or 2 diabetes. Pramlintide is also associated with weight loss in patients with and without diabetes. Its chief side effect is nausea.
- Zonisamide. This drug is approved for use in epilepsy. It is a carbonic anhydrase inhibitor, and as with other antiepileptic agents, it has been associated with psychomotor slowing and depression. It is sometimes used off-label to aid in weight management and usually started at 100 mg and titrated up to 600 mg. Zonisamide can be used in a manner similar to topiramate (i.e., in combination with a stimulant agent such as phentermine or diethylpropion).

NEW AND EMERGING PHARMACOLOGIC APPROACHES

Gelesis100: a Capsule FDA-Cleared as a Device[32]

In 2019, the FDA approved a new device for weight management. Gelesis100 is a nonsystemic, water-soluble gel. In the stomach, the capsule releases the cellulose microgel which forms a matrix and occupies about 25% of the stomach, with the consistency of food. In the large intestine, it is broken down by enzymes, and the cellulose is excreted. Gelesis100 and placebo were evaluated[32] over 24 weeks in patients with BMI 27 to ≤40 kg/m² and fasting plasma glucose 90 to 145 mg/dL. Gelesis100 treatment caused greater weight loss over placebo (6.4% vs. 4.4%, $P = .0007$), and 59% of Gelesis100-treated patients achieved weight loss of 5%, and 27% achieved 10% versus 42% and 15% in the placebo group, respectively. For unclear reasons, the capsules appeared to be more effective in patients with prediabetes or drug-naive T2D. Gelesis100 treatment had no apparent increased safety risks. The capsules are available by mail order prescription for patients with a BMI of at least 25 kg/m², with or without comorbidities.

Combination Approaches; Using Multiple Medications or Using Medications With Surgery and Devices

Following bariatric surgery, failure to achieve adequate weight loss or weight regain are frequent problems. About 25% of patients fail to achieve and sustain 10% weight loss. Obesity specialists approach this problem by initiating medications for patients who are not losing weight successfully as early as 6 months postoperatively. Similarly, obesity specialists are using multiple medications concomitantly, sometimes off-label.[33,34] Since obesity is a complex, heterogeneous disease, it makes sense to use multiple therapeutic approaches together to maximize weight loss. HCPs should view this as a specialty approach and refer to obesity specialists for these more complicated scenarios.

WHEN TO REFER?

The HCP needs to know when it is appropriate to refer a patient to another clinician with specific expertise in pharmacologic management of obesity. Below are some suggested criteria:

- Lack of familiarity with antiobesity medications
- Complicated medication regimen, including drug-drug interactions or polypharmacy
- Complicated patient with multiple comorbid conditions
- Insufficient staff to monitor weight and other parameters (blood pressure) monthly at the start of therapy

Investigational Approaches

There are three phase III compounds under study, as follows:

1. Setmelanotide, a melanocortin-4 receptor agonist being evaluated for rare genetic obesity syndromes. This will be the first "personalized obesity therapy" since it will require specific genetic alterations for its use.
2. Semaglutide 2.4 mg, a GLP-1 receptor agonist that is given once weekly by subcutaneous injection. This drug produces about twice as much weight loss as is currently being achieved with liraglutide 3.0 mg. The compound also impacts glycemia. This will mark the second generation of GLP-1 targeted agents and will usher in a new era of achievable weight loss.
3. Tirzepatide, a single-molecule dual-action compound. This molecule targets both the GLP-1 receptor and the GIP receptor. In a phase 2 trial, it produces mean weight loss in the range of ~12% and has potent effects on glycemia.

In addition to these exciting phase 3 drugs on the horizon, the earlier drug discovery field is also promising. Most interesting are the development and alteration of peptides to target multiple receptors in the glucagon superfamily (GLP-1, GIP and glucagon). These altered physiologic compounds will have remarkable pharmacologic effects, producing more weight loss and perhaps impacting not only food intake, but also energy expenditure. Pharmaceutical companies are also exploring combination approaches, particularly with other biologic agents such as pramlintide and PYY.

Dietary Supplements for Obesity

Due to the challenges of long-term adherence with behavioral intervention and patients' frustration with high rates of weight regain, many patients revert to dietary supplements that have been touted to lead to weight loss. Manufacturers often advocate that their supplements reduce appetite, alter body composition, reduce body fat, and increase thermogenesis. The supplement industry is not regulated by the FDA, and many studies have shown that what is reported to be active ingredients often is not. Common ingredients in dietary supplements for weight loss include herbs and other plant components, dietary fiber, caffeine, and minerals.[35] There have been instances of dietary supplements surreptitiously having amphetamines or other stimulants in them which has caused dangerous side effects in consumers.[36] Fifteen percent of Americans report trying a dietary supplement for weight loss, and the supplement industry in the United States is a $2.1 billion business due to advertising of unrealistic expectations and unproven benefits. When a patient is evaluated for management of overweight or obesity in the primary care setting, a physician should ask about over-the-counter dietary supplements that the patient is using to fully reconcile medications. Patients should be advised not to take non–FDA-approved supplements for weight loss without consulting their physician.

SUMMARY

Every HCP knows that patients struggle to lose weight and maintain weight loss. It is common for HCPs to point out one's overweight or obesity but not prescribe structured interventions on how to lose weight. One component of comprehensively managing patients with obesity includes knowing the currently available medications that can be prescribed as an adjunct to lifestyle modification. HCPs can have confidence that several medicines have been rigorously evaluated for efficacy and safety and learn to use these in practice. Understanding the indications, basic mechanisms, contraindications and scenarios of appropriate use is important to increase prescriber confidence and competence. Effective weight management can mitigate and remediate many of the chronic diseases that are addressed in primary care. Medications are tools for effective weight management. This chapter gives practical advice and useful tips for maximizing successful weight loss with medications used as an adjunct to lifestyle intervention.

QUIZ QUESTIONS

1. A 30-year-old male presents to his primary care provider for an annual visit. His BMI has increased from 30 to 32 kg/m² since his last visit 1 year ago. The patient has a history of major depression and reports a recent worsening of his mood. He was started on a trial of fluoxetine by his psychiatrist and told to address his weight with his primary provider with the hope that weight loss could improve his mood. The patient previously was very active and did yoga regularly. He says he has been trying to address portion size and snacking but finds sweets comforting. He is interested in hearing more about any medication that can help control his weight gain and cravings for sweets. Medically, he uses tramadol on an intermittent basis for low-back pain. Upon your evaluation, he denies suicidal ideation and his vital signs, physical examination,

and laboratory studies are normal. The patient is on governmental insurance and has limited medication coverage. In addition to optimizing his nutrition, sleep, stress, and physical activity, which antiobesity medication would be most appropriate?

A. Phentermine

B. Naltrexone/bupropion

C. Liraglutide

D. Phentermine/topiramate

E. Orlistat

Answer: A. *Phentermine is the most appropriate choice due to its lowest out of pocket cost and no contraindications. Naltrexone is contraindicated with use of opiates or with tramadol. Orlistat does not affect appetite, and the patient says appetite is a problem. Liraglutide and phentermine/topiramate would also be appropriate, but given the higher cost, would be considered as second-line agents in this context.*

2. A 28-year-old female, with a BMI of 34 kg/m², comes to you for help with weight loss. She has been following a commercial weight loss program for several months and has lost about 15 pounds but feels as though she is at a plateau and is feeling hungry. Her past medical history is significant for anxiety and a seizure disorder managed on levetiracetam. She has two children and has had a tubal ligation. The patient is particularly interested in medication that might help control her appetite, especially as she tries to move forward without using the packaged meals her previous weight loss program provided. Her BP is 125/80, HR 70 bpm, and the rest of her physical examination is normal. Her only abnormal laboratory value is a hemoglobin A1c of 6.1%. In addition to working with you to optimize her lifestyle, which of the following options would be preferred in this patient?

A. Phentermine/topiramate ER

B. Naltrexone ER/bupropion ER

C. Liraglutide

D. Phentermine

E. Orlistat

Answer: C. *Liraglutide is the best answer due to no effect on seizure threshold and improvement in glucose. Anything with a stimulant effect such as phentermine or bupropion may exacerbate her anxiety. She meets criteria for antiobesity pharmacotherapy based on her BMI alone, but she also has comorbidities of her obesity.*

PRACTICAL RESOURCES

- *Obesity* patient handouts (https://www.obesity.org/information-for-patients/); the journal *Obesity* developed patient handouts that are available at this source. They describe a variety of approaches and can be downloaded and printed.
- Full Guideline: Pharmacological Management of Obesity (https://www.endocrine.org/guidelines-and-clinical-practice/clinical-practice-guidelines/pharmacological-management-of-obesity); the Endocrine Society provides online access and download of the Full Guideline: Pharmacological Management of Obesity from JCEM in February 2016.
- American Board of Obesity Medicine (https://www.abom.org); the American Board of Obesity Medicine is a key resource for certifying physicians.
- Obesity Medicine Association (https://obesitymedicine.org); the Obesity Medicine Association (OMA) provides an annually updated obesity treatment algorithm that includes information on medicating the patient with obesity.

REFERENCES

1. Hales CM, Carroll MD, Fryar CD, Ogden CL. *Prevalence of Obesity Among Adults and Youth: United States, 2015-2016. NCHS Data Brief, No 288.* National Center for Health Statistics; 2017.

2. Jensen MD, Ryan DH, Donato KA, et al. Guidelines (2013) for managing overweight and obesity in adults. *Obesity (Silver Spring).* 2014;22(S2):S1-S410.

3. Apovian CM, Aronne LJ, Bessesen DH, et al; Endocrine Society. Pharmacological management of obesity: an Endocrine Society clinical practice guideline. *J Clin Endocrinol Metab.* 2015;100(2):342-362. Erratum in: *J Clin Endocrinol Metab.* 2015;100(5):2135-2136.

4. Garvey WT, Mechanick JI, Brett EM, et al; Reviewers of the AACE/ACE Obesity Clinical Practice Guidelines. American Association of Clinical Endocrinologists and American College of Endocrinology Comprehensive clinical practice guidelines for medical care of patients with obesity. *Endocr Pract.* 2016;22(7):842-884.

5. Garvey WT, Mechanick JI, Brett EM, et al. American Association of Clinical Endocrinologists and American College of Endocrinology comprehensive clinical practice guidelines for medical care of patients with obesity. *Endocr Pract.* 2016;22(suppl 3):1-203.

6. Berthoud HR, Munzberg H, Morrison CD. Blaming the brain for obesity: Integration of hedonic and homeostatic mechanisms. *Gastroenterology.* 2017;152:1728-1738.

7. The Look AHEAD Research Group. Reduction in weight and cardiovascular disease risk factors in individuals with type 2 diabetes: one-year results of the Look AHEAD trial. *Diabetes Care.* 2007;30(6):1374-1383.

8. Look AHEAD Research Group; Wing RR. Long-term effects of a lifestyle intervention on weight and cardiovascular risk factors in individuals with type 2 diabetes mellitus: four-year results of the Look AHEAD trial. *Arch Intern Med.* 2010;170(17):1566-1575.

9. Wadden TA, Butrin ML, Hong PS, Tsai AG. Behavioral treatment of obesity in patients encountered in primary care settings: a systematic review. *J Am Med Assoc.* 2014;312(17):1779-1791.

10. Ryan DH, Yockey SR. Weight loss and improvement in comorbidity: Differences at 5%, 10%, 15%, and over. *Curr Obes Rep.* 2017;6(2):187-194.

11. Phentermine/topiramate (Qsymia) prescribing information. Accessed June 19, 2019. https://www.accessdata.fda.gov/drugsatfda_docs/label/2012/022580s000lbl.pdf

12. Naltrexone SR/Bupropion SR (Contrave®). FDA prescribing information. Accessed June 20, 2019. https://www.accessdata.fda.gov/drugsatfda_docs/label/2014/200063s000lbl.pdf

13. Saxenda® prescribing information. Accessed June 19, 2019. https://www.novo-pi.com/saxenda.pdf

14. Accessed February 24, 2020. https://www.accessdata.fda.gov/drugsatfda_docs/label/2012/022529lbl.pdf

15. Cadegiani FA, Diniz GC, Alves G. Aggressive clinical approach to obesity improves metabolic and clinical outcomes and can prevent bariatric surgery: a single center experience. *BMC Obesity.* 2017;4:9.

16. Erdmann J, Lippi F, Klose G, Schusdziarra V. Cholesterol lowering effect of dietary weight loss and orlistat treatment – efficacy and limitations. *Aliment Pharmacol Ther.* 2004;19(11):1173-1179.

17. Lomaira (phentermine) 8 mg prescribing information. Accessed June 19, 2019. https://lomaira.com/Prescribing_Information.pdf

18. Phentermine (ADIPEX-P) prescribing information. Accessed June 19, 2019. https://www.accessdata.fda.gov/drugsatfda_docs/label/2012/085128s065lbl.pdf

19. Aronne LJ1, Wadden TA, Peterson C, Winslow D, Odeh S, Gadde KM. Evaluation of phentermine and topiramate versus phentermine/topiramate extended release in obese adults. *Obesity (Silver Spring).* 2013;21(11):2163-2171.

20. Hirsch J1, Mackintosh RM, Aronne LJ. The effects of drugs used to treat obesity on the autonomic nervous system. *Obes Res.* 2000;8(3):227-233.

21. https://www.fda.gov/drugs/drug-safety-and-availability/safety-clinical-trial-shows-possible-increased-risk-cancer-weight-loss-medicine-belviq-belviq-xr

22. Bohula EA, Wiviott SD, McGuire DK, et al; on behalf of the CAMELLIA–TIMI 61 Steering Committee and Investigators. Cardiovascular safety of lorcaserin in overweight or obese patients. *N Engl J Med* 2018;379:1107-1117.

23. Bohula EA, Scirica BM, Inzucchi SE, McGuire DK, et al; CAMELLIA-TIMI 61 Steering Committee Investigators. Effect of lorcaserin on prevention and remission of type 2 diabetes in overweight and obese patients (CAMELLIA-TIMI 61): a randomized, placebo-controlled trial. *Lancet.* 2018;392:2269-2279.

24. Sharretts J, Galescu O, Gomatam S, et al. Cancer risk associated with lorcaserin—The FDA's review of the CAMELLIA-TIMI 61 trial. *N Engl J Med.* 2020;383:1000-1002.

25. Le Roux CW, Astrup A, Fujioka K, et al; SCALE Obesity Prediabetes NN8022-1839 Study Group. 3 years of liraglutide versus placebo for type 2 diabetes risk reduction and weight management in individuals with prediabetes: a randomized, double-blind trial. *Lancet.* 2016;389(10077):1399-1409.

26. Marso SP, Daniels GH, Brown-Frandsen K, et al; LEADER Steering Committee; LEADER Trial Investigators. Liraglutide and cardiovascular outcomes in type 2 diabetes. *N Engl J Med.* 2016;375:311-322.

27. Wadden TA, Hollander P, Klein S, et al; NN8022-1923 Investigators. Weight maintenance and additional weight loss with liraglutide after low-calorie-diet-induced weight loss: the SCALE Maintenance randomized study. *Int J Obes (Lond).* 2013;37(11):1443-1451.

28. Orlistat (Xenical) prescribing information. Accessed June 20, 2019. https://www.accessdata.fda.gov/drugsatfda_docs/label/2009/020766s026lbl.pdf

29. Cavaliere H, Floriano I, Medeiros-Neto G. Gastrointestinal side effects of orlistat may be prevented by concomitant prescription of natural fibers (psyllium mucilloid). *Int J Obes Relat Metab Disord.* 2001;2(7):1095-1099.

30. Chanoine JP, Hampl S, Jensen C, Boldrin M, Hauptman J. Effect of orlistat on weight and body composition in obese adolescents: a randomized controlled trial. *J Am Med Assoc.* 2005;293(23):2873-2883.

31. Khera R, Murad MH, Chandar AK, et al. Association of pharmacological treatments for obesity with weight loss and adverse events. A systematic review and meta-analysis. *J Am Med Assoc.* 2016;315, 2424-2434.

32. Greenway FL, Aronne LJ, Raben A. et al. A randomized, double-blind, placebo-controlled study of gelesis100: a novel nonsystemic oral hydrogel for weight loss. *Obesity (Silver Spring).* 2019;27:205-216.

33. Fox CK, Kelly AS. The potential role of combination pharmacotherapy to improve outcomes of pediatric obesity: a case report and discussion. *Front Pediatr.* 2018;6:361.

34. Wilding JP. Combination therapy for obesity. *J Psychopharmacol.* 2017;31(11):1503-1508.

35. Sharpe PA, Granner ML, Conway JM, Ainsworth BE, Dobre M. Availability of weight-loss supplements: results of an audit of retail outlets in a southeastern city. *J Am Diet Assoc.* 2006;106:2045-2051.

36. U.S. Food and Drug Administration. *Tainted Weight Loss Products.* 2017. Accessed March 22, 2020. https://www.fda.gov/drugs/medication-health-fraud/tainted-weight-loss-products

9

METABOLIC AND BARIATRIC SURGERY

Wayne J. English, Vance L. Albaugh

CASE STUDY 1

Ms. Jane M is a 45-year-old woman and has been your patient for 20 years. She comes in annually for routine evaluations and has no major medical problems. She had overweight when you first started seeing her, but her weight has slowly increased yearly despite multiple behavioral and dietary interventions prescribed by you in the past. She now has a diagnosis of class 3 obesity with a body mass index (BMI) of 41 kg/m² and you are considering referring her for a surgical weight loss consultation.

CLINICAL SIGNIFICANCE

Obesity is a disease that affects the entire patient, both physically and psychologically, and requires a multidisciplinary treatment approach for long-term success. Despite an increased focus on identifying and developing more effective treatments for obesity, an increased awareness of its associated comorbid conditions, and increasing costs on the healthcare system, its prevalence continues to rise. It is predicted that obesity will affect almost 50% of American adults by the year 2030.[1] For some patients, bariatric surgery is a good treatment option.

METABOLIC AND BARIATRIC SURGERY AS AN EFFECTIVE OBESITY TREATMENT OPTION

Numerous clinical studies have demonstrated beneficial effects of bariatric surgery on weight loss, mostly compared with lifestyle intervention.[2,3] More recent data has demonstrated that in addition to weight loss, bariatric surgery is also associated with decreased incidence of cancer and decreased risk of cardiovascular mortality compared to nonsurgical control subjects.[4,5] All of these studies demonstrate the combined impact of bariatric surgery on weight loss along with decreased cardiovascular mortality.

Metabolic and bariatric surgery continues to become increasingly recognized (a 60% increase in the number of procedures performed has been noted since 2011) as the most effective and sustained treatment available for patient with moderate to severe obesity with associated medical conditions. These procedures are typically performed using minimally invasive techniques that result in short hospital stays and minimal postoperative pain. The advances the bariatric surgical field has continued to make in terms of patient safety and outcomes will no doubt continue to fuel the growth of this field.

The American Association of Clinical Endocrinologists (AACE) Task Force on Obesity in 2011 recommended that surgery is indicated in high-risk patients with obesity and that significant evidence exists to classify obesity as a disease. AACE updated obesity treatment guidelines in 2019, initially created in 2013, which was cosponsored by the American College of Endocrinology, The Obesity Society (TOS), American Society for Metabolic & Bariatric Surgery (ASMBS), Obesity Medicine Association (OMA), and American Society of Anesthesiologists and subsequently endorsed by the American Society for Nutrition (ASN), the Obesity Action Coalition (OAC), and the American Society for Parenteral and Enteral Nutrition (ASPEN). These clinical practice guidelines provide valuable information pertaining to the preoperative and postoperative nutrition and metabolic and nonsurgical care for metabolic and bariatric patients.

Despite the documented benefits of bariatric surgery, healthcare professionals (HCPs) may be hesitant to recommend these procedures to their patients due to wanting to "do no harm"; questioning the long-term effectiveness of surgery; limited knowledge about surgery; not wanting to recommend surgery too early; and not knowing if insurance would cover surgery.[6] This chapter will address some of these knowledge gaps and review primary procedures commonly performed in the United States, indications, contraindications, and psychological and other special considerations when electing to refer a patient for metabolic and bariatric surgery in the primary care setting. This chapter will also discuss risks, as well as the short- and long-term results, that can be expected for the overwhelming majority of patients. Commonly held misconceptions will also be addressed, specifically through case examples that demonstrate the decision-making during the evaluation of the patient with obesity considering metabolic and bariatric surgery.

TYPES OF PROCEDURES

Sleeve Gastrectomy

The vertical sleeve gastrectomy (VSG) is the most common procedure performed in the United States, representing approximately 61% of all metabolic and bariatric procedures performed in 2018. In this procedure, gastric volume is reduced by approximately 75% to 80%. This is accomplished by removing the greater curvature segment of the stomach with the pylorus being preserved. An intraluminal bougie is placed along the lesser curvature of the stomach and gastric resection begins approximately 5 to 6 cm proximal to the pylorus along the greater curvature. The stomach is then transected vertically toward, but not including, the angle of His (Figure 9.1).

Initially, the VSG was thought to be purely restrictive, but it is now known that endocrine cells responsible for producing ghrelin, a gastrointestinal hunger hormone, are primarily distributed with the stomach and are removed with the gastric segment. Subsequently, decreased hunger and improved glucose metabolism are seen after VSG. The stomach also empties faster after VSG, leading to rapid exposure of nutrients within the small intestines and earlier neurohormonal activity leading to alteration of hunger and satiety.[7]

When compared to Roux-en-Y gastric bypass (RYGB), the VSG has a slight safety advantage, namely avoiding the risks of bowel obstruction or marginal ulcers. Chronic nonsteroidal anti-inflammatory drugs (NSAIDs) and aspirin (ASA) use after gastric bypass are thought to cause marginal ulcers; therefore, a VSG may be a better option for patients requiring these medications. However, a low-dose ASA daily appears to be well tolerated by gastric bypass patients without major risks of marginal ulceration.[8] The main disadvantages of VSG is that gastroesophageal reflux disease (GERD) may

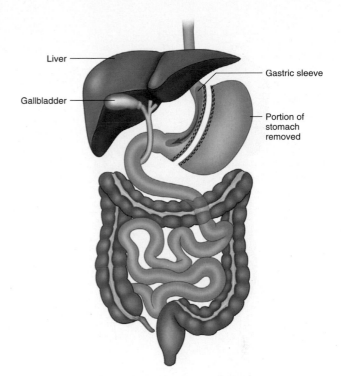

Liver

Gallbladder

Gastric sleeve

Portion of stomach removed

FIGURE 9.1 Vertical sleeve gastrectomy.

significantly worsen in approximately 30% of patients, and resolution of type 2 diabetes mellitus (T2DM) is not experienced as often with an odds ratio of 2.11, compared with 3.51 seen after RYGB.[9,10]

Roux-en-Y Gastric Bypass

RYGB involves creating a small gastric pouch measuring approximately 15 to 30 mL, causing a restriction in food intake. Additionally, malabsorption is seen due to the rearrangement of the small intestine and diversion of nutrient flow to the small intestine away from the duodenum and proximal jejunum. The jejunum, approximately 50 cm distal to the ligament of Treitz, is divided and the proximal end is reconnected to the small intestines after measuring an additional 100 to 150 cm distally. A jejunojejunostomy is created to re-establish bile and pancreatic enzyme flow into the distal small intestine. The gastrojejunostomy is then created by attaching the initial distal end divided to the gastric pouch.

The small intestine from the ligament of Treitz to the jejunojejunostomy is referred to as the biliopancreatic, or nonalimentary, limb. The segment of the intestine between the gastric pouch and jejunojejunostomy is the Roux, or alimentary, limb and the remaining small intestine from the jejunojejunostomy to the ileocecal valve is the common channel (Figure 9.2).

In addition to causing nutritional malabsorption, the gastric bypass diverts gastric secretions and bile immediately into the mid-jejunal segment resulting in

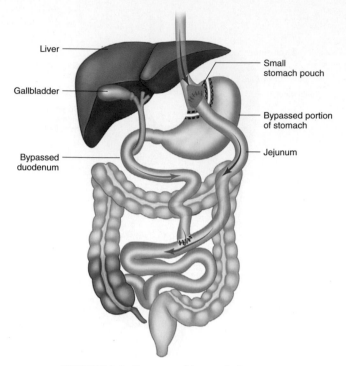

FIGURE 9.2 Roux-en-Y gastric bypass.

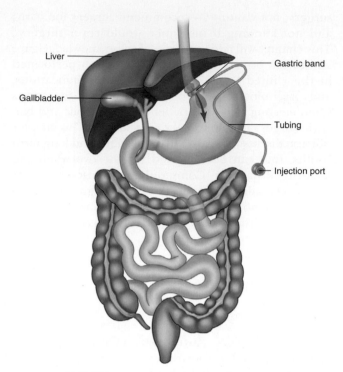

FIGURE 9.3 Adjustable gastric band.

complex neurohormonal, bile acid, and microbiome alterations that affect hunger, satiety, insulin sensitivity, and glucose homeostasis.[11]

Gastric Banding

Adjustable gastric banding (AGB) is a purely restrictive procedure, creating a compression of the proximal stomach with an adjustable balloon that reduces gastric outflow. During the procedure, a retrogastric passage is created toward the angle of His and the gastric band is pulled through, wrapped around the proximal stomach, and buckled closed. Fixation sutures are placed anteriorly to secure the band into position. The tubing is pulled through one of the laparoscopic port sites and attached to the AGB subcutaneous port, which is then sutured to the rectus muscle fascia to stabilize it for future access. Changing the aperture of the band alters gastric outflow and is accomplished by accessing the port with a specialized needle to inflate or deflate the band (Figure 9.3).

Earlier studies demonstrated effective weight loss and comorbidity resolution, but it has been shown to be relatively ineffective for producing sustained weight loss and resolution of comorbidities. Furthermore, interventions to address complications or weight loss failure represented up to 77% of insurance payments related to AGB. Complication rates reported are as high as 56% and include gastric prolapse, band slippage, erosion, dysphagia, GERD, and esophageal dysmotility.[12] These complications can occur any time from weeks to even many years (>5 to 10+ years) from AGB placement and can have an indolent course. For example, reflux, heartburn, and epigastric pain can slowly progress over years. Additionally, cellulitis at the subcutaneous port is many times the earliest sign of an eroded AGB, which necessitates surgical consultation for removal. A referral to the bariatric surgeon is strongly recommended if there are any questions whether symptoms are being caused by the AGB.

The AGB was approved by the Federal Drug Administration in 2001. The procedures performed annually reached its peak in the United States in 2009, when it comprised over 40% of all metabolic and bariatric procedures. Conversely, in 2018, it represents only 1.1% of all metabolic and bariatric procedures performed and the trend appears to be steadily declining.

Biliopancreatic Diversion With Duodenal Switch

Biliopancreatic diversion with duodenal switch (BPD/DS) represented only 0.8% of all metabolic and bariatric procedures performed in the United States in 2018. While it is infrequently performed compared to the VSG and RYGB, it delivers the best results when considering durable weight loss and comorbidity resolution.[9]

Bile and pancreatic secretions to the distal small intestine are diverted, considerably further distally than gastric bypass. The procedure was initially performed with a partial gastrectomy and pyloric resection and

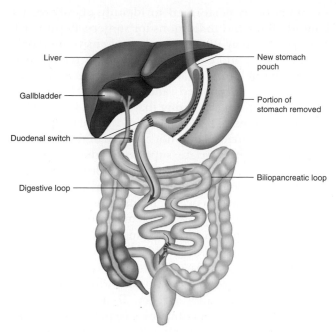

FIGURE 9.4 Biliopancreatic diversion with duodenal switch.

Labels: Liver, Gallbladder, Duodenal switch, Digestive loop, New stomach pouch, Portion of stomach removed, Biliopancreatic loop

was known as the BPD. However, a pylorus-preserving technique was adopted and is now the most common technique performed today. This adaptation is known as the duodenal switch.

The pylorus-preserving DS procedure involves a VSG as the initial component of the procedure, but a larger sized bougie is used. The second component of the procedure involves dividing the ileum and duodenum. The distal stapled end of the ileum is then connected to the proximal stapled end of the duodenum, creating a duodenoileostomy. The proximal stapled end of the ileum is attached more distally toward the terminal ileum, creating an ileoileostomy, effectively diverting all bile and pancreatic enzymes to the distal ileum. The common channel often measures between 50 and 100 cm in length, but one of the main disadvantages of this procedure is a greater potential for electrolyte abnormalities and protein malabsorption compared to the RYGB. As a result, some surgeons have increased the common channel lengths to 200 cm or more (Figure 9.4). In comparison to other metabolic and bariatric procedures, BPD/DS is associated with the highest resolution of type 2 diabetes (T2D).[9]

INDICATIONS AND CONTRAINDICATIONS

Indications for metabolic and bariatric surgery endorsed by the National Institutes of Health (NIH) are outlined in the publication "Clinical Guidelines

on the Identification, Evaluation, and Treatment of Overweight and Obesity in Adults." The NIH specified that surgery is an effective obesity treatment option for patients with a BMI of 40 kg/m² or 35 kg/m² with obesity-related comorbidities, primarily hypertension, T2D, dyslipidemia, and obstructive sleep apnea (http://www.nhlbi.nih.gov/guidelines/obesity/ob_gdlns.pdf). Additionally, metabolic and bariatric surgery has been shown to be of value in patients with class 1 obesity (BMI between 30 and 35 kg/m²) and severe uncontrolled diabetes. While only a few insurance companies in the United States authorize surgery for patients in this category, it is fully supported within the European guidelines for metabolic and bariatric surgery.[13] The center in which you refer your patient will know if class 1 obesity is a covered insurance benefit for your patient.

Absolute contraindications for metabolic and bariatric surgery may include, but are not limited to:

- Uncontrolled depression
- Uncontrolled anxiety
- Uncontrolled bipolar disorder
- Active substance abuse (drugs/alcohol)
- Suicidal ideation
- Borderline personality disorder
- Schizophrenia
- Significant eating disorder
- Acute psychosis
- Defined noncompliance with previous medical or psychological care
- Unwilling to comply with necessary guidelines following bariatric surgery
- Hormonal causes of obesity that can be medically treated
- Severe cardiopulmonary disease

Some surgeons may not consider schizophrenia as an absolute contraindication, but a relative contraindication depending on whether the patient is highly functional and has readily available psychiatric and psychological support in the postoperative period. Additionally, advanced cardiopulmonary disease may be considered a relative contraindication by some surgeons. It is imperative that you refer patients with increased risk to centers that are experienced in dealing with these types of complex issues.

Relative contraindications for metabolic and bariatric surgery in which a decision to proceed with surgery will be made on an individual basis include, but is not limited to:

- History of cancer within previous 5 years
- Hepatic cirrhosis
- Collagen vascular disease
- Inflammatory bowel disease (IBD)
- Down syndrome or intellectual disability

Decisions to operate on patients are typically based on available resources at the metabolic and bariatric center and the discretion of the surgeon. Many surgeons will consider performing metabolic and bariatric surgery on patients with cancer prior to 5 years from their diagnosis if the cancer is associated with a low recurrence risk and are no longer receiving treatment. Advanced cirrhosis with portal hypertension would be considered an absolute contraindication by most surgeons. Furthermore, severe active ulcerative colitis or Crohn's disease may be considered an absolute contraindication by most surgeons as it is preferable to perform surgery under conditions in which symptoms are stabilized (a case study below reviews a patient with IBD).

PREOPERATIVE EVALUATION

It is essential that patients receive preoperative education, medical and psychological evaluations, and dietary preparation (Table 9.1). The preoperative evaluation must be comprehensive to identify potential treatable causes of obesity and determine factors that will increase risks for potential complications. The goal is to optimize, or prehabilitate, a patient's health and modify risk factors to ensure surgery is performed under optimal conditions. A complete history and physical examination is performed to identify obesity-related comorbidities and indications for surgery. Routine laboratory tests may include a comprehensive metabolic profile (CMP) and complete blood count (CBC), lipid profile, thyroid function, urinalysis, prothrombin time/international normalized ratio (PT/INR), blood type, and micronutrient screening that includes iron studies, ferritin, vitamin B12, folic acid, and 25-OH vitamin D. Insurance companies may not cover all of these lab tests without the appropriate supporting diagnoses and, at a minimum, a CBC and CMP should be obtained. The nutrient screening is essential in the postoperative period and is usually covered by insurance with the supporting diagnosis of postsurgical malabsorption.

Dietary and psychological evaluations are vital in the preoperative assessment to identify possible areas of concern, such as binge eating disorder, night eating syndrome, or undiagnosed depression, which could compromise outcomes after surgery. To accomplish these goals, most insurance companies require that patients undergo a dietary and psychological assessment prior to bariatric surgery and are typically performed within the comprehensive bariatric surgical center. Furthermore, most centers have preoperative protocols that mandate attendance at one more group classes. Patients are taught how they will need to eat following surgery and learn coping strategies when faced with behavioral and dietary challenges. Understanding your patient's

---

TABLE 9.1 Preoperative Checklist

PREOPERATIVE CHECKLIST FOR METABOLIC AND BARIATRIC SURGERY

• Comprehensive history and physical	• Identify treatable causes of obesity and treat, if present
	• Look for inclusion criteria meeting the National Institutes of Health and insurance criteria
	• Note contraindications for surgery, if present
	• Document medical necessity for surgery including obesity-related comorbidities, weight, body mass index
	• Assess patient level of commitment
	• Identify history of cancer, if present
	• Assess for nicotine use (smoking, vaping, patch, chewing, etc.) and require nicotine cessation; refer for counseling if needed
• Routine labs	• Complete blood count and comprehensive metabolic profile, including fasting blood glucose and liver function tests, are routine during initial consultation
	• Other recommended labs, if indicated, include thyroid function, lipid profile and glycated hemoglobin, urinalysis, prothrombin time, and partial thromboplastin time
	• Type and screen just prior to surgery
• Additional nutrition labs, if indicated	• Iron, TIBC, ferritin, vitamin B12, folic acid, 25-OH vitamin D, parathyroid hormone levels
• Dietary evaluation	• Educate about dietary behavior required postsurgery
	• Educate about potential for vitamin and mineral deficiencies in the postoperative period
	• Review body composition and energy balance
	• Set weight loss goals and manage discrepancies

TABLE 9.1 Preoperative Checklist (Continued)

PREOPERATIVE CHECKLIST FOR METABOLIC AND BARIATRIC SURGERY

• Psychological evaluation (includes lifestyle assessment)	• Assess healthy eating index and identify binge eating and night eating disorder, and treat if present • Assess overall mood and identify untreated depression, and treat if present • Assess for substance and alcohol abuse, and treat if present • Identify medications that may contribute to suboptimal weight loss • Assess overall support structure • Identify need for further behavioral support and counseling
• Cardiology evaluation, if indicated	• Electrocardiogram • Echocardiogram • Stress testing • Cardiac catheterization • Optimization of hypertension

• Pulmonary evaluation, if indicated	• Sleep apnea screening
	  • STOP-BANG questionnaire
	  • Epworth Sleepiness Scale
	• Optimization of COPD, asthma

• Gastrointestinal (GI) evaluation, if indicated	• Esophagogastroduodenoscopy • Upper GI contrast study • *Helicobacter pylori* testing • Gallbladder ultrasound • Colonoscopy
• Endocrine evaluation, if indicated	• Optimization of diabetes mellitus • Glycated hemoglobin • Dexamethasone test • 24-Hour urinary cortisol • Thyroid-stimulating hormone • Testosterone • Dehydroepiandrosterone
• Insurance prerequisites, if applicable	• Confirm patient has benefits covering metabolic and bariatric surgery • Preoperative weight management documentation • Documented weight loss prior to surgery

goals is important to the overall success after surgery as there may be discrepancies between a patient's weight loss goals and the realistic weight loss potentially realized after surgery. Numerous factors may influence a patient's ability to achieve an optimal result after surgery, including psychological profiles as described above, comorbidities, medications that may lead to suboptimal weight loss, age and metabolism, body composition, and energy balance. A comprehensive metabolic and bariatric surgery center is committed to identifying variations in any of these factors which may predispose a patient to insufficient weight loss outcomes or weight regain after experiencing a satisfactory weight nadir.

Cardiopulmonary evaluation is often required in patients interested in having metabolic and bariatric surgery. Cardiology evaluations for risk assessment should follow standards of practice for perioperative evaluation and management of patients undergoing noncardiac surgery, which may include electrocardiogram, echocardiogram, stress testing, and cardiac catheterization as indicated.[14] Patients with previous history of unprovoked deep vein thrombosis or pulmonary embolism should undergo a formal hematology evaluation to rule out a hypercoagulable state. Pulmonary clearance should be obtained in patients with significant chronic obstructive pulmonary disease in order to optimize patients prior to surgery. Chest x-rays are not routinely obtained unless clinically indicated. A sleep study is indicated in patients with significant snoring, witnessed apnea episodes, morning headaches, daytime sleepiness, and significant oxygen desaturation on overnight pulse oximetry. Screening using the Epworth Sleepiness Scale or STOP-BANG questionnaire may help to identify at-risk patients to refer for an overnight polysomnogram (Table 9.2).[15,16] Patients newly diagnosed with obstructive sleep apnea should implement continuous positive airway pressure (CPAP) treatment to optimize their pulmonary status for at least 1 month prior to surgery.

Gastrointestinal (GI) evaluations are often obtained as clinically indicated. Some centers routinely obtain esophagogastroduodenoscopy (EGD) on all patients, while others are more selective and perform preoperative EGDs only when indicated, such as a history of dyspepsia, reflux, dysphagia, or previous ulcer disease. *Helicobacter pylori* screening is not routinely performed but should be considered in regions of high prevalence and treated with triple antibiotic regimen if tested positive. A gallbladder ultrasound may be obtained routinely by some surgeons but is usually ordered selectively as clinically indicated. If cholelithiasis is present, surgeons may elect to perform a cholecystectomy concurrently with the metabolic and bariatric procedure.

TABLE 9.2 Epworth Sleepiness Scale and STOP-BANG Questionnaire Used for Obstructive Sleep Apnea Screening

Epworth Sleepiness Scale	Use the following point tabulation for each question
0-10: Normal range 10-12: Borderline 12-24: Abnormal	0: No chance of dozing 1: Minimal chance of dozing 2: Moderate chance of dozing 3: High chance of dozing
	How likely are you to doze off or sleep during the following? **1.** Sitting or reading? **2.** Watching television? **3.** Sitting inactive in a public space? **4.** As a passenger in a car for an hour without a break? **5.** Lying down to rest when circumstances permit? **6.** Sitting and talking to someone? **7.** Sitting quietly after lunch without alcohol? **8.** In a car, while stopped for a few minutes in traffic?
STOP-BANG Questionnaire	Use the following point tabulation for each question
0-2: Low risk 3-4: Intermediate risk 5-8: High risk	0: No 1: Yes S: Snore loudly? T: Feel tired during the day? O: Observe apnea while sleeping? P: Treated for high blood pressure? B: Body mass index ≥ 35 kg/m^2 A: Age ≥ 50 years N: Neck circumference • Male ≥ 17 inches • Female ≥ 16 inches G: Gender—male

Endocrine evaluations for patients with severe uncontrolled diabetes despite taking multiple medications should be considered since hyperglycemia is associated with increased risk for infection, poor wound healing, and extended hospitalization. A preoperative glycated hemoglobin level of ≤8% should be achieved, if possible. A serum thyroid-stimulating hormone level should be obtained if clinical evidence of hypothyroid is present and treated accordingly. Screening for PCOS and Cushing syndrome should be only be conducted if clinically indicated.

PSYCHOLOGICAL CONSIDERATIONS

The principal goal for the preoperative psychosocial evaluation in patients preparing for metabolic and bariatric surgery is to ensure patients are committed to the necessary lifelong changes after surgery, but most importantly to identify those with increased risk for potential relapse of preexisting depression or behavioral eating disorders and subsequently address potential issues that may contribute to a poor postoperative outcome.

Patients with class 2 (BMI 35.0 to 39.9 kg/m^2) and 3 (BMI ≥40 kg/m^2) obesity often carry a diagnosis of depression, anxiety, and other stress-related conditions including eating disorders. They also often battle with body image and poor self-esteem issues. The psychologist can help patients develop coping strategies to ensure a more positive outcome after surgery. To underscore the importance of having continued behavioral health services available in the postoperative period, patients with a diagnosed psychological health disorder were noted in one study to have 34% increased odds of 30-day readmission when compared with patients who did not have a mental health disorder diagnosis. The odds were even greater (46%) in patients diagnosed with depression or bipolar disorder. Careful consideration must be given to patients with depression taking antidepressants who undergo an RYGB procedure as medication malabsorption may exacerbate symptoms.

An awareness of the potential for excessive alcohol and illicit substance use following surgery is critical as patients may seek substitutes to attain the dopaminergic reward previously achieved with food. Obesity-induced dysregulation of dopamine reward processing, in theory, can result in compensatory overeating, and this process is thought to be reversed after RYGB.

Finally, there are some studies suggesting that there are potentially increased risks for self-harm and suicide after metabolic and bariatric surgery. However, other studies argue the increased risks were already present prior to surgery and that patients need to be monitored carefully in the postoperative period.[17] A number of psychosocial issues that might potentially attribute to suicide include the lack of improvement in quality of life, physical limitation, sexual dysfunction, relationship, or low self-esteem. Additional factors to consider include a prior history of being abused or perceived postoperative failure due to insufficient weight loss or weight regain.

WEIGHT LOSS REQUIREMENTS PRIOR TO SURGERY

Preoperative medical weight management requirements with mandatory weight loss in the preoperative period is often imposed by many insurance companies, and patients may be denied surgery benefits if weight loss is not observed during this time period. However, there is no evidence to support that insurance-mandated preoperative weight loss results in decreased complication rates or improved outcomes after surgery and these practices should be abandoned as it causes unnecessary delays in receiving treatment, contributes to patient attrition, and leads to the progression of obesity-related comorbidities.[18] A preoperative very low calorie diet (VLCD) treatment is prescribed by many surgeons for up to 2 to 4 weeks prior to surgery to achieve substantial liver size reduction, which allows for better exposure of the gastroesophageal region during surgery. A 5% to 20% reduction in liver volume has been demonstrated in patients completing a preoperative VLCD. Additionally, one study demonstrated that greater than 3.5% total weight loss in patients completing VLCD 4 weeks preoperatively was associated with significantly greater weight loss at 12 months postoperatively compared with patients who lost less weight.[19]

PROCEDURE TRENDS

In 2018, approximately 252,000 metabolic and bariatric procedures were performed in the United States, noting a 60% increase in the number of procedures performed compared with 2011. VSG is currently the most common procedure, representing 61% of procedures performed in the United States. The number of RYGB and AGB procedures performed annually has been steadily declining since 2011 and currently account for 17% and 1.1% of all procedures, respectively. But there was slight increase in RYGB noted in 2017 and 2018 in which RYGB represented approximately 17% of all procedures. Revisions of previous metabolic and bariatric procedures, which will be briefly reviewed later in this chapter, continue to rise as increasing numbers of AGB are removed and may soon surpass the number of RYGB procedures being performed annually (Figure 9.5).

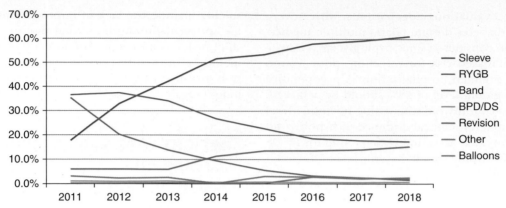

FIGURE 9.5 Metabolic and bariatric surgery procedure trends: 2011-2018. RYGB, Roux-en-Y gastric bypass; BPD/DS, biliopancreatic diversions with duodenal switch.

SAFETY AND EFFICACY OF METABOLIC AND BARIATRIC SURGERY

Metabolic and bariatric surgical procedures are now among the safest performed in the United States. This extraordinary achievement is principally due to the introduction of laparoscopic techniques and national accreditation with a long-standing emphasis on patient safety and continuous quality improvement efforts.

Leading the way in quality improvement efforts is the Metabolic and Bariatric Surgery Accreditation and Quality Improvement Program (MBSAQIP), a joint effort between the American College of Surgeons (ACS) and the American Society of Metabolic and Bariatric Surgery (ASMBS) developed standards that are designed to optimize patient safety and requires centers to enter patient demographic and outcomes data into a national data registry. This data registry allows a comprehensive analysis of safety and outcomes data on a large scale in which centers can use as an opportunity to improve structural and process deficiencies. (See Clinical Highlights for information on how you can refer your patient to an accredited center.)

Moreover, recovery and hospital stay have significantly decreased with the use of enhanced recovery programs designed to decrease postoperative nausea, vomiting, and pain. Nerve blocks lasting for up to 24 hours are administered in the upper abdomen, which allows for a substantial reduction in postoperative opiate use for pain control. Quality and safety improvement efforts utilizing enhanced recovery programs have driven down length of stay, even for patients undergoing the most complex operations. Postoperative patients are typically discharged the first or second postoperative day, most of the time without any necessary laboratory or radiologic testing.

After discharge, the HCP's role in the immediate postoperative period is to manage medications adjustments, especially for T2DM and hypertension, but most importantly to identify emergencies and refer to the surgeon for further evaluation. It is important to refer your patient to the bariatric surgeon for immediate evaluation, or the emergency department, if you suspect an emergency in the initial postoperative period, typically within the first 7 to 10 days after surgery. Signs of a potential emergency include tachycardia, which is the first sign of a potential leak, fever >101.5°F, dyspnea, chest pain, leg pain and swelling, persistent nausea and vomiting, and oral intake intolerance.

Comparative analysis of metabolic and bariatric procedures demonstrates a lower mortality rate than that which is seen with cholecystectomy or hip replacement (0.1%, 0.7% and 0.93%, respectively). Aminian et al reviewed the ACS National Surgical Quality Improvement Program (NSQIP) database to determine the safety of RYGB in patients with T2D compared with patients who underwent other commonly performed nonbariatric laparoscopic procedures. A lower mortality rate, as well as a lower complication rate, was seen in patients undergoing RYGB compared with patients undergoing laparoscopic cholecystectomy, appendectomy, and colectomy (Figures 9.6 and 9.7).[20]

ADVERSE OUTCOMES AFTER METABOLIC AND BARIATRIC SURGERY

The MBSAQIP participant use data file, based on data from approximately 200,000 metabolic and bariatric operations performed in 2018, demonstrates an extremely low morbidity and mortality rates in RYGB and VSG patients. The results show that complications were quite rare for both VSG and RYGB, with most early complications having an incidence of less than

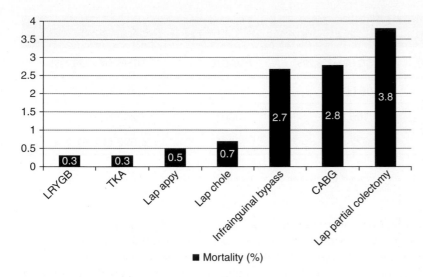

FIGURE 9.6 Comparative 30-day mortality rate between different procedures. Appy, appendectomy; CABG, coronary artery bypass grafting; Chole, cholecystectomy; Lap, laparoscopic; LRYGB, laparoscopic Roux-en-Y gastric bypass; TKA, total knee arthroplasty. (Adapted from Aminian A, Brethauer SA, Kirwan JP, Kashyap SR, Burguera B, Schauer PR. How safe is metabolic/diabetes surgery? *Diabetes Obes Metab.* 2015;17(2):198-201.)

1%. VSG was less likely to experience most of the early complication types (Table 9.3). It should be noted that the venous thromboembolism rate was one of the few perioperative complications that was similar between the two procedures and that portomesenteric and splenic vein thrombosis, although a rare adverse event, has been shown to be more common following VSG (0.4%) than after RYGB (0.2%). The portal vein was the most common vessel involved.

Most potential long-term complications after VSG and RYGB are minor and treatable, such as constipation and dumping syndrome. A few complications are more unfavorable but extremely rare, such as hyperinsulinemic hypoglycemia and autonomic dysfunction. The relatively more common late complications and the corresponding reported incidence rates are listed in Table 9.4. It should be noted that although GERD symptoms may improve with weight loss after VSG and RYGB, worsening symptoms are reported in up to one-third of patients undergoing VSG, whereas GERD symptoms are shown to improve in greater than 95% of patients undergoing RYGB.[21]

Medication malabsorption may occur, especially after RYGB, and consideration must be given when managing comorbidities long-term postoperatively. Undertreatment of medical conditions may occur when prescribing medications with the same dose or preparation that patients were receiving preoperatively. Keep in mind, however, decreased dosing of medication may be required as patients lose weight and their comorbidities resolve or improve.

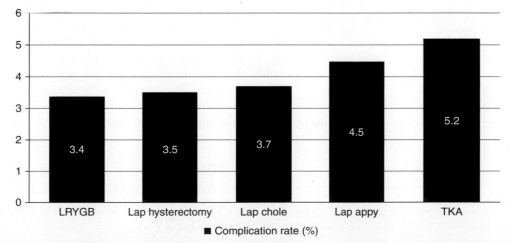

FIGURE 9.7 Comparative 30-day complication rate between different procedures. Appy, appendectomy; Chole, cholecystectomy; Lap, laparoscopic; LRYGB, laparoscopic Roux-en-Y gastric bypass; TKA, total knee arthroplasty. (Adapted from Aminian A, Brethauer SA, Kirwan JP, Kashyap SR, Burguera B, Schauer PR. How safe is metabolic/diabetes surgery? *Diabetes Obes Metab.* 2015;17(2):198-201.)

TABLE 9.3 30-Day Outcomes for Primary RYGB and VSG in the MBSAQIP Database, 2018

	RYGB (N = 48,527)	VSG (N = 128,209)	P VALUE	TOTAL (N = 176,736)
30-Day mortality n (%)	61 (.1)	105 (.08)	.0036	166 (.09)
30-Day reoperation n (%)	1,139 (2.3)	1,106 (.9)	<.0001	2,245 (1.3)
30-Day readmission n (%)	2,963 (6.1)	3,627 (2.8)	<.0001	6,590 (3.7%)

n, number of patients; RYGB, Roux-en-Y gastric bypass; VSG, vertical sleeve gastrectomy.
Adapted from American College of Surgeons. Metabolic and Bariatric Surgery Accreditation and Quality Improvement Program. Accessed October 20, 2019. www.facs.org/quality-programs/mbsaqip

Lifetime monitoring of vitamin and mineral levels is essential following metabolic and bariatric surgery, and deficiencies need to be corrected when identified in the postoperative period. Iron, calcium, vitamin B_{12}, thiamine, and vitamin D deficiencies are among the most commonly seen after metabolic and bariatric procedures. Parathyroid hormone levels are checked to ensure adequate calcium intake, as actual serum calcium levels will remain normal, potentially at the expense of skeletal reabsorption. Due to fat malabsorption after RYGB, periodic monitoring for fat-soluble vitamin deficiencies (particularly A and D) is part of

TABLE 9.4 Late Complications After Metabolic and Bariatric Surgery

RYGB	Incidence
Gastrojejunostomy anastomotic stricture	5.4%-7.3%
Gastrojejunostomy anastomotic (marginal) ulceration	2.3%-4%
Internal hernia	0.2%-2.6%
Small bowel obstruction	1.4%-5.2%
Cholelithiasis requiring cholecystectomy	3%-13%
Nephrolithiasis	7.7%-11%
VSG	**Incidence**
Luminal stenosis	0.1%-1.0%
Staple line leak (after 30 days)	1.1%-3.3%
Symptomatic GERD	28%-33%
Refractory GERD (requiring revision to RYGB)	1.4%-2.9%
New-onset Barrett esophagus	4%-17%

GERD, gastroesophageal reflux disease; RYGB, Roux-en-Y gastric bypass; VSG, vertical sleeve gastrectomy.

routine postoperative care. For patients on warfarin, vitamin K deficiencies may result in excess anticoagulation, so the PT/INR must be closely monitored. Long-term management of nutritional deficiencies is addressed in Chapter 10.

SUSTAINED AND DURABLE WEIGHT LOSS AFTER METABOLIC AND BARIATRIC SURGERY

Weight loss after metabolic and bariatric surgery can be sustainable with the proper multidisciplinary team available, including registered dietitian nutritionists, psychologists, and advance practice providers. One representative study analyzed metabolic and weight loss outcomes in over 400 patients who underwent RYGB, with greater than 90% follow-up at 12 years. At year 12, compared to baseline, 93% maintained at least 10% total body weight loss (TBWL), 70% maintained at least a 20% TBWL, and 40% maintained at least a 30% TBWL (Figure 9.8). In contrast, control patients did not experience significant weight loss over the 12-year follow-up period.[22]

An ongoing randomized controlled trial, the Surgical Treatment and Medications Potentially Eradicate Diabetes Efficiently (STAMPEDE) trial, compares metabolic and bariatric surgery to medical therapy for the treatment of T2D and other cardiovascular risk factors.[23] The 5-year results of this trial demonstrated weight loss trends over time, showing RYGB and VSG were superior compared to intensive medical therapy.[2]

COMORBIDITY RESOLUTION AND CARDIOVASCULAR RISK REDUCTION AFTER METABOLIC AND BARIATRIC SURGERY

Significant reduction, or complete resolution, of obesity-related comorbidities is noted after metabolic and bariatric surgery (Figure 9.9). Metabolic and bariatric surgery has proven to be exceptionally successful at

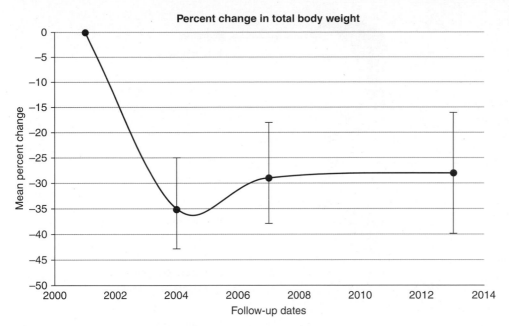

FIGURE 9.8 Total body weight changes 2, 6, and 12 years after Roux-en-Y gastric bypass. (Adapted from Adams TD, Davidson LE, Litwin SE, et al. Weight and metabolic outcomes 12 years after gastric bypass. *N Engl J Med.* 2017;377(12):1143-1155.)

treating T2D, resulting in a significant complete remission rate for more than 5 years and decreased mortality due to diabetes by 92%.[22] It is worth noting that in the previously mentioned STAMPEDE trial, all of the patients had uncontrolled diabetes, with a mean hemoglobin A1C level of greater than 9% and mean duration of T2D for greater than 8 years. Approximately half of the patients required a treatment regimen requiring at least three medications, and 44% of the patients required insulin.[23]

Patients in both of the surgery cohorts were more likely to achieve the glycated hemoglobin levels of 6% or less while no longer taking diabetes medications. If patients did not achieve a glycated hemoglobin of 6%, but decreased to 7% or less, they were more likely to achieve better control of their T2D without the use of insulin. Patients in both surgery groups experienced T2D control on fewer medications. Most notably, 45% of the RYGB patients and 25% of the VSG patients were able to discontinue all T2D medications. The percentage of patients requiring insulin therapy decreased in the RYGB and VSG cohorts, from 47% to 12% and 45% to 11%, respectively. The reductions in insulin requirement in both surgery cohorts were statistically significant when compared with the medical therapy group. Clinical resolution or improvement of T2D is more likely realized in patients with a shorter duration of T2D (less than 8 years), lower preoperative glycated hemoglobin levels, and an intestinal diversion procedure. Patients with a long history of T2D (>10 years) or with severe T2D (requiring insulin) were less likely to achieve complete resolution.[24]

Mortality due to cardiovascular disease (CVD) and cancer has been shown to be significantly lower in patients who underwent RYGB. Risk factors associated with increased CVD risk include hypertension, T2D, and dyslipidemia. Adams et al. demonstrated that T2D, low levels of high-density lipoprotein cholesterol, and high triglyceride levels were practically eradicated from the surgery group. All-cause mortality was decreased 40% in the gastric bypass group, while mortality due to diabetes decreased by 92%, and mortality due to coronary artery disease decreased by 56%.[22] CVD outcomes in surgery patients are shown to be superior, compared to nonoperative patients with class 2 and 3 obesity. A significant number of patients who underwent surgery were able to completely discontinue all CVD medications, but a small percentage of patients in the surgery group continue to require three or more CVD medications. Of note, no significant reduction in CVD medications is seen in the medical therapy group.[2] Surgery patients experience a 53% risk reduction in CVD deaths and a 33% risk reduction in first-time CVD events such as myocardial infarction or stroke.[25]

Looking at the association between metabolic and bariatric surgery with major adverse cardiovascular events in patients with T2D, Aminian et al. reported a significant 39% reduction in first occurrence of all-cause mortality, coronary artery events, cerebrovascular events, heart failure, nephropathy, and atrial fibrillation. Additionally, a 41% risk reduction was noted in the surgical cohort when using myocardial infarction, ischemic stroke, and mortality as endpoints.[5]

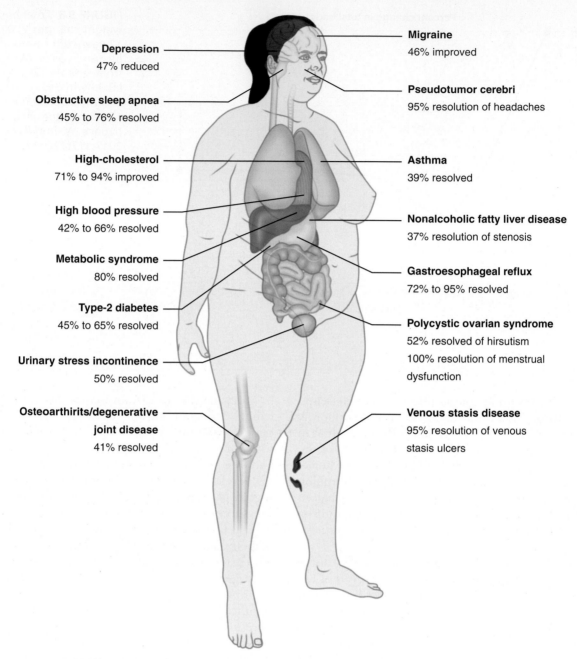

Depression
47% reduced

Obstructive sleep apnea
45% to 76% resolved

High-cholesterol
71% to 94% improved

High blood pressure
42% to 66% resolved

Metabolic syndrome
80% resolved

Type-2 diabetes
45% to 65% resolved

Urinary stress incontinence
50% resolved

Osteoarthirits/degenerative joint disease
41% resolved

Migraine
46% improved

Pseudotumor cerebri
95% resolution of headaches

Asthma
39% resolved

Nonalcoholic fatty liver disease
37% resolution of stenosis

Gastroesophageal reflux
72% to 95% resolved

Polycystic ovarian syndrome
52% resolved of hirsutism
100% resolution of menstrual dysfunction

Venous stasis disease
95% resolution of venous stasis ulcers

FIGURE 9.9 Comorbidity resolution following metabolic and bariatric surgery.

CANCER RISK REDUCTION

Obesity-related cancers include breast, prostate, colorectal, endometrial, ovarian, kidney, esophageal adenocarcinoma, liver, pancreas, thyroid, non-Hodgkin lymphoma, and leukemia. Weight loss after metabolic and bariatric surgery is associated with a significant reduction in overall cancer incidence and occurrence of obesity-related cancer. It also appears to be protective for the development of breast cancer.[26]

REVISIONS AND REOPERATIVE BARIATRIC SURGERY

Approximately 14% of all metabolic and bariatric procedures performed in the United States are revision of previous procedures. While insufficient weight loss may play a significant role in reoperative bariatric surgery, many of the reoperative procedures are indicated for corrective action of acute and chronic complications. Indications for reoperative surgery after RYGB include leaks, bleeding, ulcers, gastrogastric fistulas, gastrojejunostomy stenosis, jejunojejunostomy stenosis, bowel obstructions, and internal hernias. Indications for VSG revision include staple line leaks, bleeding, sleeve migration into the mediastinum, gastric stenosis, and chronic intractable GERD. Indications for AGB revision include perforation, band intolerance, band slippage with gastric prolapse, band erosion, and port and tubing complications. BPD/DS revision indications are similar to VSG as well as chronic protein calorie malnutrition. Metabolic and bariatric revisional procedures to address insufficient weight loss are considered only when there is an anatomical cause, such as a gastrogastric fistula. An upper GI x-ray is used to confirm this diagnosis. Most importantly, reoperative bariatric procedures should be performed by experienced surgeons at centers in which resources are available to manage the challenges of these complex procedures.

Patients may elect to undergo body contouring procedures after losing a significant amount of weight. A weight loss plateau should be realized before considering a referral to a plastic surgeon, which in general is ≥18 months postoperatively. Many insurance companies will not readily cover body contouring unless there are specific medical issues related to the overhanging pannus, such as severe intertrigo and skin maceration despite efforts to correct this with conventional topical treatments and skin care, and a low-lying overhanging pannus that interferes with normal daily activity.

CASE STUDIES—PREOPERATIVE AND POSTOPERATIVE CONSIDERATIONS

Discussion of Case Study 1

As introduced at the beginning of the chapter, Jane is a 45-year-old woman who is a long-standing patient of yours with no major medical problems. Jane has had overweight for many years; however, her weight continues to slowly increase despite multiple behavioral and dietary interventions, and she is appropriately concerned. She currently has class 3 obesity (BMI 41 kg/m^2) and you are considering referring her for a surgical weight loss consultation.

Jane is the average type of patient who undergoes consideration for bariatric surgery. Without any major medical problems, her operative risks are very low, and depending on her goals for weight loss and surgical evaluation, she would likely be an excellent candidate and benefit greatly from bariatric surgery. Overall, there are many caveats and misconceptions about what is feasible or prohibitive surgically. The following cases are representative of patients who are commonly referred for bariatric surgery and raise important management issues.

CASE STUDY 2

PATIENT WITH CARDIAC DISEASE

Mary is a 62-year-old woman with a medical history significant for hypertension, hyperlipidemia, mild osteoarthritis, and a previous myocardial infarction 10 years ago, who also has known congestive heart failure with an ejection fraction of 40%. Previous cardiac catheterizations show stable coronary artery disease not amenable to intervention. Her blood pressure is controlled on two medications (i.e., beta blocker, angiotensin-converting enzyme [ACE] inhibitor), and she takes two lipid lower medications (i.e., statin, bile acid sequestrant). She has impaired fasting glucose and has recently started on metformin (500 mg BID). Her BMI is 43 kg/m^2 and her weight has continued to slowly increase over the last few years, which is not secondary to worsening of her well-controlled heart failure. At one time she was interested in bariatric surgery, but a healthcare provider once told her that she would be ineligible because of her heart failure diagnosis.

Discussion of Case Study 2

A common misconception is that heart failure is a prohibitive risk for elective metabolic and bariatric surgery. If not severe, heart failure is not prohibitive and heart function has been shown to improve following bariatric surgery. In a systematic review of 23 studies looking at patients with preserved systolic function, metabolic and bariatric surgery had a number of beneficial effects, including decreased left ventricular (LV) mass and relative wall thickness, improved LV diastolic function, and decreased left atrium diameter.[27] Obviously, performing surgery on patients with severe obesity and end-stage heart failure, requiring mechanical circulatory support, presents formidable challenges. Thus, it is important to note that not all metabolic and bariatric surgeons will feel comfortable accepting this patient as a viable surgical candidate, and it is critical that a patient with increased risks is referred to a center that is capable of handling complex cases with appropriate intensive resources available. Regardless, metabolic and bariatric surgery should be explored as it can potentially provide a bridge for patients with advanced heart failure to cardiac transplantation who would not otherwise be eligible based on their severe obesity. Increasing numbers of advanced centers providing comprehensive clinical support, involving a multidisciplinary team approach, have shown that metabolic and bariatric surgery can be performed safely, with patients achieving sufficient weight loss postoperatively to eventually undergo cardiac transplantation.[28] Careful collaboration between the bariatric surgery center and cardiologist experienced in caring for advanced heart failure patients is critical for optimizing treatment and minimizing postoperative complications.

CASE STUDY 3

PATIENT WITH DEPRESSION/ BIPOLAR DISORDER

Ms. B is a 25-year-old woman with a history of suicide attempt related to severe depression as a teenager and is currently being treated with risperidone and topiramate daily, which has been a stable treatment regimen for the last 6 years. She is otherwise well, except for suffering from class II obesity (BMI 35.8 kg/m²) and T2D. She takes metformin daily to treat her T2D. She has tried to lose weight through caloric restriction and exercise over the last several years and has tried many fad diets as well, but long-term weight loss has been unsuccessful. She currently is interested in metabolic and bariatric surgery because she has a strong family history of severe obesity.

Discussion of Case Study 3

Patients must be psychologically stable for at least 1 year after an attempted suicide. This patient has a history of an attempted suicide 6 years ago and is currently psychologically stable. Therefore, she is considered a suitable candidate for metabolic and bariatric surgery. Psychiatric illness may prolong the preoperative planning for metabolic and bariatric surgery but should not be viewed as an absolute contraindication for surgery. In fact, many psychotropic medications have been linked to weight gain and make it even more difficult to lose weight. A number of studies have demonstrated that bariatric surgery is safe in patients with psychiatric disease, including patients with bipolar disorder, as long as the patients are stable on their medication regimens prior to surgery. In some patients on multiple medications, it may be prudent to proceed with VSG instead of RYGB because of concerns of medication malabsorption but increasing numbers of centers are offering bariatric surgery successfully in psychiatric patients. Mental health should not be a barrier to weight loss surgery in this patient population that clearly benefits in terms of quality of life.[29]

CASE STUDY 4

PATIENT TAKING DIRECT ORAL ANTICOAGULANTS OR WARFARIN

Mr. M is a 55-year-old man with a medical history significant for a mechanical mitral valve replacement 11 years ago requiring lifelong anticoagulation with a vitamin K antagonist (i.e., warfarin, goal INR 2 to 3). His other medical conditions include severe obstructive sleep apnea requiring CPAP, hypertension, hyperlipidemia, T2D requiring three medications (i.e., metformin, sulfonylurea, long-acting insulin), and obesity (BMI 49 kg/m²). His endocrinologist started liraglutide 1.8 mg daily 4 months ago and he has seen a six-pound weight loss with that added therapy. He has struggled with obesity his entire adult life and his weight past slowly increased over the last several years.

Discussion of Case Study 4

Even though taking medications for anticoagulation increases the perioperative risk of bleeding, this should not preclude surgical consultation for consideration of metabolic and bariatric surgery. Many surgeons are familiar with bridging patients who take lifelong anticoagulation for numerous reasons (e.g., pulmonary embolus, deep venous thrombosis, presence of a mechanical valve), which is done regularly in elective surgery. Bridging may be done with vitamin K antagonists or other novel anticoagulants, but studies examining the efficacy are limited but suggest the efficacy may be similar to nonsurgical patients. Conservative approaches using traditional vitamin K analogs may be safer until further studies examine the pharmacokinetic and pharmacodynamic parameters in patient's postbariatric surgery.[30]

As mentioned previously, patients undergoing RYGB and requiring warfarin are likely to experience a decrease in vitamin K levels due to fat malabsorption and antibiotic administration at the time of surgery. Warfarin is discontinued 5 days prior to surgery and bridging with heparin begins, if indicated, 2 to 3 days prior to surgery. Warfarin is typically restarted within 48 hours postoperatively and PT/INR levels are drawn approximately 1 week later. An enhanced warfarin response should be anticipated after RYGB due to decreased vitamin K antagonism. Therefore, a lower dose than what was prescribed preoperatively should be given when resuming warfarin postoperatively. Dosing adjustments can be made accordingly based on PT/INR results.

CASE STUDY 5

PATIENT ON IMMUNOSUPPRESSANT THERAPY

Ms. B is a 48-year-old woman with a long-standing history of steroid use (prednisone 10 mg/day) and methotrexate for rheumatoid arthritis and subsequent development of obesity (BMI 42 kg/m²). She has a strong family history of obesity as well as T2D and CVD. She continues to struggle with her weight, which she feels is limiting her lifestyle even though her arthritis pain is well-controlled on chronic steroids. She wants to lose weight but has been told that her risks for surgery are too high.

CASE STUDY 6

PATIENT WHO BECOMES PREGNANT AFTER BARIATRIC SURGERY

Ms. S is a 28-year-old woman with no obesity-associated medical conditions except for hypertension that is controlled with an ACE inhibitor. Her previous pregnancy was successful only after multiple rounds of fertility treatments, and she states that her husband and she are not planning on any additional children. She underwent a laparoscopic RYGB 3 months ago primarily for weight loss to be able to be more active with her child. Her preoperative BMI was 46 kg/m². In the last 3 months she has lost 80 pounds and had new onset of nausea. Upon further workup, she was found to be 6 weeks pregnant.

Discussion of Case Study 5

Although long-standing steroid use and other immunosuppressant medications can negatively affect healing and predispose to infection, these medications should not be seen as contraindications to surgical weight loss. Large national data analyses have examined outcomes of patients on immunosuppressants at the time of bariatric surgery. Patients were at slightly increased risk of infections and anastomotic leak; however, there were no changes in 30-day mortality, and the overall risk profile at 30 days remained acceptable despite having elevated risks compared with patients not taking immunosuppressant medications. It is commonly known that immunosuppressant medications cause weight gain and greatly impede successful weight loss as well as worsening T2D. Metabolic and bariatric surgery is appropriate to consider in patients taking immunosuppressants, especially as thoughtful perioperative planning and procedure selection can decrease these risks to even lower rates.[31] Immunosuppressants are typically discontinued at least 7 to 14 days prior to surgery, if possible, and can be resumed approximately 2 to 4 weeks after surgery. Resuming medications postoperatively will be at the discretion of the surgeon, but expert specialty recommendations (i.e., rheumatology) should be considered when deciding when to discontinue and resume medications. There are studies suggesting it is safe to continue methotrexate in the perioperative period to reduce the risk of flare-ups.[32] Additionally, it is safe to continue hydroxychloroquine in the perioperative period. Biologic agents are typically stopped 2 weeks prior to surgery, while nonbiologic agents have more flexibility based on patient's history and symptomatology.

Discussion of Case Study 6

Many women with obesity struggle with fertility, as the hormonal milieu of obesity can affect and even lead to cessation of normal menstruation. It is not infrequent that surgeons see a patient within the first several months following metabolic and bariatric surgery become pregnant unexpectedly. This scenario is becoming increasingly common as younger women are increasingly utilizing metabolic and bariatric surgery for obesity treatment. A joint statement from the ASMBS and the American College of Obstetricians and Gynecologists identify that oral contraception may not have the same efficacy in a patient postoperatively, and alternative methods (e.g., intrauterine devices, subcutaneous implants) that might have more reliable pharmacokinetic profiles should be considered for use.[33] Given that pregnancy in a time of rapid weight loss is not ideal, most surgeon and centers recommend avoiding pregnancy for at least 12 to 18 months, at which time most patients have stabilized body weight. As in the scenario above, the patient who becomes pregnant unexpectedly presents with an increased need for follow-up and consultation with maternal fetal medicine specialists for frequent monitoring of pregnancy. A number of considerations related to ensuring that the fetus has optimal nutritional resources for development is the highest priority, as fetal development and experience with pregnancy during the rapid weight loss phase has not been well studied. However, resources exist based on expert consensus given the increasing frequency of this scenario.

PATIENT WITH CURRENT HISTORY OF ACTIVE TOBACCO USE

Ms. Y is a 32-year-old woman with obesity (BMI 36 kg/m^2) as well as T2D, hypertension, and hypercholesterolemia. She not only takes metformin (1 g BID) for her T2D but also takes an ACE inhibitor and a statin. She has a strong family history of vascular disease and diabetes and is interested in bariatric surgery to help her lose weight and better control her diabetes. She admits to smoking one pack of cigarettes daily and is reluctant to quit because she fears that she will gain 10 pounds.

Discussion of Case Study 7

The patient with active tobacco use presents a management challenge in which the risks associated with perioperative and postoperative complications are prohibitive. Smoking has been shown to be associated with pulmonary and wound healing complications, such that many surgeons will not perform elective operations in patients with active tobacco use.[34] Similarly, the risks associated with active tobacco use include marginal ulceration and perforation. In the above case, even though tobacco cessation would likely lead to a slight increase in body weight per the patient, the risks of continued tobacco use would outweigh the risk of a small increase in body weight preoperatively. Preoperatively it is critical that patients stop using tobacco; however, the length of time between cessation and surgery would be an individualized decision between the patient and surgeon. It is likely that increased smoking cessation is beneficial, but the minimal time prior to bariatric surgery to mitigate risk is not well studied.

PATIENT REQUIRING LONG-TERM USE OF NONSTEROIDAL ANTI-INFLAMMATORY DRUGS

Mr. M is a 52-year-old man with a long-standing history of osteoarthritis (mostly knees and hips bilaterally) that has been worsening over the past decade for which he takes diclofenac regularly as well as muscle relaxers and acetaminophen. His past medical history is otherwise significant for obesity (BMI 46 kg/m^2), hypertension, and prediabetes. He recently saw his primary care physician who coordinated a consultation with an orthopedic surgeon who agreed that he had severe osteoarthritis and would likely benefit from bilateral knee arthroplasty. However, the orthopedic surgeon stated that Mr. M would need to lower his weight to a BMI of ≤40 before he would consider performing elective joint replacement—his group practice's new policy.

Discussion of Case Study 8

With the continued rise in obesity prevalence, the above scenario is becoming increasingly common. Mr. M is currently taking NSAIDs (i.e., diclofenac) and is having a good response to that therapy, but the natural history of his osteoarthritis is that it will continue to worsen with time and likely require increased pharmacotherapy unless he undergoes joint replacement. There are several possible outcomes for Mr. M if he undergoes weight loss surgery. Typically, patients on preoperative NSAIDs for arthritis pain may be able to discontinue all medications within months of surgery, as a loss of >50 pounds of weight greatly improves arthritis pain and medication requirements. This is less likely, though, given that Mr. M's joints are already meeting the threshold for replacement. Since he has multiple joints that may need replacement, it would likely be prudent to proceed with VSG for weight loss since patients can safely resume NSAIDS typically >1 month postoperatively as needed. In this case, as VSG and RYGB have similar weight loss in the first 5 years postoperatively, Mr. M can lose weight with a VSG safely and continue his NSAIDs as needed.

Alternatively, another common scenario is a patient requiring long-term low-dose ASA used most likely for cardioprotection or other indications. Similarly, these patients can more safely undergo VSG instead of RYGB and continue prophylaxis with ASA as long term as necessary. Thus, long-term NSAID/ASA use should not be considered prohibitive for bariatric surgery as there are options available for these patients for treatment of obesity as well.

PATIENT WITH INFLAMMATORY BOWEL DISEASE

Mr. A is a 42-year-old man with a history of Crohn disease limited to his colon and is s/p laparoscopic total abdominal colectomy with end ileostomy. He denies any other previous operations and currently does not take any medications or corticosteroids. He has class 3 obesity (BMI 42.5 kg/m^2), T2D, osteoarthritis, and hypertension.

Discussion of Case Study 9

The patient with IBD presents several challenges to surgical management of obesity, though IBD should not be considered contraindication for metabolic and bariatric surgery. IBD, typically thought of as Crohn disease and ulcerative colitis, exists on a spectrum, and these patients frequently have obesity related to long-term use of corticosteroids and other immunomodulatory medications. Surgeons will not operate on patients with acutely active disease and would prefer to see treatment regimens stabilize for a prescribed period of time before considering patients a suitable surgical candidate.

RYGB is not necessarily a desirable option in Crohn disease as it can involve any portion of the GI tract and is associated with increased risk of stenosis, leak, and fistula formation along the staple lines. Many surgeons would only consider VSG in patients with IBD; however, consideration must be given to the fact that gastric involvement can be seen in approximately 5% to 15% of patients with Crohn disease. Another consideration for patients with obesity and Crohn disease aside from fistula and leak is that it would likely be desirable to avoid RYGB due to increased risk of malabsorption with more rapid intestinal transit.

For patients presenting with ulcerative colitis, VSG and RYGB are both reasonable options. Preoperatively, it would be prudent to perform an EGD to rule out the presence of active disease in the stomach. It is also preferable that the patient has had quiescent disease for at least 5 years. Interestingly, bariatric surgery in patients with obesity and IBD is increasingly being studied and it has been shown that these patients may benefit from surgery and weight loss in terms of IBD remission. A systematic review in particular cites almost 50% IBD remission rate in these patients after surgery.[35]

CASE STUDY 10

PATIENT WITH END-STAGE RENAL DISEASE REQUIRING DIALYSIS

Mr. J is a 50-year-old man with a BMI of 46.8 kg/m² and a history of long-standing hypertension, prediabetes, and hypertensive nephropathy requiring hemodialysis three times weekly via an upper extremity fistula. He has struggled with obesity his entire life and has a strong family history of diabetes and hypertension. He is pursuing metabolic and bariatric surgery because he was told he needs to lose 100 pounds to be eligible for a kidney transplant. Additional medical problems include a small hiatal and umbilical hernia, both of which are asymptomatic. He has lost varying amounts of weight in the past, but never greater than 50 pounds with diet and exercise alone.

Discussion of Case Study 10

With the steady rise in the diabetes epidemic over the past 30-plus years, the incidence of diabetes-related kidney disease continues to increase as well, with many patients developing end-stage renal disease. Additionally, many of these patients have concurrent obesity that presents challenges to transplant programs as obesity significantly increases the technical challenges of the operation as well as the risk of delayed graft function. Given that lifestyle change and pharmacotherapy produce minimal to moderately sustained effects on weight loss, metabolic and bariatric surgery is increasingly being performed on patients with end-stage renal disease with or without dialysis in anticipation of future transplant. Surgical weight loss in these patients is safe with an acceptable risk/benefit ratio and produces results that improve quality of life and allow patients to undergo successful transplantation.[36] Interestingly, it is not uncommon for patients to experience an improvement in renal function postbariatric surgery, an observation whose mechanisms is not well understood, but nonetheless welcomed. Patients undergoing surgery need to be closely monitored and managed by the nephrology team.

CASE STUDY 11

ADOLESCENT PATIENT

Joseph is a 16-year-old boy who has always been a "bigger kid" according to family but his parents have become increasingly concerned with his weight recently. Obesity is common in his family with his mother and father both having obesity with a BMI >40 kg/m² as well as several obesity-associated medical conditions, including T2D, hypertension, severe osteoarthritis, and hyperlipidemia. Joseph is currently in the 99th percentile for body weight/BMI and has borderline hypertension but currently with no other medical conditions. Joseph's parents have tried structured lifestyle and dietary interventions for Joseph (as well as themselves), but nothing has significantly improved Joseph's weight. They are both interested in bariatric surgery for themselves and are curious to know what/when Joseph might be able to have surgery too—as they have heard that increasing numbers of adolescents are undergoing bariatric surgery. They are presenting with him to your office because they both do not want Joseph to become as sick as they have become over time.

Discussion of Case Study 11

The prevalence of adolescent obesity, similar to adult obesity, continues to increase over time. Adolescents with obesity are at high risk to become adults with obesity with significant end-organ dysfunction even as young adults. The proportion of adolescent bariatric surgery has increased over time, with the largest study being the Longitudinal Assessment of Bariatric Surgery in Teens (Teen-LABS), which demonstrated that adolescent bariatric surgery is safe and effective.[37]

Operative indications in adolescent patients are similar to those in adults, with class 2 obesity and an obesity-associated medical condition being indications for metabolic and bariatric surgery and class 3 obesity alone being an indication for surgical intervention. In adolescent patients, these categories are defined as having a BMI ≥35 kg/m² or ≥120% of the 95th percentile for age and sex for class 2 obesity, while class 3 obesity is a BMI ≥40 or ≥140% of the 95th percentile for age and sex.

Considerable evidence and current robust best practice guidelines developed and endorsed by the American Academy of Pediatrics support the safety and effectiveness of surgical weight loss for children and adolescents, acknowledging that the surgical management of adolescent obesity, similar to adults, continues to be more efficacious than pharmacologic or lifestyle interventions.[38]

If visual disturbances and headaches were added to this case scenario, metabolic and bariatric surgery may be considered more urgent considering the possible association of pseudotumor cerebri (PTC) that could possibly lead to permanent blindness. It has been well-documented that PTC significantly improves after metabolic and bariatric surgery, thus averting the possibility of developing permanent blindness.[39]

CLINICAL HIGHLIGHTS

Determining risks for, and comorbidity resolution after, metabolic and bariatric surgery.

It is important to refer patients to nationally accredited metabolic and bariatric surgery centers that are meeting and maintain high standards to promote patient safety and best outcomes. Centers are required to have pathways designed to educate patients and staff, follow preoperative and postoperative care pathways and protocols that include availability to behavioral health providers, and must offer support groups to enhance the value of the patient experience. To find an accredited center near you, please use the MBSAQIP website.

A validated risk calculator tool using risk-adjusted MBSAQIP data is available to assist centers with determining appropriate patient selection. The bariatric surgical risk/benefit calculator was built using data collected from more than 775,000 operations from 925 centers participating in MBSAQIP from January 1, 2013 to June 30, 2018.[40] See Figure 9.10 for an example of the information obtained from the MBSAQIP risk/benefit calculator that can be shared with your patients in determining which procedure may be considered the best treatment.

The Escape Diabetes risk calculator tool developed by the Cleveland Clinic can also be used to compare surgical versus nonsurgical treatment outcomes in patients with obesity and diabetes.[41] This risk calculator has been validated using approximately 14,000 Cleveland Clinic patients with T2D and obesity to predict the 10-year risk of developing major adverse cardiovascular outcomes. See Figure 9.11 for an example patient using this calculator tool.

WHEN TO REFER?

- Patients with a BMI of 40 kg/m², or 35 kg/m² with obesity-related comorbidities.
- Consider patients with class 1 obesity (BMI between 30 and 35 kg/m²) and severe uncontrolled diabetes.

PRACTICAL RESOURCES

Resources to consider using when referring a patient include the following:

- MBSAQIP website (https://www.facs.org/search/bariatric-surgery-centers); this resource will help you find a nationally accredited metabolic and bariatric surgery center.
- Clinical practice guidelines for the perioperative nutrition, metabolic, and nonsurgical support of patients undergoing bariatric procedures—2019 update (https://journals.aace.com/doi/10.4158/GL-2019-0406?url_ver=Z39.88-2003&rfr_id=ori:rid:crossref.org&rfr_dat=cr_pub%3dpubmed); this resource provides valuable recommendations for metabolic, nutrition, and nonsurgical management of metabolic and bariatric patients.
- MBSAQIP bariatric surgery risk/benefit calculator (https://www.facs.org/quality-programs/mbsaqip/calculator); this resource will determine your patient's potential operative risk, weight loss outcomes, and comorbidity resolution.
- Escape Diabetes calculator tool on the ASMBS website (https://asmbs.org/escape-diabetes); this resource will help you determine your patient's potential diabetes resolution outcomes and reduction of cardiovascular risks.
- MBSAQIP Standards Manual (https://www.facs.org/quality-programs/mbsaqip/standards); this resource explains the requirements of being a nationally accredited metabolic and bariatric surgery center.
- ASMBS website (https://asmbs.org/); this resource can provide valuable consensus guidelines pertaining to metabolic and bariatric surgery.

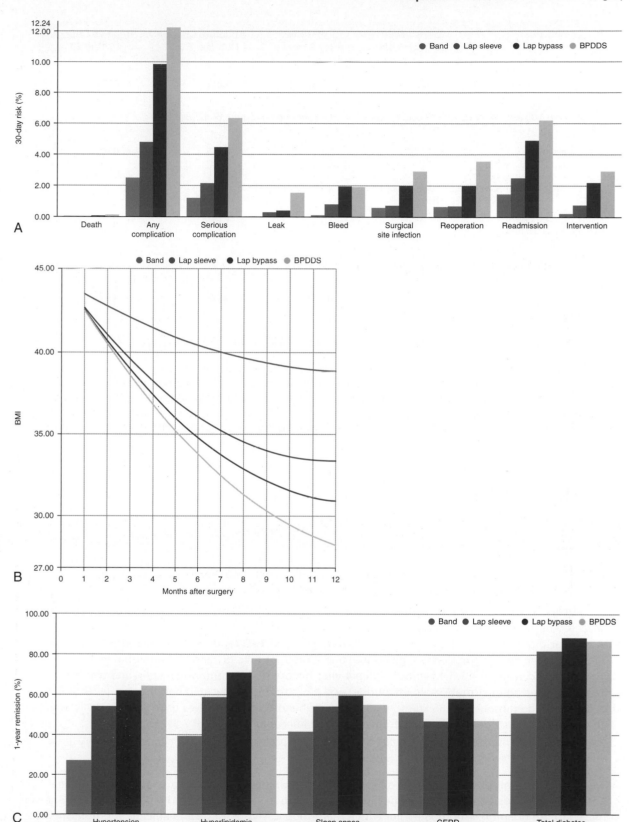

FIGURE 9.10 Example using the MBSAQIP risk/benefit surgical risk calculator to determine risks associated with metabolic and bariatric surgery in a 45-year-old Caucasian woman with hypertension, type 2 diabetes, hyperlipidemia, gastroesophageal reflux disease, and obstructive sleep apnea. Height 65 inches, weight 270 pounds, and body mass index (BMI) 44.93 kg/m². A, Predicted risks associated with metabolic and bariatric surgery. B, Predicted BMI change 1 year after metabolic and bariatric surgery. C, Predicted comorbidity resolution 1 year after surgery. BPDDS, biliopancreatic diversions with duodenal switch; GERD, gastroesophageal reflux disease. (Adapted from American College of Surgeons. Bariatric Surgical Risk/Benefit Calculator. Accessed October 20, 2019. https://www.facs.org/quality-programs/mbsaqip/calculator)

Complication	Your Current 10-Year Risk	10-Year Risk After Surgery	Absolute Change in 10-Year Risk	Relative Change in 10-Year Risk
Death (all-cause)	3.2%	1.7%	▼ 1.5%	▼ 46%
Your 10-year risk of death (all-cause) would be 46% lower after surgery for diabetes.				
Heart failure	7.0%	2.3%	▼ 4.7%	▼ 67%
Your 10-year risk of heart failure would be 67% lower after surgery for diabetes.				
Coronary heart disease	4.4%	2.9%	▼ 1.6%	▼ 35%
Your 10-year risk of coronary heart disease would be 35% lower after surgery for diabetes.				
Diabetic kidney disease	34.8%	10.8%	▼ 24.0%	▼ 69%
Your 10-year risk of diabetic kidney disease would be 69% lower after surgery for diabetes.				

FIGURE 9.11 Example using the Escape Diabetes risk calculator to predict the 10-year cardiovascular risks with and without metabolic and bariatric surgery in a 45-year-old African American woman with hypertension, type 2 diabetes on metformin, and hyperlipidemia requiring medication. Body mass index 45 kg/m², blood pressure 140/85, HbA1C 6.5%, creatinine level 1.1, and triglyceride level 100. (Adapted from American Society for Metabolic and Bariatric Surgery. Escape Diabetes Risk Calculator. https://asmbs.org/escape-diabetes/risk-calculator)

QUIZ QUESTIONS

1. Which of the following patients is most likely to experience complete resolution of type 2 diabetes (T2D) within the first year after laparoscopic Roux-en-Y gastric bypass?

   A. A 25-year-old woman (BMI 41 kg/m²) with a 3-year history of T2D on metformin and a preoperative glycated hemoglobin level of 6.9%

   B. A 55-year-old man (BMI 44 kg/m²) with a 11-year history of T2D requiring insulin and two oral hypoglycemic agents (metformin, glyburide) and a preoperative glycated hemoglobin level of 6.5%

   C. A 40-year-old woman (BMI 43 kg/m²) with a 4-year history of T2D requiring insulin and two oral hypoglycemic agents (metformin, glyburide) and a preoperative glycated hemoglobin level of 8.2%

   D. A 60-year-old woman (BMI 38 kg/m²) with a 10-year history of T2D on two oral hypoglycemic agents (metformin, glyburide) and a preoperative glycated hemoglobin level of 7.8%

   Answer: A. *Patients with shorter duration of diabetes and better glycemic control prior to surgery are more likely to experience complete resolution of T2D.*

2. A 39-year-old woman presents to your office for a routine annual physical examination. Her medical history includes obesity, gastroesophageal reflux, obstructive sleep apnea, and bipolar disorder. She was admitted to the hospital 6 months earlier with a major depressive episode and suicide attempt. She has made a marked improvement since being discharged from the hospital and is currently being followed by a psychiatrist. She has gained 10 pounds in the last 6 months and wants to undergo bariatric surgery to help

in contact with the bariatric surgeon for management. This condition is a surgical emergency and requires a high level of suspicion.

> The cardinal **signs** of an anastomotic leak include
>
> - tachycardia greater than 120 beats per minute
> - respiratory rate greater than 22 per minute
> - fever
> - extravasation of contract on computed tomography (CT) scan or upper gastrointestinal series
>
> The cardinal **symptoms** of an anastomotic leak include
>
> - shoulder pain
> - feverishness
> - abdominal pain
> - shortness of breath

While the suggested workup for a suspected anastomotic leak should be to obtain a CBC with differential and comprehensive metabolic panel and order a CT scan of the abdomen with contrast, the most important next step, if an anastomotic leak is suspected or diagnosed, is prompt communication and transfer to the bariatric surgeon. With early detection, conservative management with endoscopic stenting and parenteral antibiotics is often sufficient in managing these patients. This again underscores the need for the HCP's collaboration with the bariatric surgery team to ensure the best possible outcomes for their patients.

Nausea and Vomiting

Nausea and vomiting can occur following any of the bariatric surgery procedures.[5] Although most commonly unrelated to obstruction or anatomical defect of the surgery, if the patient is not able to keep anything down by mouth for 24 hours, an evaluation is warranted. Nausea alone is most common. It can most often be managed by antiemetic agents such as ondansetron hydrochloride 4 mg orally and hydration. Similar to suspicion of an anastomotic leak, patients with persistent nausea or vomiting should be evaluated by the bariatric surgery team.

One important sequela of persistent nausea and vomiting is Wernicke encephalopathy.[6] This is truly the only "medical emergency" that the HCP should be familiar with and facilitate treatment even before referring to the surgical team. Patients with persistent vomiting may deplete their thiamine stores in just a few days. The signs and symptoms of thiamine deficiency (Wernicke encephalopathy) are

- Ataxia (unsteady gait)
- Nystagmus (repetitive, uncontrolled movements of the eyes)
- Mental confusion (disoriented, hard time focusing or making decisions)

Due to altered GI anatomy from the metabolic and bariatric surgery as well as persistent vomiting, vitamin B1 (thiamine) levels fall. Moreover, with the common addition of dextrose in intravenous hydration, vitamin B1 is driven intracellularly which further depletes stores. The HCP should have a high index of suspicion for Wernicke encephalopathy and a low threshold for treatment. If left untreated, Wernicke encephalopathy can lead to an irreversible pontine stroke. If treated early, symptoms should resolve quickly without sequelae. Depending on the severity of deficiency, treatment should consist of[7]

- Intravenous (IV) administration of 200 mg of thiamine three times per day, or
- Oral administration 500 mg once or twice daily for 3 to 5 consecutive days followed by 250 mg for the next 3 to 5 days, or
- Intramuscular (IM) administration of 250 mg daily for 3 to 5 days or 100 to 150 monthly.

Once the patient can tolerate oral intake, 100 mg of thiamine supplementation is recommended for at least 30 days. Of note, often Wernicke encephalopathy is mistaken for vitamin B12 deficiency due to ataxia, but unfortunately, vitamin B12 supplementation will have no effect on treating Wernicke encephalopathy. The bottom line, anytime a bariatric surgery patient presents with persistent nausea and vomiting, thiamine supplementation should strongly be considered.

> Thiamine deficiency is a medical emergency. Any bariatric surgical patient who presents with persistent vomiting and signs/symptoms of Wernicke-Korsakoff syndrome should be empirically treated with thiamine supplementation.

INTERMEDIATE MEDICAL MANAGEMENT AFTER BARIATRIC SURGERY (<6 MONTHS)

As discussed in Chapter 9, metabolic and bariatric surgery is the most effective long-term treatment approach for patient with severe obesity or moderate obesity with a medical complication. As a result of the weight loss and associated anatomical and physiological changes, there is an improvement or resolution of the patients' chronic obesity-related medical problems such as diabetes mellitus, obstructive sleep apnea, fatty liver disease, hypertension, and dyslipidemia. This section will review optimal medical management following metabolic and bariatric surgery.

Diabetes Management

Metabolic and bariatric surgery has been shown to be a safe and effective treatment option for patients with type 2 diabetes mellitus (T2D). For reasons not entirely clear, improvements in insulin sensitivity can occur immediately after metabolic and bariatric surgery and even before any appreciable weight loss has occurred.[8] For this reason, the dose of any preoperative antidiabetic medications must be reduced or discontinued early after surgery in order to avoid hypoglycemia. For patients who are managed with insulin, the daily insulin regimen can be often held and replaced by using a sliding correction factor as needed, particularly for patients who undergo RYGB or BPD. Moreover, since dietary intake is significantly reduced both in volume and time of consumption, longer acting agents like insulin glargine are usually better tolerated if post-op insulin is needed.

Depending on the level of preoperative glycemic control, patients adequately controlled with only oral agents may require little, if any, glucose-lowering medication, especially in the immediate postoperative period (7 to 10 days). If an RYGB patient requires resumption of oral medications, regular release and crush or liquid rather than sustained release/extended release formulations are recommended in order to maximize absorption.[3] Patients undergoing an SG may not require changes in their formulation. Metformin, both regular and extended release, may not be well tolerated due to its GI intolerance with either procedure within the first 30 days of surgery. The thiazolidinediones (TZDs) may be better tolerated than metformin; however, because of their propensity to cause weight gain or retard weight loss, they should be prescribed judiciously. Sulfonylureas, although better tolerated from the GI standpoint, can produce significant hypoglycemia and therefore should be either discontinued entirely or used at a lower dose with frequent monitoring of blood glucose. Newer classes of medications have been approved for the treatment of T2D. These medications typically do not cause hypoglycemia, are relatively well tolerated, and may also augment weight loss. The glucagon-like peptide-1 (GLP-1) agonists and the sodium glucose co-transporter 2 (SGLT2) inhibitors are both approved for glycemic control, and some agents in these therapeutic classes have been shown to reduce cardiovascular events.[9-11]

Antihypertensive Management

For a variety of reasons, blood pressure routinely is decreased in the immediate postoperative period. This, in turn, necessitates using reduced doses of antihypertensive medications. Usually medication dosages can be cut in half, and angiotensin-converting enzyme (ACE) inhibitors and angiotensin II receptor blockers (ARBs) that are held 48 hours prior to surgery can be restarted postoperatively at a reduced dose. Diuretic agents are typically discontinued following surgery to avoid dehydration and electrolyte abnormalities. As discussed previously, medications that are prescribed in RYGB patients should be in the regular release and crushed/liquid formulation to ensure maximum absorption.

Depression Management

Due to the potential withdrawal effect with abruptly stopping psychotropic medications (particularly antidepressant drugs), they should be continued postoperatively as soon as the patient is able to tolerate p.o. intake. Similar to other medications, they should also be prescribed in the regular release, crushed/liquid form for RYGB patients. Medications that may cause weight gain, such as tricyclic antidepressants and mirtazapine, should be discontinued if possible and replaced with an alternative drug if possible.

Depression and quality of life usually improves in the weeks to months following metabolic and bariatric surgery. However, the HCP should continuously reassess the patient for a recurrence of depression or development of new-onset depression. Untreated depression can contribute to postoperative weight gain. Patients exhibiting major depressive symptoms should be considered for referral to a mental health specialist. In a recent meta-analysis, metabolic and bariatric surgery patients were about four times more likely than matched controls to commit suicide or attempt self-harm.[12]

Cholesterol Management

Although not as immediate as the improvement in insulin sensitivity/glycemic control, blood lipid profiles have been shown to significantly improve from 3 to 12 months after metabolic and bariatric surgery. Since statin agents may cause nausea in the immediate postoperative period and liver transaminase levels may increase with rapid weight loss, consideration for holding lipid-lowering medications for the first 12 weeks after surgery and reevaluating their need may outweigh the risk of restarting in the immediate postoperative period. However, for patients who are prescribed statin agents for secondary prevention of acute coronary events, the medication should be continued in the immediate postoperative period.

Aspirin and Nonsteroidal Anti-Inflammatory Management

Due to the increased risk of postoperative ulcers, strictures, and bleeding, the chronic use of nonsteroidal anti-inflammatory drugs (NSAIDs) should be avoided in RYGB patients.[3] Numerous studies have demonstrated increased complications, especially with concomitant tobacco use. If chronic anti-inflammatory use cannot be avoided, consideration for a bariatric procedure without the risk of marginal ulceration, such as the SG, may be in the patient's best interest. In RYGB patients, short courses (3 to 10 days) of anti-inflammatory therapy such as ibuprofen or naproxen for acute gouty attacks, migraine headaches, and acute musculoskeletal strain are usually well tolerated but should be taken with food to lessen the effect of direct mucosal irritation. It is generally considered safe for patients to resume low-dose aspirin therapy for anti-platelet cardioprotective benefits after the first 30 days of their surgery.

Oral Contraceptive Management

Due to improvement in insulin sensitivity and estrogen metabolism immediately after metabolic and bariatric surgery, ovulatory rates often improve soon after the bariatric surgical procedure despite little, if any, weight loss. However, pregnancy is not recommended for at least 12 months after surgery due to the increased catabolism and increased risk of nutritional deficiencies.[13] Like other medications, oral contraception absorption may be inconsistent in RYGB patients, and therefore, an alternative barrier method of birth control should be recommended. This becomes an important issue to discuss with patients, particularly for those who have polycystic ovarian syndrome (PCOS) or amenorrhea with resultant infertility for many years prior to surgery and are under the mistaken impression that they will not be able to conceive.

Medications such as medroxyprogesterone acetate (Depo-Provera) injections may be effective to prevent pregnancy, but also can inhibit weight loss after surgery and should be avoided if possible. Intrauterine devices may be a consideration as an alternative method of birth control. Also, the use of patches for contraception in women with a BMI greater than 35 kg/m² should be used with caution due to the significant loss of effectiveness and unreliability.

Obstructive Sleep Apnea Management

Obstructive sleep apnea (OSA), as measured by the apnea-hypopnea index (AHI) and daytime sleepiness, often improve after bariatric surgery. Many patients may need the face mask readjusted as the contours of their face change with weight loss. While many patients simply stop using continuous positive airway pressure (CPAP) or oral devices, it is recommended that a repeat sleep study be performed prior to the decision of discontinuing CPAP to ensure that treatment is no longer necessary.[14] Changing the prescription to AutoPAP, which detects the lowest amount of inhalation pressure needed throughout the night and adjusts accordingly, may be an option as well. Although there is no specific guidelines for the timing of reevaluation, several high-volume bariatric surgery programs recommend a repeat sleep study after 30% to 40% weight loss or 6 to 8 months after surgery.

LONG-TERM CONSEQUENCES OF METABOLIC SURGERY (>6 MONTHS)

Metabolic Bone Disease After Bariatric Surgery

Obesity was originally felt to strengthen bone because of the long-term weight-bearing burden on bone. However, more recent evidence suggests that obesity may not be as protective on bone health. Factors which contribute to the site-specific fracture risk in obesity include adipokine effects on bone physiology, systemic inflammation, reduced mobility, and vitamin D deficiency.

The prevalence of vitamin D deficiency in individuals with obesity varies from 20% to 85%. Mechanisms include lack of sufficient sun exposure to convert 7-dehydrocholesterol (7-DHC) to vitamin D_3 and sequestration of vitamin D in adipose tissue.[15] In patients with overweight and obesity, modest weight loss has been shown to result in small decreases in bone density of the hip with sparing of the spine. With greater degree of weight loss, metabolic and bariatric surgery is associated with a deterioration in bone health with specific effects shown in Table 10.1.

TABLE 10.1 Clinical Findings Showing the Deterioration in Bone Health After Metabolic Surgery

EFFECTS OF METABOLIC SURGERY ON BONE HEALTH

- Alterations in bone remodeling with increase in markers of remodeling
- Increased rates of bone loss
- Bone loss by quantitative imaging (DEXA)
- Alterations in bone strength
- Microarchitectural deterioration related to increased PTH levels
- Increase in fracture risk with time after surgery

DEXA, dual-energy x-ray absorptiometry; PTH, parathyroid hormone.

Due to greater malabsorption, the RYGB and BPD procedures are associated with the greatest risk of bone loss and fracture risk compared to the SG or the AGB. The pathogenesis of bone loss after metabolic and bariatric surgery is multifactorial. Malabsorptive surgery results in reduced intestinal absorption of calcium and vitamin D. Reduced gastric acid production related to surgery and antacid use will further reduce calcium absorption, leading to hypocalcemia which is a stimulus for parathyroid hormone (PTH) release and a diagnosis of secondary hyperparathyroidism. This in turn increases bone loss. Evidence also suggests that bone loss after bariatric surgery correlates with the amount of weight loss and the rate at which it occurs due to increased activation of the calcium-PTH axis. Surgery has also been shown to increase the bone turnover markers, N-terminal telopeptide of type I collagen (NTX), bone-specific alkaline phosphatase (BSAP), and osteocalcin. One important marker, sclerostin, is produced in osteocytes, and its main function is to inhibit bone formation. Mechanical unloading of bone after weight loss has been associated with an increased level of sclerostin resulting in significant loss in bone mineral density (BMD). Monitoring of bone health in postoperative patients undergoing all types of bariatric procedures is critical for its preservation. Guidelines for monitoring are summarized in Table 10.2.[16]

Biochemical indices for diagnostic testing for metabolic bone disease include serum calcium, phosphorus, magnesium, 25(OH)D (and 1,25(OH)D if renal function is compromised), BSAP or osteocalcin, PTH, and a bone marker of resorption such as urine n-telopeptide (NTX), 24-hour urinary calcium excretion, and albumin and prealbumin. Routine monitoring should include only PTH, 25(OH)D every 3 to 6 months for the first year and annually thereafter for patients undergoing AGB, SG, or RYGB. For those who have undergone BPD with or without switch, the following are recommended: PTH and 24-hour urine calcium monitoring every 6 to 12 months, urine N-telopeptide annually, and osteocalcin as needed[3] (Table 10.3).

Dual-energy x-ray absorptiometry (DEXA) is the gold standard for measuring bone density; the results are reported in T- and Z-score. The Z-score should be used for premenopausal women and men younger than 50 years. This score is the patient's BMD expressed in standard deviations (SDs) from the mean in an age- and sex-matched reference population. A low Z-score (below -2.0) is a concern for less bone mass compared to similar aged matched individual. Whereas the T-score is also calculated as an SD from the mean, the comparison group is that of young healthy adults. The World Health Organization (WHO) classifies T-scores above -1 SD as normal, between -1 and -2.5 SD as osteopenia, and below -2.5 SD as osteoporosis. Guidelines recommend DEXA 2 years postoperatively for both men and women after any type of metabolic and bariatric surgery. HCPs should evaluate each postoperative surgical patient based on risk factors which include age, baseline vitamin D and PTH status, weight loss trajectory, and activity level for decisions related to assessment of bone density.[17]

An abnormal DEXA scan may be indicative of both primary and secondary disease. In the post–bariatric

---

TABLE 10.2 Laboratory Screening and Monitoring for Bone Health After Surgery

GUIDELINES FOR MONITORING BONE HEALTH AFTER METABOLIC SURGERY

Laboratory tests used in the evaluation of bone health

- Calcium, phosphorous, magnesium
- 25(OH) vitamin D (and 1,25(OH) vitamin D if renal function is impaired)
- Bone-specific alkaline phosphatase or osteocalcin
- Parathyroid hormone (PTH)
- 24-hour urinary calcium excretion
- Vitamin A and K_1 levels
- Albumin, prealbumin
- DEXA at baseline and 2-year follow-up

DEXA, dual-energy x-ray absorptiometry.

TABLE 10.3 Routine Monitoring for Metabolic Bone Disease for Bariatric Surgery Patients

SG/RYGB	BPD w/wo DS
Every 3-6 months for the first year and annually thereafter:	Every 3 months for the first year, every 3-6 months thereafter:
25(OH)D	25(OH)D
Optional:	Albumin/prealbumin
PTH	Every 6-12 months:
DEXA monitoring may be indicated at baseline and at about 2 years	Parathyroid hormone (PTH) 24-hour urine calcium
	Annually:
	Urine N-telopeptide
	As needed:
	Osteocalcin DEXA monitoring may be indicated at baseline and at about 2 years

BPD w/wo DS, biliopancreatic diversion with or without duodenal switch; DEXA, dual-energy x-ray absorptiometry; RYGB, Roux-en-Y gastric bypass; SG, sleeve gastrectomy.

surgery patient, one should first suspect secondary bone disease due to nutritional deficiencies. The etiology of confirmed vitamin D deficiency, hypocalcemia, hypomagnesemia, hypophosphatemia, elevated alkaline phosphatase, secondary hyperparathyroidism, and even protein or vitamin B12 deficiency should be clearly defined and appropriately treated. Treatment should also include weight-bearing exercise and resistance training to mitigating bone loss after surgery.

For treatment of vitamin D deficiency, The Endocrine Society recommends a dose two to three times higher (6,000 to 10,000 IU/day) for patients with obesity, patients with malabsorptive syndromes, and patients on medications affecting vitamin D metabolism. A maintenance therapy of at least 3,000 to 6000 IU/day is recommended. Correction of vitamin D deficiency in bariatric surgery patients generally requires higher doses, particularly in the malabsorptive procedures. Repletion has been recommended for as high as 50,000 to 150,000 IU of D_2 or D_3 daily for one to 2 weeks. A maintenance dose of up to 50,000 IU one to three times per week may be required. Cholecalciferol (D3) has demonstrated superiority at maintaining 25(OH)D levels and has been recommended particularly if dosing is less than once weekly. It is recommended that both D_2 and D_3 be taken with a meal containing some fat to maximize absorption.

For patients with persistently low bone density on DEXA with clinical and biochemical evidence of bone disease, additional pharmacologic treatment with a bisphosphonate should be considered. Current recommendations include intravenous therapy with zoledronic acid, 5 mg once a year, or ibandronate, 3 mg every 3 months, due to higher risk of anastomotic ulceration and decreased absorption in RYGB patients. Patients without concerns for risk of ulceration or lack of absorption can be supplemented by mouth using alendronate 70 mg/week, risedronate 35 mg/week (or 150 mg/month), or ibandronate 150 mg/month.

Nephrolithiasis After Bariatric Surgery

An increase in the incidence of nephrolithiasis after metabolic and bariatric surgery has been clearly established, particularly in BPD and RYGB patients, where the calcium oxalate stone risk is threefold that of age-matched controls. A recent study also revealed a 7.6% incidence of nephrolithiasis after any bariatric surgery with a post-RYGB kidney stone incidence at 8.1%. Stone development after malabsorptive (BPD/RYGB) and restrictive (SG) bariatric procedures are largely caused by changes in 24-hour urine profiles, such as increased urinary oxalate, decreased urine volume, and reduced urinary citrate levels leading to increased risk of kidney stones.[18] Increased oxalate absorption and a hyperoxaluric state is facilitated by increased colonic oxalate related to increased colonic fatty acid and bile salts as well as alterations in the gut microflora.

The most important factor in preventing stone formation is increasing fluid intake since a greater urinary volume provides a dilutional effect leading to decreased supersaturation ratios. Patients should strive to maintain a daily urine production of at least 2 L by increasing fluid intake, limit dietary oxalate (<150 mg/day) and fat intake (<40 g/day), and consume the Recommended Daily Allowance of calcium (1,000 to 1,200 mg/day).[19] Supplemental calcium is also recommended as it binds oxalate, leading to excretion in feces. Postoperative patients who develop symptomatic stones should have an evaluation and intervention by a urologist.

Postprandial Hyperinsulinemic Hypoglycemia

An important unintended metabolic complication which has become increasingly recognized is postprandial hyperinsulinemic hypoglycemia (also called post-bypass hypoglycemia or PBH), which is characterized by hypoglycemic symptoms developing 1 to 3 hours after a meal, in association with a low blood glucose level of <54 mg/dL and relieved by the ingestion of carbohydrate. PBH is distinct from a condition called dumping syndrome where vasomotor symptoms occur within minutes to 1 hour after a meal of calorie-dense food, caused by rapid hyperosmotic food entry into the jejunum which induces fluid shifts into the small intestine.[20] Dumping usually occurs early after surgery, most commonly after RYGB, whereas classic PBH commonly develops between 1 and 4 years after surgery.

As PBH has become increasingly recognized, additional studies with larger patient numbers suggest that this condition is most commonly associated with RYGB but has been described after BPD with DS and GS as well. The exact prevalence of this disorder remains unclear, but with increased number of patients undergoing bariatric surgeries, HCPs will likely encounter such patients.

The precise mechanism for the changes in glucose homeostasis occurring with PBH remains unclear and likely has multiple contributing factors.[21] The proposed mechanism includes the rapid entry of ingested glucose into the jejunum as a result of the altered foregut anatomy after RYGB, which causes a rapid spike in glucose concentration. In conjunction with the rapid rise in glucose, there is a marked increase in meal induced levels of GLP-1 leading to an enhanced incretin effect and an abrupt rise in insulin levels. In addition, it appears that the suppression of insulin release in response to a falling level of glucose may be altered in patients with PBH. The presentation of PBH can be wide ranging and include the neuroglycopenic signs and symptoms of confusion, weakness, lightheadedness, dizziness, blurred vision, disorientation and loss of consciousness, and indications of adrenergic stimulation including sweating, tachycardia, and tremor. If the HCP is suspicious of the diagnosis, but cannot confirm it, referral to an endocrinologist should be considered for provocative testing with a mixed meal tolerance test and/or continuous glucose monitoring looking for exaggerated glucose excursions in symptomatic patients.

The variability of signs and symptoms, lack of patient awareness of hypoglycemia, and the absence of a clear pathophysiology make the management of this condition challenging. The consumption of complex carbohydrates such as brown rice, cereals, sweet potatoes, peas, and corn are useful if patients can recognize oncoming symptoms. Efforts to educate patients and family members regarding recognition of the condition and to have glucagon available for administration when patients are unable to take oral carbohydrate are important strategies to be considered.

Dietary adjustment with supervision by a registered dietitian nutritionist (RDN) should be the first line of treatment for PBH. Frequent small mixed meals with low–glycemic index carbohydrates have been successful, and the supervised use of a low-carbohydrate diet has been recently reported in a randomized controlled trial to lower glycemic peaks, increase glucose nadirs, and reduce insulin levels. The basic components of the first-line dietary approach involve a mixed diet which limits high-glycemic carbohydrate foods and emphasizes protein (Table 10.4). The dietary approach can be more aggressive if symptoms persist despite dietary changes, which consists of greater restriction of carbohydrate foods and enhancement of protein intake.

If symptoms persist despite supervised dietary changes, HCPs may consider acarbose, which decreases glucose absorption by inhibiting intestinal α-glucosidase. A referral to a board-certified obesity medicine specialist or endocrinologist should be considered if additional pharmacological treatment is necessary, which may include a trial of diazoxide or octreotide which inhibit insulin secretion.

When dietary and pharmacological treatments are unsuccessful, surgical treatment is a consideration. Placement of a feeding gastrostomy tube in the remnant stomach after RYGB allows liquid feedings to pass through the duodenum and proximal jejunum which normalizes glycemic responses. The rapid transit of ingested food from the small gastric reservoir to the jejunum can be altered by creating outflow restriction by banding or an endoscopic approach. If symptomatically necessary, surgical reversal of the bariatric procedure may be required. In the past, partial pancreatectomy was utilized, but this procedure is no longer recommended because of morbidity and risk of recurrent symptoms.

Postoperative Substance Use/Abuse

Bariatric surgical patients, particularly those who underwent an RYGB procedure, are more likely than those in the general population to die of drug- or alcohol-related causes according to a recent meta-analysis.[22] Although the exact reason is for the increase in mortality among RYGB patients is unclear, the absorption and metabolism of alcohol is augmented due to altered anatomy after the RYGB. In addition, all patients with a history of alcohol or drug use/abuse prior to surgery have a higher rate of recidivism postoperatively. HCPs should be aware of this concern and substance abuse education should be discussed with all post–bariatric surgery patients.

Postoperative Abdominal Pain

While there can be several etiologies for abdominal pain after metabolic and bariatric surgery, the most common causes are gallstones, smoking, use of NSAIDs, and internal hernias in RYGB patients.

With any rapid weight loss, gallstone formation can occur and cause right upper quadrant (RUQ) pain or discomfort with or without eating. An RUQ ultrasound and complete metabolic profile are the preferred tests to diagnosis cholelithiasis. With any procedure, chronic smoking can cause microvascular changes leading to ulcer or stricture formation. If smoking cessation and 2 to 4 weeks of proton-pump inhibitor therapy does not relieve one's symptoms, an upper endoscopy (also known as esophagogastroduodenoscopy, EGD) may be warranted. NSAIDs use such as ibuprofen or naproxen in RYGB patients may cause gastric ulcer or anastomotic strictures causing abdominal pain. If refraining from NSAIDs and 2 to 4 weeks of proton-pump inhibitor therapy does not relieve symptoms, like in smokers, an EGD may be warranted.

TABLE 10.4 Approach to Dietary Treatment of Hypoglycemia

Principles of Dietary Treatment of Postprandial Hypoglycemia

- Avoid high-glycemic carbohydrate food and beverages (cereal, sweets, rice, soda, juices)
- Prioritize protein at every meal and snack (chicken, fish, eggs, meat)
- Small portions of low-glycemic carbohydrate foods (quinoa, nonstarchy vegetables, berries)
- Carbohydrate foods should be consumed last and in small portions

---

Courtesy of Nicole Rubenstein, RD, Kaiser Permanente Colorado.

Another cause of intermittent or chronic abdominal pain in postoperative laparoscopic RYGB patients is an internal hernia. An internal hernia is the protrusion of intestines through a mesenteric defect which can result in a small bowel obstruction, ischemia, or infarction. Most of the internal hernias occur between 6 and 24 months postoperatively when appreciable fat mass is lost, and defects can occur. If suspected, a CT scan of the abdomen and urgent surgical evaluation is recommended.

NUTRITIONAL CONSEQUENCES AFTER METABOLIC SURGERY

Protein Malnutrition

Protein malnutrition is an important nutritional complication of metabolic and bariatric surgery resulting from the anatomic and physiologic changes from surgery. The overall incidence of this complication is lowest after purely restrictive operations (AGB) and increases directly with the amount or foregut alteration and malabsorption. Despite these surgical changes, no study has demonstrated protein malabsorption after RYGB, and there is evidence that protein absorption is preserved after this procedure.[23] The small gastric reservoir, postoperative anorexia, vomiting, alterations in taste and olfactory function, as well as food aversions all may contribute to reduced dietary protein intake. Protein malnutrition is recognized by a serum albumin level <3.5 g/dL (normal: 3.5 to 5 g/dL) in the absence of severe liver disease, protein loss from the gastrointestinal tract, or protein loss from renal disease. Severe hypoalbuminemia (albumin <2.5 g/dL) is associated with increased morbidity and mortality.

Adequate protein intake after surgery is important for the preservation of lean body mass. Additional benefits of adequate protein intake include a modest increase in energy expenditure and enhanced satiety. Current guidelines state that protein intake should be individualized and monitored by an RDN with attention to gender, age, and weight. A minimal protein intake of 60 g/day and up to 1.5 g/kg of ideal body weight (IBW) should be adequate.[3] However, higher protein intake up to 2.1 g/kg IBW may be needed as recommended on an individual basis. Despite these recommendations, numerous studies have demonstrated that a large percentage of postoperative patients have protein intakes less than 60 g/day during the first year after surgery and, in turn, results in reductions in lean body mass leading to sarcopenic obesity.

Patients with normal nutrition can usually tolerate short-term protein catabolism without consequence. However, chronic protein malnutrition can have serious consequences.[24] For this reason, ongoing patient education and supervision by an RDN is an essential component of postoperative care. Liberal use of easily digested and absorbed modular protein supplements is recommended to ensure a protein intake between 60 to 120 g/day. Patients who demonstrate increasing protein malnutrition during the postoperative period should be considered for referral for more intensive nutritional interventions which include nasojejunal feeding, gastrostomy feedings via the excluded gastric remnant, or total parenteral nutrition.

Micronutrient Deficiencies

Micronutrients, also referred to as vitamins and minerals, are substances needed by the body in only small amounts. However, they are essential for development, growth, and overall health. Micronutrients are not produced naturally by the body and must be provided from dietary or supplemental sources. Micronutrient absorption following metabolic and bariatric surgery can be limited by decreased exposure to gastric acid, decreased volume of food intake, and the surgical alteration of the gastrointestinal tract. As demonstrated in Figure 10.1, micronutrient absorption occurs in different sections of the intestinal tract.[1] The risk of micronutrient deficiencies increases with the extent of foregut anatomic changes affecting absorption. A patient with a BPD or RYGB procedure is at greater risk for deficiencies than a patient who underwent an SG or AGB procedure. Of note, patients with an AGB that is too tight or malpositioned can have protracted vomiting that can result in micronutrient deficiencies.

Bariatric surgery patients should undergo life-long nutritional surveillance and follow-up care. The following is a review of each micronutrient and recommendations regarding perioperative clinical evaluation, routine postoperative micronutrient supplementation (Table 10.5), recommendations for micronutrient monitoring (Table 10.6), signs and symptoms of deficiency (Table 10.7), and treatment of deficiency states.[7] The prevalence of micronutrient deficiencies pre– and post–bariatric surgery will be reviewed. Of note, thiamine and vitamin D deficiencies were previously addressed as underlying causes of Wernicke-Korsakoff syndrome and metabolic bone disease, respectively.

Iron

One of the most important and common nutritional complications of metabolic and bariatric surgery is iron deficiency, resulting both from the permanent anatomic and physiologic changes in foregut anatomy. Iron is essential for health because of its major role in oxygen transport and storage as a constituent of hemoglobin and muscle myoglobin, respectively. In addition, its ability to shift between the ferrous (Fe^{2+}) and ferric

TABLE 10.5 Recommended Vitamin and Mineral Supplementation After Bariatric Surgery[a]

	AGB	SG	RYGB	BPD/DS
Vitamin B1[b]	• Minimum 12 mg/d • At risk: at least 50-100 mg/d			
Vitamin B12[b]	• 300-500 µg/d oral, disintegrating tablet, SL or nasal or • 1,000 µg/mo IM			
Folate[b]	• 400-800 µg/d oral • 800-1,000 µg/d F childbearing age			
Calcium	1200-1500 mg/d	1200-1500 mg/d	1200-1500 mg/d	1800-2,400 mg/d
Vitamin A	5000 IU/d	5,000-10,000 IU/d	5,000-10,000 IU/d	10,000 IU/d
Vitamin E[b]	15 mg/d			
Vitamin K	90-120 µg/d	90-120 µg/d	90-120 µg/d	300 µg/d
Vitamin D[b]	At least 3000 IU/d to maintain D, 25 (OH) > 30 ng/mL			
Iron	At least 18 mg/d	M and nonmenstruating F 18 mg/d from multivitamins from multivitamins	At least 65-60 mg/d in F with menses after SG,	RYGB, BPD/DS, and patients with history of anemia
Zinc	8-11 mg/d	8-11 mg/d	8-11 mg/d	16-22 mg/d
Copper	1 mg/d	1 mg/d	1-2 mg/d	2 mg/d

AGB, adjustable gastric banding; BPD/DS, biliopancreatic diversion with duodenal switch; d, daily; F, female; IM, intramuscularly; M, male; mo, monthly; RYGB, Roux-en-Y gastric bypass; SG, sleeve gastrectomy; SL, sublingual.

There are several specialized multivitamin preparations available for bariatric surgery patients. These preparations have higher levels of vitamin B12, iron, and vitamin D in comparison to many standard complete multivitamins in order to meet the supplemental guidelines set forth by the ASMBS. Multivitamins specifically for BPD/DS patients also have additional fat-soluble vitamins (A, D, E, and K). Using such products can help ensure the patient is getting the recommended doses, decrease pill burden, and increase compliance.

[a]Adapted from Parrott J, Frank L, Rabena R, Craggs-Dino L, Isom KA, Greiman L. American society for metabolic and bariatric surgery integrated health nutritional guidelines for the surgical weight loss patient 2016 update: micronutrients. Surg Obes Relat Dis. 2017;13(5):727-741.

[b]Recommended vitamin supplementation same in all bariatric procedures.

(Fe^{3+}) state underlies its important role in electron transport and mitochondrial energy generation. These functions collectively explain the common association between iron deficiency and refractory fatigue.

The pathogenesis of iron deficiency complicating metabolic and bariatric surgery is multifactorial. A marked reduction in gastric acid in the small gastric reservoir along with use of antacid medications limits the solubility of ingested iron. Additionally, bypass of the duodenum and proximal jejunum in the RYGB procedure eliminates food contact with the major sites of iron absorption. Other contributing factors include a reduction in consumption of foods containing heme iron, food aversions, and anorexia.

The diagnosis of iron deficiency in the absence of inflammation is based on the association of the circulating level of ferritin with iron stores. A ferritin level <30 ng/mL is diagnostic of absolute iron deficiency in the absence of inflammation. The presence of inflammation is easily detected by measuring the circulating level of C-reactive protein (CRP), a well-recognized

marker of inflammation. A CRP level >3 mg/L indicates that inflammation is present, and thus ferritin is no longer an accurate predictor of iron stores. In association with a CRP level >3 mg/L, ferritin levels between 30 and 100 ng/mL or a normal ferritin level together with a transferrin saturation (Tsat) < 20% are also consistent with iron deficiency. HCPs should be aware that inflammation slowly resolves during surgical weight loss and that the presence of iron deficiency is a strong stimulus to enhance iron absorption. The diagnosis of iron deficiency usually requires several laboratory tests in combination including ferritin, CRP, and transferrin saturation.

Iron absorption after metabolic and bariatric surgery is reduced by all current procedures, and the reported prevalence of iron deficiency in short- to intermediate-term follow-up after surgery is 20% to 50%.[26] Several studies have shown that the prevalence increases with time after surgery. Patients with the greatest risk for postoperative deficiency and iron deficiency anemia (IDA) include menstruating females,

TABLE 10.6 Recommended Nutritional Monitoring after Metabolic and Bariatric Surgery[a]

	SCREENING (ADDITION TESTING)	PREOPERATIVELY	3 MO. POSTOPERATIVELY	6 MO. POSTOPERATIVELY	ANNUALLY
Vitamin B1	Whole blood thiamine	X	Any time N/V-	–	–
Vitamin B12	Serum B12 (MMA, homocysteine)	X	RYGB SG BPD/DS	RYGB SG BPD/DS	X
Folate	Folate (RBC folate, homocysteine, MMA)	X	X	X	X
Vitamin A	Plasma retinol (RBP-retinol binding protein)	X		BPD/DS	X
Vitamin D	25(OH)D	X	X	X	X
Vitamin E/K	Plasma α-tocopherol/ Plasma phylloquinone (PT-prothrombin time)	X			X
Iron[b]	Ferritin (serum iron, TSAT, TIBC, CBC)	X	X	X	X
Zinc[b]	plasma or serum zinc (RBC zinc, urine zinc)	X			RYGB SG BPD/DS
Copper[b]	Serum copper (ceruloplasmin, Erythrocyte superoxide dismutase)	X			RYGB SG BPD/DS
PTH	Serum PTH, serum calcium	X	X	X	X
Calcium	Combination: vitamin D25(OH), ALP, serum P, 24 hour urinary calcium in comparison to dietary calcium	X	X	X	X
DEXA		X			Every 2 yrs

X = all bariatric procedures.

ALP, alkaline phosphatase; BPD/DS, biliopancreatic diversion with duodenal switch; CBC, complete blood count; DEXA, dual-energy x-ray absorptiometry; MMA, methylmalonic acid; mo, month; N/V, nausea and vomiting; P, phosphorus; PTH, parathyroid hormone; RBC, red blood cell; RYGB, Roux-en-Y gastric bypass; SG, sleeve gastrectomy; TIBC, total iron binding capacity; TSAT, transferrin saturation; yrs, years.

[a]Adapted from Parrott J, Frank L, Rabena R, Craggs-Dino L, Isom KA, Greiman L. American society for metabolic and bariatric surgery integrated health nutritional guidelines for the surgical weight loss patient 2016 update: micronutrients. Surg Obes Relat Dis. 2017;13(5):727-742.

[b]Ferritin, zinc, and copper are acute phase reactant. Levels fluctuation with infection, inflammation, and age.

older males (>40 years), and those with a low level of ferritin before surgery. Presenting signs and symptoms of IDA include fatigue, shortness of breath, pale conjunctiva, and a microcytic anemia. Current guidelines recommend that all postoperative patients should receive supplemental iron at a dose of 45 to 60 mg/day.[7] Oral supplements should be taken in divided doses and separately from calcium supplements. Adherence to taking supplements is a major concern

as oral iron treatment can induce GI side effects, most notably constipation. Laboratory screening for iron status should be performed at least annually and more frequently if deficiency is present to assess treatment efficacy.

The first-line treatment for iron deficiency is oral iron in doses of 150 to 200 mg daily.[27] Oral iron can be increased to 300 mg two to three times daily as tolerated. Absorption can be enhanced with the addition of

TABLE 10.7 Clinical Findings of Vitamin/Mineral Deficiencies[a]

	SIGNS AND SYMPTOMS OF DEFICIENCY
Vitamin B1 (thiamine)	Muscle weakness, ataxia, loss of reflexes Oculomotor dysfunction (nystagmus/ophthalmoplegia), paresthesia, confusion, heart failure/edema (wet beriberi) Wernicke encephalopathy triad: mental status change, oculomotor changes, gait ataxia
Vitamin B12 (cobalamin)	Sensory distal neuropathy Loss of proprioception, ataxia Macrocytic anemia Dementia, depression Glossitis
Folate	Macrocytic anemia, neural tube defects Mild pancytopenia
Iron	Microcytic anemia, fatigue, decrease work performance, glossitis, nail spooning or ridges, pica, restless legs
Calcium	Bone disease, secondary hyperparathyroidism
Vitamin D	Osteomalacia, muscle weakness and pain, cramps, tingling sensation, bone pain, hypocalcemia, tetany
Vitamin A	Bitot spots, night blindness Skin hyperkeratosis Blindness
Vitamin E	Neuropathy (sensor and motor) Ataxia Hemolysis
Vitamin K	Impaired coagulation Osteoporosis
Zinc	Decreased taste/smell, impaired healing, Skin rash, hair loss, glossitis, diarrhea
Copper	Hypochromic anemia, neutropenia, ataxia, paresthesia, myeloneuropathy

[a]Adapted from Parrott J, Frank L, Rabena R, Craggs-Dino L, Isom KA, Greiman L. American society for metabolic and bariatric surgery integrated health nutritional guidelines for the surgical weight loss patient 2016 update: micronutrients. Surg Obes Relat Dis. 2017;13(5):727-743.

ascorbic acid. During the postoperative period, systemic inflammation lessens and the impaired erythropoiesis accompanying iron deficiency will enhance absorption. Failure to respond to oral iron is an indication for parenteral iron infusion. There are currently no guidelines for the treatment of preoperative patients with iron deficiency. These patients should be treated before surgery in order to restore more normal iron stores and reduce the risk of postoperative anemia. The decision to treat with intravenous iron is a function of the presence and severity of anemia, efficacy of oral iron, the development of GI side effects, patient adherence with oral supplementation, chronic blood loss, and cost and safety of infusion protocols.

Vitamin B12

Vitamin B12 (cobalamin) is a water-soluble vitamin needed for proper function of many hematologic and neurologic processes. Gastric acid, intrinsic factor, and proteolytic enzymes present in gastric secretions are needed to utilize vitamin B12 from dietary sources. Bariatric surgeries that limit exposure to gastric secretions increase risk of deficiency.

Preoperative screening for vitamin B12 deficiency is recommended for all patients. Deficiency is seen in 2% to 18% of patients with obesity and increases to 6% to 30% if taking proton-pump inhibitors. Vitamin B12 deficiency is also seen with chronic use of metformin.

Serum B12 levels alone, especially when at the lower end of the normal range, may be inadequate to diagnosis deficiency. Elevated methylmalonic acid (MMA) level is a better test since it is specific for metabolic changes seen in vitamin B12 deficiency. The prevalence of vitamin B12 deficiency at 2 to 5 years postoperatively has been reported as <20% in RYGB and 4% to 20% in SG. Routine supplementation after bariatric surgery is recommend by one of the following methods:

- 300 to 500 µg orally via disintegrating tablet, sublingual, or liquid formulation,
- 1,000 µg intramuscularly (IM) monthly, or
- intranasal (dose per manufacture's recommendation).

Vitamin B12 deficiency can manifest as macrocytic anemia, glossitis, distal sensory neuropathy, loss of proprioception, ataxia, and neuropsychiatric changes. Treatment of vitamin B12 deficiency without neurologic symptoms is 1,000 µg/mL IM weekly for 8 weeks. For those with neurologic symptoms, treatment is 1,000 µg/mL IM daily for 5 days, followed by monthly for life.

Vitamin B1 (Thiamine)

Thiamine (B1) is a water-soluble vitamin that is essential for carbohydrate metabolism. It also plays a role in muscle contraction and nerve conduction. Thiamine diphosphate is the active form of thiamine and is best measured in whole blood, as it has low concentration in the plasma. Thiamine plasma levels reflect recent intake, not body stores. Albumin is the carrier for thiamine; therefore, hypoalbuminemia will reflect decreased thiamine levels.

The prevalence of vitamin B1 deficiency in patients prior to bariatric surgery has been reported as high as 29%, whereas the prevalence after bariatric surgery has been reported to be < 1 to 49% varying by surgical procedure and the amount of time since surgery. Postoperative screening is recommended for any high-risk surgery patient which includes those with chronic nausea and vomiting, small intestinal bacterial overgrowth, or history of cardiac failure receiving loop diuretic therapy (such as furosemide). The presence of malnutrition, rapid weight loss, and excessive alcohol consumption increases the risk of deficiency.

The minimal daily dose for vitamin B1 supplementation postoperatively is 12 mg for all surgery patients. This amount is higher than the typical 1.5 mg contained in over-the-counter multivitamin-mineral supplements. Accordingly, a B-complex supplement containing 50 mg of B1 is often advised.

In addition to the acute presentation described earlier in the chapter, signs and symptoms of B1 deficiency include muscle weakness, paresthesia, gait and ocular disturbances, change in mental status (confusion/impaired memory), and heart failure (also called wet beriberi). In the bariatric surgery patient, B1 deficiency can present as a constellation of neurological symptoms including encephalitis, oculomotor dysfunction, and gait disturbance (Wernicke encephalopathy).

Folic Acid

Folic acid is a water-soluble vitamin needed by every cell in the body. Its roles include DNA synthesis, cell division and growth, and red blood cell formation. The prevalence of folic acid deficiency in patients with obesity is as high as 54%. The postoperative prevalence of folic acid deficiency after the RYGB and SG procedures has been reported as high as 65% and 18%, respectively. Recommended supplementation following metabolic and bariatric surgery is 400 to 800 µg daily (women of childbearing age should take 800 to 1,000 µg daily to decrease risk of neural tube defects). Folic acid deficiency can present with findings similar to B12 deficiency including macrocytic anemia, angular stomatitis, glossitis, and neurologic symptoms (more common in B12 deficiency, rarely in folic acid deficiency). Oral treatment of folic acid deficiency is 1,000 µg daily. Higher doses of folic acid are not advised as it may mask vitamin B12 deficiency. Therefore, checking for and correcting vitamin B12 deficiency is recommended.

Vitamin A

Vitamin A is a fat-soluble vitamin that plays a vital role in vision, immune function, bone growth, cell growth and repair, reproduction, and embryonic/fetal development. Vitamin A status is measured with a plasma retinol and retinol binding protein (RBP) level. Presurgery deficiency is reported at a prevalence of 14%, whereas postoperative deficiency is seen in 8% to 11% of RYGB patients and up to 70% of BPD/DS patients within 4 years. Current guidelines recommend routine vitamin A supplementation after bariatric surgery at a daily dose of 5,000 IU for AGB, 5,000 to 10,000 IU for SG and RYGB, and 10,000 IU for BPD/DS.

Vitamin A deficiencies can initially present with night blindness, impaired healing, decreased taste, and skin hyperkeratinization. Bitot spots, patches of hyperkeratinization on the conjunctiva, may also be observed. As vitamin A deficiency persists, it may lead to corneal damage and blindness.

Treatment of vitamin A deficiency is based on the presence of corneal findings. When present, vitamin A should be administered at a dose of 50,000 to 100,000 IU intramuscularly for 3 days followed by 50,000 IU IM for 2 weeks. When corneal involvement is absent, repletion dose of 10,000 to 25,000 IU should be given daily until improvement is seen. Iron, copper, and zinc status should be evaluated when a vitamin A deficiency is present since vitamin A can affect the metabolism of these minerals. Concomitant deficiencies will impair correction of vitamin A deficiency.

Vitamin D

Vitamin D plays essential roles in bone health, calcium/phosphorus homeostasis, immune function, and reduction of inflammation. Presurgery assessment of vitamin D status is recommended for all patients as the prevalence for deficiency has been reported as high as 90%. Postoperative deficiency has been reported as high as 100%. Vitamin D deficiency can cause muscle cramping and pain, tingling, tetany, hypocalcemia, and secondary hyperparathyroidism, increasing the risk for metabolic bone disease. The supplementation dose for all surgery patients is 3,000 IU D3 daily in order to maintain a 25(OH)D level > 30 ng/mL.

Treatment of vitamin D deficiency includes a daily dose of D3 at 3,000 to 6000 IU or a one to three times per week dose of D2 at 50,000 IU. Higher levels of 25(OH)D may be needed to suppress PTH levels. In one study of RYGB patients, a lower incidence PTH elevation and secondary hyperparathyroidism were seen with patient who had a 25 (OH) D level >40 ng/mL.

Calcium

Calcium is needed in the body for bone health, muscle contraction, nerve conduction, and other metabolic processes in the body. Calcium absorption is dependent on vitamin D. Long-term deficiency of calcium intake can lead to metabolic bone disease and secondary hyperparathyroidism. Persistent PTH elevation has been reported in bariatric patients. However, there is no solid evidence that this is associated with bone loss or turnover. In the presence of normal serum calcium and sufficient vitamin D levels, there is no evidence to support aggressive supplementation attempts to lower the PTH level. Recommended calcium supplement following bariatric surgery depends on the surgical procedure.[7] Patients who undergo AGB, SG, and RYGB should take 1,200 to 1,500 mg daily. The recommended dose for BPD/DS patients is 1,800 to 2,400 mg daily. Calcium supplementation should be divided into at least two daily doses to improve absorption. The formulation of calcium is important. Calcium carbonate is not well absorbed in low acidic environments and should be taken with meals. In contrast, calcium citrate absorption is independent of gastric acid and can be taken with or without meals. Calcium citrate is recommended for patients who undergo a surgical procedure that reduces gastric acid and anyone taking acid reducing medications, such as H2 blockers and proton-pump inhibitors.

Vitamin E

Vitamin E functions in the body as an antioxidant protecting cells from damage from free radicals. Vitamin E is needed for proper development of red blood cells and immune system function. Presurgery deficiency is reported at a prevalence of 2.2%. Postoperative deficiency is uncommon, and recommended supplementation is 15 mg daily. In breastfeeding women, the dose should be increased to 19 mg daily. Malabsorptive procedures (BPD/DS) may require higher doses to maintain levels.

Vitamin K

Vitamin K is a fat-soluble vitamin and has an important role in coagulation factor synthesis, bone metabolism, and the regulation of blood calcium. The presurgery prevalence of vitamin K deficiency has not been thoroughly studied. However, one study reported 40% of preoperative bariatric surgery patients had insufficiency of vitamin K independent of concurrent vitamin deficiencies. Vitamin K levels were lower in patients with diabetes and higher BMI. Although postoperative deficiency is uncommon. vitamin K deficiency presents as a sequela of impaired coagulation (easy bruising, mucosal bleeding, hematuria) and metabolic bone disease. The recommended supplementation dose for AGB, SG, and RYGB is 90 to 120 μg daily (most complete multivitamins provide this amount). For BPD/DS patients, the requirement is 300 μg daily which requires a vitamin K supplement in addition to a standard multivitamin. Many specialized bariatric vitamins are formulated to meet the vitamin K requirements.

Treatment recommendation for vitamin K deficiency caused by acute malabsorption is 10 mg vitamin K parenterally. In cases of chronic malabsorption, treatment options include a daily oral dose of vitamin K at 1 to 2 mg or a weekly parenterally dose of 1 to 2 mg.

Zinc

Zinc is necessary for proper function of many of the body systems, including immune, reproductive, endocrine, integumentary, and digestive system. Patients with obesity have lower levels of zinc in serum, plasma, and in erythrocytes when compared with lean controls. Zinc is a negative acute phase reactant, and in states of illness or inflammation, zinc levels will be lower. Treatment with zinc supplements are used for severely depleted levels and in those with signs and symptoms of deficiency. Zinc plays an important role in iron metabolism, and IDA can be seen secondary to zinc deficiency. Zinc deficiency is seen in 24% to 28% of patients prior to all bariatric surgery procedures and increases to 70% after BPD/DS, 40% after RYGB, 19% after SG, and 34% after AGB.

The recommended supplementation of zinc is 8 to 11 mg for AGB and SG patients, 8 to 22 mg for RYGB patients, and 22 mg for BPD/DS patients. Most complete multivitamin-mineral supplements will provide adequate zinc. When using a multivitamin-mineral to supplement zinc, it is advised to use a compound that has a ratio of 8 to 15 mg of zinc per 1 mg of copper. Early zinc deficiency can present with altered sense of taste and smell, skin rash, increased infection from immune dysfunction, and infertility. In states of severe deficiency, additional symptoms including diarrhea, hypogonadism, alopecia, acrodermatitis enteropathica (eczematous type rash), delayed wound healing, and night blindness (from secondary vitamin A deficiency) may be present. Treatment with zinc supplements are used for severely depleted levels and in those with signs and symptoms of deficiency. Recommended treatment includes 60 mg zinc orally twice daily until improvement of levels occurs. Zinc supplements should be given separately from other vitamins and minerals (especially iron, calcium and copper).

Copper

Copper is needed for normal function of the nervous system, production of red and white blood cells, and iron transport. The prevalence of copper deficiency prior to bariatric surgery has been reported as high as 70% of pre-BPD women. The American Society for Metabolic and Bariatric Surgery (ASMBS) recommends screening with serum copper and ceruloplasmin levels prior to RYGB and BPD/DS. Care must be taken with interpretation, as both are positive acute phase reactants that can be elevated due to inflammation or illness. The preferred test for determining copper deficiency is erythrocyte superoxide dismutase, but use may be limited by availability and cost. The prevalence of postoperative deficiency ranges from 10% to 20% after RYGB to 90% after BPD/DS.

Copper gluconate or sulfate are the recommended sources for copper supplementation. A dose of 1 mg/day is recommended for AGB and SG patients and a dose of 2 mg/day for RGYB and BPD/DS patients. Symptoms of copper deficiency manifest with hematologic (hypochromic anemia, neutropenia, pancytopenia) and neurologic findings (neuropathy, paresthesia, gait disturbance, spasticity). Hypopigmentation of hair, skin, and nails along with hypercholesterolemia may be observed.

Treatment for mild or moderate deficiency includes 3 to 8 mg daily until levels normalize. Severe deficiencies may require IV copper administration at 2 to 4 mg daily for 6 days or until neurologic symptoms resolve. With any history of copper deficiency, levels should be monitored every 3 months.

WEIGHT REGAIN FOLLOWING BARIATRIC SURGERY

Weight regain can occur following all the bariatric procedures.[28] In addition to changes in diet and physical activity, the biological defense of our adiposity through several adaptive physiologic and metabolic pathways strive to restore body weight. Although these metabolic processes occur with both medical and surgical weight loss, they are thought to be less prominent following surgical weight loss, therefore making it a more powerful tool for long-term weight management. All patients who experience weight regain or inadequate weight loss following metabolic and bariatric surgery should undergo a comprehensive evaluation for

1. Anatomical defects
2. Dietary indiscretion
3. Reduced physical activity and exercise
4. Nonsuicidal depression
5. Weight-promoting medication
6. Biologic and physiologic pathways

Anatomical Defects

Though uncommon, some patients experience more rapid weight gain following surgery due to an anatomical complication. These include formation of a gastrogastric (G-G) fistula, an overly dilated anastomosis, or a larger than expected stomach remnant after an SG. Anatomical defects can often be detected by obtaining a contrast upper gastrointestinal (UGI) x-ray, upper endoscopy, or CT scan with contrast. These should be reviewed by a bariatric surgeon who is familiar with bariatric procedures.

Dietary Indiscretion

Dietary "indiscretion" is the most common cause of weight regain following bariatric surgery. Between 12 to 16 months postoperative, patients often change from eating two to three structured meals per day to more of a "grazing" pattern. Moreover, total caloric intake increases and the macronutrient composition can change to include more energy-dense foods and liquids.

Exercise and Physiologic Influences

Like diet, patient's adherence to their recommended physical activity may tend to dwindle in the postoperative months/years. Robust physical activity and exercise is a crucial part of weight maintenance. Following rapid weight loss, patients can experience decreases in muscle mass and resultant decreased resting energy expenditure. Resistance training along with adequate protein intake helps maintain muscle mass which, in turn, maintains one's metabolic rate.

Depression and Weight Regain

Depression is another cause of weight regain that can occur in the immediate postoperative period (~6 to 8 months). It can cause some patients to "self-medicate" with food, especially carbohydrates, often falling into the grazing eating pattern. It is important to screen patients for depression using an objective depression inventory and initiate treatment if warranted.

Weight-Promoting Medications

Another consideration for weight regain are medications. It is important to take a thorough medication history to ensure that the medications that patients are taking are not causing weight gain or inhibiting weight loss. Examples of medications promoting weight loss or inhibiting weight loss are included in Chapter 2. While there may or may not be an identifiable cause for weight regain following bariatric surgery, antiobesity medication should be considered in patients with inadequate weight loss or weight gain following bariatric surgery. Please refer to Chapter 8 on antiobesity medications for further information and indications.

Biologic and Physiologic Pathways

An individual's weight is influenced by several factors, including genetics, environment, and hormonal regulation. The "set point" is the weight range in which our bodies are programmed to function optimally. When body weight is lowered by reduced caloric intake, hormone levels and adipocytes signal the brain to increase appetite. Because of these processes, it is often difficult for people to maintain a significant weight loss over a long period of time without some weight regain.

SUMMARY

As the awareness and beneficial outcomes of metabolic and bariatric surgery for obesity continue to increase, more patients will be electing to undergo these procedures as a long-term approach to obesity management. Accordingly, HCPs will be expected to monitor and manage these patients for metabolic and nutritional complications. Close collaboration between the multidisciplinary surgical program and the primary care network is essential in order to improve patient engagement and the quality of medical and nutritional care after surgery.

Iron deficiency is the most common nutritional deficiency following bariatric surgery.

- As a result of chronic systemic inflammation, obesity is associated with abnormal iron sequestration.
- Iron deficiency is seen in up to 40% of candidates for metabolic surgery.
- After surgery, the prevalence is higher because the surgical procedures interfere with iron absorption.

Because systemic inflammation alters the levels of the usual laboratory markers of iron nutrition, the diagnosis of iron deficiency in obesity is challenging.

- Laboratory tests needed include ferritin, transferrin saturation, hemoglobin, and CRP (marker of inflammation).
- When inflammation is absent (CRP normal), ferritin< 30 ng/mL is diagnostic of iron deficiency.
- In the presence of inflammation (CRP elevated), ferritin level up to 100 ng/mL reflects iron deficiency when transferrin saturation < 20%.
- The primary treatment for iron deficiency is oral iron at 100 to 200 mg/day in divided doses.
- During iron therapy, close follow-up with frequent laboratory testing is essential.
- Oral iron absorption is variable after surgery types.
- Gastrointestinal side effects resulting in poor patient compliance are common.
- A poor response to treatment and/or significant GI side effects are considerations for intravenous iron therapy.

CLINICAL HIGHLIGHTS

Metabolic Bone Disease

Obesity, once felt to strengthen bone because of the long-term increased weight bearing and increased bone density, may not be protective on bone health.

Factors which contribute to obesity-related fracture risk include

- Inflammatory proteins secreted by adipose tissue
- Obesity-associated systemic inflammation
- Reduced mobility
- Vitamin D deficiency

The prevalence of vitamin D deficiency in individuals with obesity ranges from 20% to 85%. Contributing factors include

- Lack of sun exposure required to convert to vitamin D3
- Sequestration of vitamin D in adipose tissue

Healthcare providers should evaluate each patient based on risk factors which include

- Age
- Baseline vitamin D and PTH status
- Weight loss trajectory
- Activity level

The primary treatment to mitigate bone loss:

- Maintain normal calcium and vitamin D levels
- Regular routine monitoring
- Encourage regular physical activity and especially resistance training

WHEN TO REFER?

Referral to the multidisciplinary bariatric surgery center should be considered for

- Postoperative nausea, vomiting, and suspected obstruction
- Suspected postprandial hyperinsulinemic hypoglycemia
- Concerns about macronutrient and micronutrient deficiencies
- Dietary nonadherence
- Development of behavioral or psychological distress
- Postoperative weight regain

CASE STUDIES

Discussion of Case Study 1—Development of Iron and Vitamin B12 Deficiency

Bariatric surgery is associated with development of several micronutrient deficiencies that are predictable based on the surgically altered anatomy and the imposed dietary changes. The patient's fatigue and exercise intolerance is most likely due to IDA and possibly vitamin B12 deficiency. Patients who undergo an RYGB procedure are at particular risk for developing iron deficiency and IDA due to reduced iron absorption, decreased iron intake, and, for menstruating women, increased iron losses. Diagnostic workup should include a CBC, ferritin level, iron, and total iron-binding capacity. Serum ferritin is the most sensitive indicator of iron status. The concentration of serum ferritin reflects the size of the storage iron compartment.

The patient's neurological sensory disturbances in the lower extremities of clumsiness and numbness may be due to several vitamin deficiencies, most notably vitamin B12. Although B12 deficiency is predictable, onset of signs and symptoms are typically delayed for months to years due to prolonged hepatic storage of the vitamin. Clinical effects of deficiency are similar to those of pernicious anemia—hematological and neurological. Hypersegmented polymorphonuclear leukocytes and macrocytic erythrocytes can be seen on peripheral blood smear along with a macrocytic anemia. Vitamin B12 status is most commonly assessed by serum or plasma vitamin levels. However, a more sensitive biochemical indicator of deficiency is elevation of serum homocysteine and methylmalonic acid, levels which rise when the supply of B12 is low and virtually confirms the diagnosis. In this patient, a combined deficiency of iron and vitamin B12 would result in a normal MCV.

Treatment would consist of oral supplementation with an iron salt preparation containing ferrous sulfate, gluconate, or fumarate. Typical dosing of iron therapy is 150 to 300 mg/day po given in two to three divided doses for 4 to 6 months or until the serum ferritin normalizes. Coadministration with ascorbic acid (vitamin C), the best known reducing agent, is recommended to increase iron absorption. Replenishment of vitamin B12 may be provided by prescribing oral crystalline B12 500 µg daily, as a once weekly nasal spray 500 µg cyanocobalamin gel, or by intramuscular injection 100 µg monthly. The route of delivery is based on patient preference and monitoring of vitamin B12 status.

CASE STUDY 2

WEIGHT REGAIN LATE AFTER SUCCESSFUL SURGERY

Mary is a 48-year-old woman who previously underwent an uneventful laparoscopic RYGB procedure 5 years ago. She has a past medical history of diabetes, depression, migraine headaches, and seasonal allergies. Her preoperative weight was 320 pounds. She reached a nadir weight of 224 pounds 15 months after surgery, representing a 30% weight loss. She presents today seeking a "surgical redo" as she has regained 48 pounds.

The patient was last seen 2 years ago. She stated she was doing well and did not think it was necessary to return. When she started to regain weight, she was embarrassed and thought it was her fault. She stated that "life got in the way," and she just got off track with her prescribed diet and regular physical activity. She states her hunger has increased over the last 6 months.

Her current medications include metformin 500 mg BID, propranolol 160 mg QD, paroxetine 37.5 mg QD, and diphenhydramine 25 mg at bedtime. On examination, her weight is 272 pounds, height 65″, BMI 45.4 kg/m², BP 120/82, and HR 76 BPM. The remainder of examination is notable for well-healed abdominal laparoscopic scars. Blood glucose is 88 mg/dL and HbA1c 5.6%

Discussion of Case Study 2

Mary's story is very typical of postoperative weight gain. The salient points are that she was doing well for the first 2 years after surgery and did not think regular follow-up was necessary. When she did start to experience weight regain, she was embarrassed and was hesitant to come back for assistance as she thought it was her fault. The fact is, although metabolic and bariatric surgery is the most effective treatment for long-term weight management, weight regain is common among all the various procedures. The key in dealing with postoperative weight gain is early intervention.

In evaluating a patient with postoperative weight gain, there are several key areas to consider. Occasionally, anatomical defects can contribute to weight regain. Although relatively uncommon, a G-G fistula can occur where there is a communication between the new pouch and the gastric remnant. Nonetheless, a UGI or upper endoscopy should be considered to rule out a G-G fistula or an enlarged anastomosis. If this is the case, and the surgeon believes it is large enough to be an important factor in the patient's weight gain, a surgical revision may be warranted. Often a UGI or endoscopy is important for the patient to objectively see there is no indication for surgical intervention and that medical management should be the focus to combat one's weight regain.

Once an anatomical defect has been ruled out, several other causes for weight regain need be considered. The first evaluation should be a thorough medication review to determine if the patent is taking any medications promoting weight gain or inhibiting weight loss. In Mary's case, she is taking several medications known to cause weight gain; paroxetine, propranolol, and diphenhydramine. Alternative medications should be considered that at least are weight neutral if not assist with weight loss. In Mary's case, consideration for bupropion in place of paroxetine, an ACE inhibitor in place of propranolol, and cetirizine in place of diphenhydramine.

The next area to evaluate is dietary indiscretion. Between 12 to 16 months postoperative, patients often liberalize their diet, tolerating larger portions of food, snacking throughout the day (referred to as grazing), and consuming more energy-dense foods. As in Mary's case, dietary emphasis should focus on meeting her protein needs, including vegetables and fruits, and limiting refined carbohydrates.

Screening for depression is important in patients with postoperative weight gain. It can cause some patients to "self-medicate" with food, especially carbohydrates, often falling into the grazing eating pattern. It is important to screen patients for depression using an objective depression inventory and initiate treatment if warranted.

The next area to evaluate is physical activity and exercise. Exercise is a crucial part of weight maintenance. Physical activity along with adequate protein intake helps maintain muscle mass which, in turn, maintains one's resting energy expenditure. Mary would likely benefit from a review of how to reinitiate an exercise routine and perhaps a referral to a fitness trainer for more accountability.

Mary states her appetite has increased over the last 6 months. There are several physiologic factors that our body possesses to maintain one's adiposity and regain weight. This is referred to as the set point or weight range in which our bodies are programmed to function optimally. Patients need to be educated about the biological changes that occur with extended weight loss and hold realistic expectations.

Finally, and maybe most importantly, regular follow-up is crucial for Mary to provide guidance, monitoring, and accountability. Treatment should be directed at the underlying causes of weight regain and, if indicated, considered for adjunctive use of an antiobesity medication.

CASE STUDY 3

POSTBYPASS HYPOGLYCEMIA

Jenny is a 35-year-old female that presents to the office after experiencing a near syncopal episode at work this morning. She reported that she began to feel shaky, dizzy, and broke out in a cold sweat. She had similar episodes in the past month that resolved with a few pieces of candy. Today, she did not have candy with her, and after 5 minutes, her vision became blurry and she "started to see stars." She sat down on the floor, and her coworker grabbed her a cola from the nearby cooler. Jenny reports eating a bagel for breakfast 2 hour prior to her symptoms beginning.

Jenny has a past medical history of severe obesity. She underwent laparoscopic RYGB 2 years ago. At the time of surgery Jenny weighed 320 pounds with a BMI of 50 kg/m². Her postoperative course was uncomplicated. Her only medications are chewable complete children's multivitamins twice daily, calcium citrate with vitamin D twice daily, monthly vitamin B12 injection, and acetaminophen if needed.

On examination, her weight is 175 pounds with a BMI 27 kg/m². BP sitting is 108/68 with a HR of 70 bpm, and BP standing is 110/66 and a HR of 72 bpm. Heart sounds are normal, and her abdominal incisions are healed. Her blood sugar in clinic is 92 mg/dL.

Discussion of Case Study 3

PBH following bariatric surgery occurs with estimated overall prevalence approximating 10% to 15% of patients. PBH usually develops late (1 to 4 years) after surgery and must be distinguished from the dumping syndrome which causes vasomotor symptoms within minutes after a meal and occurs early primarily after RYGB. Neuroglycopenic symptoms follow the pattern of Whipple triad: a low plasma glucose level in association with symptoms and resolution with the administration of glucose.

PBH most commonly follows gastric bypass but has been described in patients after sleeve gastrectomy and duodenal switch. Factors associated with higher susceptibility for PBH include female sex, no history of preoperative diabetes, and longer interval from surgery.

A glucometer should be prescribed in order to document blood sugars when symptoms occur. Continuous glucose monitoring (CGM) can be helpful also to warn patients of possible impending symptoms. The mainstay of treatment for PBH is prevention through dietary modifications with close supervision by an RDN. Recommended dietary modifications include small frequent mixed meals, which include protein and fats and limiting simple carbohydrates.

For relief of severe hypoglycemia, the patient should consume 15 g of carbohydrate (glucose tablets/gel, juice). If the patient is unable to safely eat by mouth or is unconscious, a glucagon injection should be administered. For mild/moderate hypoglycemia, complex carbohydrates are recommended to avoid a "yo-yo" response (blood sugar increasing rapidly only to drop again in response to simple carbohydrates).

In summary, PBH following bariatric surgery is common and potentially dangerous for patients. Specialty referral to an Obesity Medicine Specialist or Endocrinologist is indicated for patients who continue to have symptoms despite dietary modification and education. For additional information, see the section on PBH elsewhere in this chapter.

QUIZ QUESTIONS

1. A 45-year-old woman with class III obesity, type 2 diabetes, and hypertension returns for a follow-up visit 2 months following an uneventful RYGB procedure. She has no nausea, vomiting, or abdominal pain. She is consuming three meals and two snacks daily consisting of protein shakes, eggs, cheese sticks, turkey slices, and chicken soup. Over the past week, she has noticed several episodes of lightheadedness and diaphoresis that resolve by eating a yogurt or several crackers. Medications include ramipril 5 mg/day, metformin 500 mg BID, glyburide 5 mg/day, and omeprazole 20 mg/day. Supplements include two chewable multivitamin-mineral tablets.

   On examination, weight is 220 lb (she has lost 20 lb since surgery), BP 100/68, and HR 96. She is comfortable and in no distress. Abdomen reveals well-healing laparoscopic scars, normal active bowel sounds, and no tenderness or rebound.

   What is the next most appropriate action to take to address the patient's symptoms?

   A. Add carbohydrate foods to her diet
   B. Discontinue ramipril
   C. Discontinue glyburide
   D. Increase fluid intake

   Answer: C. *The patient is presenting with symptoms consistent with hypoglycemia. Insulin secretagogues, such as sulfonylureas should be discontinued after bariatric surgery. Adding complex carbohydrate foods to her diet will also be beneficial as a secondary recommendation. The patient's blood pressure is well controlled which may warrant discontinuation of ramipril; however, her symptoms are more likely due to hypoglycemia. All patients are counseled to remain well hydrated.*

2. A 52-year-old man presents to the emergency department 3 weeks following an uneventful laparoscopic sleeve gastrectomy (SG) complaining of persistent nausea, vomiting, and double vision. He has only been able to tolerate small amounts of water and sugar free jello. He is feeling lightheaded and his urine is malodorous and dark colored. He is not taking any medications or nutritional supplements. On examination, he appears lethargic and dehydrated; afebrile; and BP 98/68, HR 108, and RR 14. HEENT: Notable for nystagmus and unilateral palsy of his extraocular muscles. Cardiac, pulmonary, and abdominal examination is unremarkable. He has weakness of the arms and legs.

   In addition to starting an IV line, what is the next most important step in his management?

   A. Infuse normal saline with 5% dextrose
   B. Inject vitamin B12 1,000 μg IM
   C. Insert a nasogastric tube
   D. Inject thiamine 200 mg IV

   Answer: D. *The patient presents with classic signs and symptoms of Wernicke syndrome, the only medical nutritional emergency that may occur following metabolic and bariatric surgery. All patients should be treated immediately with IV thiamine prior to administration of dextrose which may precipitate Wernicke encephalopathy and development of an irreversible pontine stroke. Deficiency of vitamin B12 occurs months to years following bariatric surgery due to hepatic storage. Insertion of a nasogastric tube, if indicated, needs to be done with extreme caution due to the altered anatomy and reduced volume of the stomach.*

REFERENCES

1. Rubin D, Levin M. Mechanisms of intestnal adaptation. *Best Pract Res Clin Gastroenterol.* 2016;30:237-248.

2. Bojsen-Moller K, Jacobsen S, Dirksen C, et al. Accelerated protein digestion and amino acid absorption after roux-en-Y gastric bypass. *Am J Clin Nutr.* 2015;102:600-607.

3. Mechanick J, Apovian C, Brethauer S, et al. Clinical practice guidelines for the perioperative nutritional, metabolic, and nonsurgical support of the bariatric surgery patient—2019 update: cosponsored by American Association of Clinical Endocrinologists, the Obesity Society, and American Society for Metabolic & Bariatric Surgery. *Obesity.* 2020;28(4):O1-O58.

4. Shukeri WFWM, Hassan MH, Hassan WMNW, Zaini RHM. Anastomotic leak after bariatric surgery from a critical care perspective: a lesson shared. *Malays J Med Sci.* 2018;25(5):158-159. doi:10.21315/mjms2018.25.5.15

5. Groene P, Eisenlohr J, Zeuzem C, Dudok S, Karcz K, Hofmann-Kiefer K. Postoperative nausea and vomiting in bariatric surgery in comparison to non-bariatric gastric surgery. *Wideochir Inne Tech Maloinwazyjne.* 2019;14(1):90-95. doi:10.5114/wiitm.2018.77629

6. Kushner RF, Cummings S, Herron DM. Bariatric surgery: postoperative nutritional management. In: Chen W, ed. *UpToDate.* UpToDate; 2019. Accessed October 22, 2019.

7. Parrott J, Frank L, Rabena R, Craggs-Dino L, Isom KA, Greiman L. American society for metabolic and bariatric surgery integrated health nutritional guidelines for the surgical weight loss patient 2016 update micronutrients. *Surg Obes Relat Dis.* 2017;13(5):727-741.

8. Cavin J, Bado A, Le Gail M. Intestinal adaptations after bariatric surgery: consequences on glucose homeostasis. *Trend Endocrin Metab.* 2017;28:354-364.

9. Marso SP, Daniels GH, Brown-Frandsen K, et al; LEADER Steering Committee; LEADER Trial Investigators. Liraglutide and cardiovascular outcomes in type 2 diabetes. *N Engl J Med* 2016;375:311-322.

10. Zinman B, Wanner C, Lachin JM, et al; for the EMPA-REG OUTCOME Investigators. Empagliflozin, cardiovascular outcomes, and mortality in type 2 diabetes. *N Engl J Med.* 2015;373:2117-2128.

11. Neal B, Perkovic V, Mahaffey KW, et al; on behalf of the CANVAS Program Collaborative Group. Canagliflozin and cardiovascular and renal events in type 2 diabetes. *N Engl J Med* 2017;377(7):644-657.

12. King W, Belle S, Hinerman A, Mitchell J, Steffen K, Courcoulas A. Patient behaviors and characteristics related to weight regain after roux-en-Y gastric bypass: a multicenter prospective cohort study. *Ann Surg.* 2019. doi:10.1097/SLA.0000000000003281.

13. Monson M, Jackson M. Pregnancy after bariatric surgery. *Clin Obstet Gynecol.* 2016;59(1):158-171.

14. de Raaff C, Gorter-Stam M, de Vries N, et al. Perioperative management ofobstructive sleep apnea in bariatric surgery: a consensus guideline. *Surg Obes Relat Dis.* 2017;13(7):1095-1109.

15. Gregory NS. The effects of bariatric surgery on bone metabolism. *Endocrinol Metab Clin North Am.* 2017;46(1):105-116.

16. Kushner RF, Still CD. *Nutrition and Bariatric Surgery.* CRC Press; 2014.

17. Bredella M, Greenblatt L, Eajaza A, Torriani M, Yu EW. Effects of Roux-en-Y gastric bypass and sleeve gastrectomy on bone mineral density and marrow adipose tissue. *Bone.* 2017;95:85-90.

18. Mishra T, Shapiro J, Ramirez L, Kallies KJ, Kothari SN, Londergan TA. Nephrolithiasis after bariatric surgery: a comparison of laparoscopic Roux-en-Y gastric bypass and sleeve gastrectomy. *Am J Surg.* 2020;219(6):952-957.

19. Reece J, Vosburg R, Goyal N. *Bariatric surgery and stone risk.* In: *Nutritional and Medical Management of Kidney Stones.* Springer; 2019:169-179.

20. Eisenberg D, Azagury D, Ghiassi S, Grover B, Kim J. ASMBS position statement on postprandial hyperinsulinemic hypoglycemia after bariatric surgery. *Surg Obes Relat Dis.* 2017;13:371-378.

21. Salehi M, Vella A, McLaughlin T, Patti M. Hypoglycemia after gastric bypass surgery: current concepts and controversies. *J Clin Endocrinol Metab.* 2018;103:2815-2826.

22. White G, Courcoulas A, King W. Drug- and alcohol-related mortality risk after bariatric surgery: evidence from a 7-year prospective multicenter cohort study. *Surg Obes Relat Dis.* 2019;15(7):1160-1169. doi:10.1016/j.soard.2019.04.007

23. Steenackers N, Gesquiere I, Matthys C. The relevance of dietary protein after bariatric surgery: what do we know? *Curr Opin Clin Nutr Metab Care.* 2018;21:58-63.

24. Ito MK, Goncalves V, Faria S, et al. Effect of protein intake on the protein status and lean mass of post-bariatric surgery patients: a systematic review. *Obes Surg.* 2017;27:502-512.

25. Clark SF. Vitamins and trace elements In: Mueller S, ed. *The ASPEN Adult Nutrition Support Core Curriculum.* 2nd ed. American Society for Parenteral and Enteral Nutrition; 2012:121-148.

26. McCracken E, Wood GC, Prichard W, et al. Severe anemia after roux-en-Y gastric bypass: a cause for concern. *Surg Obes Relat Dis.* 2018;14:902-909.

27. Munoz M, Botella-Romero F, Gomez-Ramirez S, et al. Iron deficiency and anaemia in bariatric surgery patients: causes, diagnosis, and proper management. *Nutr Hosp.* 2009;24:640-654.

28. Maleckas A, Gudaitytė R, Petereit R, Venclauskas L, Veličkienė D. Weight regain after gastric bypass: etiology and treatment options. *Gland Surg.* 2016;5(6):617-624. doi:10.21037/gs.2016.12.02

11

PEDIATRIC AND ADOLESCENT OBESITY

Edmond Pryce Wickham III, Melanie K. Bean

CASE STUDY

A 10-year-old girl is establishing care with you for ongoing primary care. At the visit, the patient's mother expresses concern about her daughter's increasing weight. The mother reports a steady weight gain over the past 6 years despite the daughter's regular participation in sports and is concerned that her daughter may have an underlying medical condition responsible for her weight gain. The patient has a past medical history of asthma and previously received several courses of oral steroids; however, her asthma is currently managed with intermittent use of a beta-adrenergic agonist and she has not required an oral steroid in the past 3 years. There is no history of developmental delay or a learning disability, but the mother does note worsening school performance over the past 2 years that she believes is associated with increased teasing and bullying that the patient has experienced at school. The patient's father has obesity, and there is a strong family history of type 2 diabetes mellitus (T2D). There is no family history of thyroid disease.

On physical examination, the patient's height is 147 cm, weight is 53.6 kg, with a body mass index (BMI) of 24.8 kg/m^2, and blood pressure is 119/78 mm Hg. Her examination is significant for mild acanthosis nigricans on her posterior neck, the absence of thyromegaly, and stage 3 breast and stage 2 pubic hair development. She had not had any previous laboratory testing.

CLINICAL SIGNIFICANCE

The prevalence of overweight and obesity in youth has increased dramatically, such that approximately one in five children in the United States would be classified as having obesity and one in three children having overweight.[1] Youth with obesity are at significant risk of developing weight-related comorbidities over their lifetime, and such conditions may already be present during childhood and adolescence. Thus, the prevention, identification, and effective treatment of obesity by healthcare professionals (HCPs) caring for youth is paramount. In evaluating children and adolescents with obesity, the clinical assessment and management should be modified to account for the child's specific developmental stage and physical development. This specific chapter will build on content from preceding chapters and highlight unique considerations in the assessment and treatment of pediatric obesity in the primary care setting including the appropriate classification of weight status in children, distinct components of the comprehensive pediatric obesity-focused assessment, and the importance of family-based change in behavioral weight management in the treatment of obesity in youth. In addition, the potential roles of pharmacotherapy and metabolic and bariatric surgery (MBS) in adolescents with severe obesity will be reviewed.

DEFINING PEDIATRIC OVERWEIGHT AND OBESITY

Classification of Weight Status During Childhood

As in adults, BMI is the recommended screening assessment of weight status in children aged 2 years and older.[2,3] Although not a direct measure of body fat, BMI generally correlates with more direct and robust methods for measuring body fat in children and correlates with both concurrent and future health risks, including morbidity and mortality. Consequently, the calculation, documentation, and interpretation of BMI is recommended at least annually as part of routine pediatric health care.

However, the clinical interpretation of BMI in children is more complex than in adults, as weight and height are dynamic and anticipated to change as part of a child's normal growth and development. Moreover, unlike other growth parameters, BMI does not simply increase from birth to adulthood. In fact, BMI is typically expected to decrease beginning in the second year of life, reaching a nadir at the age of 5 to 6 years, and then increase steadily throughout later childhood and adolescence. The vertex of this v- or u-shaped pattern in BMI trajectory is termed "adiposity rebound," and children who experience adiposity rebound prior to 4 years of age are at increased risk of obesity later in life.[4]

In light of these normal developmental patterns, an absolute BMI value is typically not sufficient for characterizing weight and adiposity status in children and younger adolescents, and BMI percentiles specific for age and sex should be determined for children ≥2 years of age in the United States according to the revised 2000 Centers for Disease Control and Prevention (CDC) BMI data (https://www.cdc.gov/growthcharts/cdc_charts.htm). Age- and sex-specific BMI percentiles may be calculated by plotting the child's calculated BMI on the appropriate CDC BMI chart (Figure 11.1). Alternatively, numerous online pediatric BMI percentile calculators

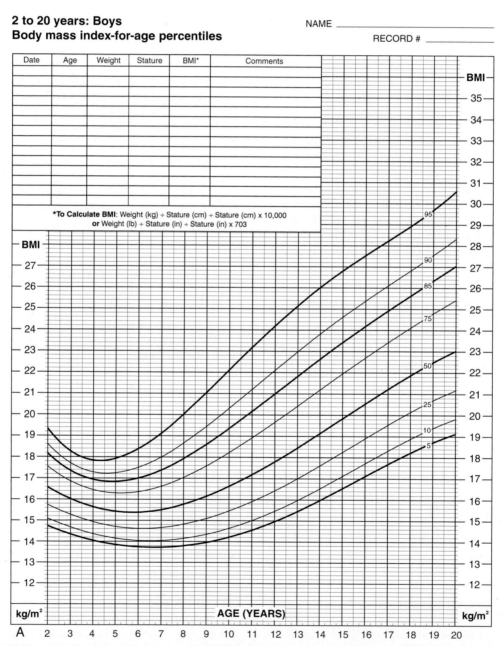

FIGURE 11.1 2002 Centers for Disease Control and Prevention body mass index-for-age growth charts. A, Boys. B, Girls. (Reprinted from Centers for Disease Control and Prevention. *Clinical Growth Charts*. https://www.cdc.gov/growthcharts/clinical_charts.htm#Set1)

2 to 20 years: Girls
Body mass index-for-age percentiles

NAME _____

RECORD # _____

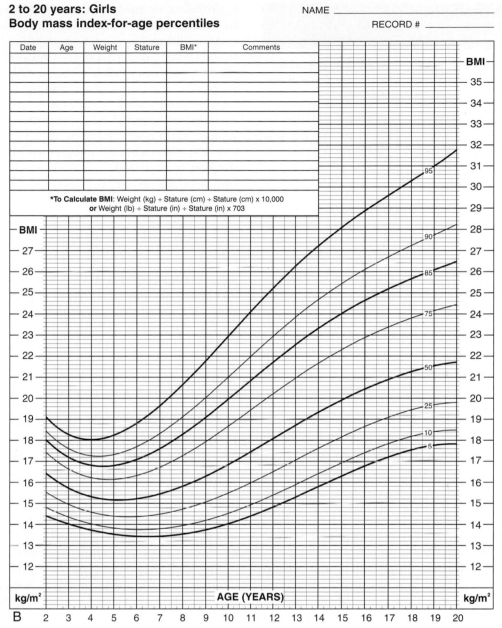

FIGURE 11.1 Cond'd

are publicly available (https://www.cdc.gov/healthy-weight/bmi/calculator.html); many electronic medical records also contain automated functions for calculating BMI percentiles for pediatric patients.

The body weight status of a child or adolescent ≥2 years of age can then be classified according to the determined age- and sex-specific BMI percentiles (Table 11.1). Specifically, a BMI that is ≥85th percentile but <95th percentile is consistent with overweight, and a BMI ≥95th percentile (*or* an absolute BMI ≥30 kg/m², whichever is lower) is consistent with obesity. Astute HCPs (and parents) may question how more than 5% of children can have obesity in light of the proposed definition (i.e., BMI ≥95th percentile). To avoid an

upward shift in the weight- and BMI-for-age growth curves as a result of the secular increases in body weight that occurred during the 1980s and 1990s, the weight data for children aged 6 years and older used in the development of the 2000 CDC curves exclude data collected after 1980.

More recently, the classification of obesity in youth has been revised to include a definition for severe obesity (BMI ≥120% of the age- and sex-appropriate 95th percentile *or* an absolute BMI ≥35 kg/m²) in order to underscore the increased health risks of severe weight gain among children and adolescents.[5] This category of severe obesity in youth has been further refined to include proposed definitions for Class 2 (BMI ≥120%

TABLE 11.1 Classification of Pediatric Body Mass Index Categories

BMI AGE- AND SEX-PERCENTILE	WEIGHT CLASSIFICATION
<5th percentile	Underweight
5th-84th percentile	Healthy weight
85th-94th percentile	Overweight
≥95th percentile *or* absolute BMI ≥30 kg/m²	Obesity
BMI ≥95th percentile *or* an absolute BMI ≥30 kg/m²	Class 1 Obesity
BMI ≥120% of the age- and sex-appropriate 95th percentile *or* an absolute BMI ≥35 kg/m²	Class 2 Obesity[a]
BMI ≥140% of the age- and sex-appropriate 95th percentile *or* an absolute BMI ≥40 kg/m²	Class 3 Obesity[a]

BMI, body mass index.
[a]*Class 2 and 3 obesity may both additionally be classified as severe obesity.*

of the age- and sex-appropriate 95th percentile *or* an absolute BMI ≥35 kg/m²) and Class 3 (BMI ≥140% of the 95th percentile *or* an absolute BMI ≥40 kg/m²) to coincide with adult definitions, as well as criteria for MBS in adolescents.[1,2,6] Figure 11.2 contains specialized growth charts that can be used to determine pediatric obesity severity and class.[5]

Although increasing data support that rapid weight gain in early life and infancy may portend an increased risk of obesity in later childhood, the importance of an elevated BMI in children <2 years of age has not been definitively established.[3] Moreover, both the CDC and the American Academy of Pediatrics (AAP) recommend using 2006 World Health Organization (WHO) growth standards (https://www.cdc.gov/growthcharts/who_charts.htm), as opposed to the 2000 CDC growth references, for assessing growth patterns for infants <2 years of age given the WHO growth standards' more robust longitudinal data and inclusion of predominantly breastfeed infants.[7] Even though the 2006 WHO growth standards include a BMI reference chart beginning at birth, the CDC-AAP expert panel does not recommend its clinical use before 2 years of age.[7] Alternatively, guidelines have proposed that in children <2 years of age, a weight-for-recumbent length ratio ≥97.7th percentile according WHO growth standards may represent an

appropriate definition of obesity[2]; however, the clinical utility of this definition remains unclear.

An additional approach that addresses the dynamic characteristics of BMI among youth is the use of BMI z-scores (or standard scores); a BMI z-score corresponds to the number of standard deviations that a given child's BMI is away from the corresponding age- and sex-specific 50th percentile. However, even though automated pediatric BMI percentile calculators may also generate z-scores and BMI z-scores are frequently reported in the research literature, the clinical utility of a BMI z-score in direct patient care is limited.

Prevalence of Overweight and Obesity in Youth

Rates of overweight and obesity among US youth have increased substantially over the past 40 to 50 years across all age and racial/ethnic groups.[1,2] According to the 2015-2016 National Health and Nutrition Examination Survey (NHANES) data, 18.5% of children in the United States aged 2 to 19 years have obesity and 35.1% have overweight.[8] Prevalence rates of obesity among children and adolescents rise with increasing age and are slightly higher in boys compared with girls across age groups (Figure 11.3).[8] Obesity also disproportionately affects African American and Hispanic youth; however, no racial/ethnic group is immune from the epidemic of pediatric obesity.[8] Even though reported rates are lowest in Asian American children, there is concern that the proposed BMI percentile definitions of pediatric obesity may underestimate the health risks associated with increasing adiposity in this population.[2]

Although overall rates of obesity may be plateauing in some pediatric age groups,[8] the prevalence of severe obesity continues to rise at alarming rates.[1] Based on 2015-2016 NHANES data, 6.0% of US children aged 2 to 19 years have severe (i.e., Class 2 or higher) obesity. Prevalence estimates of severe obesity climb with age, with an estimated 9.5% and 4.5% of US youth aged 16 to 19 years meeting proposed definitions of Class 2 and Class 3 obesity, respectively.[1]

Health Impact of Overweight and Obesity During Childhood

Children with overweight and obesity are likely to have persistent obesity as adults. Based on the current prevalence of excess weight in youth, predictive modeling suggests that ~50% to 60% of the current generation of US children will have obesity when they are 35 years old.[9] Childhood obesity is associated with significant life-long morbidity and mortality, including an increased risk of

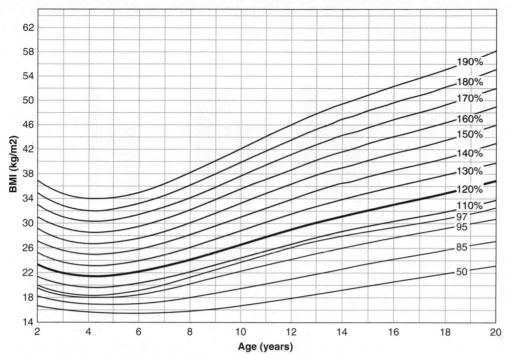

Source: BMI from CDC. BMI calculated as % of 95th percentile.

A

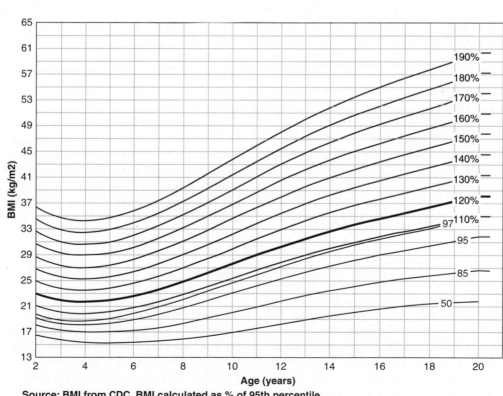

Source: BMI from CDC. BMI calculated as % of 95th percentile.

B

FIGURE 11.2 Modified Centers for Disease Control and Prevention (CDC) body mass index (BMI) growth curves for severe obesity in boys (A) and girls (B). (Reprinted with permission from Kelly AS, Barlow SE, Rao G, et al. Severe obesity in children and adolescents: identification, associated health risks, and treatment approaches. A scientific statement from the American Heart Association. *Circulation*. 2013;128:1689-1712.)

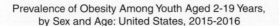

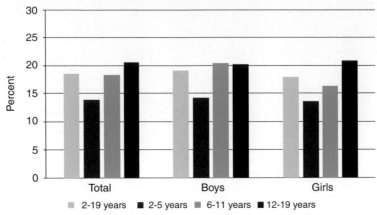

FIGURE 11.3 Prevalence of obesity among youth aged 2 to 19 years, by sex and age: United States, 2015-2016. (Adapted from Hales CM, Carroll MD, Fryar CD, Ogden CL. Prevalence of Obesity Among Adults and Youth: United States, 2015-2016. *NCHS Data Brief.* 2017;(288):1-8. Data from the National Health and Nutrition Examination Survey (NHANES).)

T2D, cardiovascular disease, and premature death in adulthood.[3,5,10] The risk for the development of many weight-related conditions in childhood (Figure 11.4) increases with obesity severity. Furthermore, pediatric obesity is associated with significant reductions in quality of life.[11] As a result of obesity and the weight-related comorbidities, a decline in life expectancy is projected, with today's youth living shorter lives than their parents.[12] Thus, the development of skills required for the compassionate and comprehensive care of youth with overweight and obesity, including an understanding of the complexities of the disease and evidenced-based treatment recommendations, is critical for all HCPs who care for children.

ETIOLOGY OF ABNORMAL WEIGHT GAIN IN YOUTH

As in adults, the etiology of the imbalance in energy metabolism that leads to excess weight gain in childhood is complex, resulting from the interactions of individual and family behaviors, environmental factors, and genetic susceptibility. Parental weight status is strongly associated with the offspring's weight status, both when the offspring is a child and subsequently an adult. In fact, if a child has one parent with obesity, the child's risk of obesity is increased three- to fourfold.[13] Having two parents with obesity is associated with greater than a 10-fold increased risk of obesity in the child.[13] The observed relation between parent and child BMI likely results from a combination of shared genetic and environmental factors; however, genetic factors appear to be the stronger contributor. Indeed,

twin studies point to a heritability of up to 70% to 80% for BMI and adiposity.[14] However, like other complex disease phenotypes, obesity results from the interplay of genetic predisposition which is most fully expressed in the setting of environmental triggers and exposures.

For the majority of youth with obesity, the genetic susceptibility toward excess weight gain is polygenic, resulting from the cumulative risk from multiple genetic loci, each accounting for relatively small variations in body weight.[14] Discussions with patients and families should acknowledge the strong genetic contributions to obesity while promoting autonomy and self-efficacy in changing modifiable behaviors and factors within the obesogenic environment, which form the foundation of effective treatments and mitigate genetic risk. As there currently are no clinically useful genetic markers for obesity, HCPs should obtain a family history for overweight and obesity among family members.

Specific Genetic Conditions Associated With Obesity

Although severe early-onset obesity may result from single gene mutations or defects in specific chromosome regions, such conditions are rare.[15] Nevertheless, providers should remain vigilant to clinical characteristics suggestive of underlying syndromic and monogenic etiologies that may be present. Specific diagnoses may convey additional health risks to affected individuals that warrant ongoing monitoring or impact clinical treatment recommendations and response. Most children with genetic syndromes associated with obesity manifest severe hyperphagia and have one or more suggestive clinical characteristics:

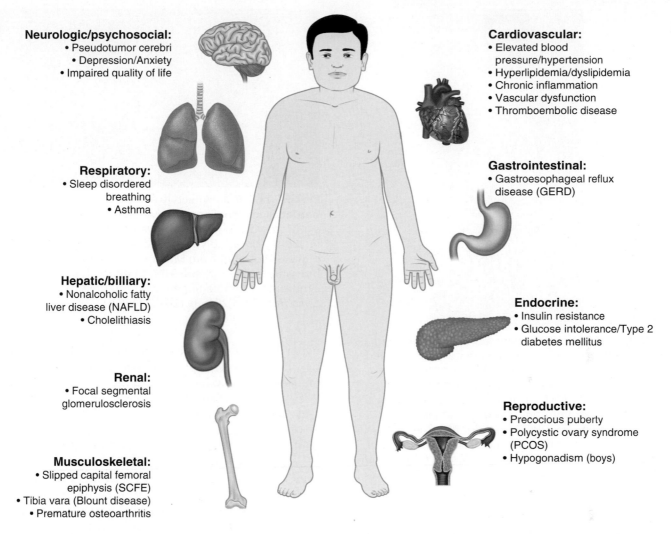

FIGURE 11.4 Health impact of obesity on children and adolescents.

- Neurodevelopmental abnormalities (e.g., developmental delay, intellectual disability, or behavioral concerns)
- Phenotypic features (e.g., short stature, dysmorphic physical features, retinal dystrophy, deafness)
- Associated endocrinopathies (e.g., hypogonadotropic hypogonadism leading to delayed puberty)

Syndromic Obesity

Prader-Willi Syndrome

The most common syndromic etiology of obesity is Prader-Willi syndrome (PWS), a multisystemic genomic imprinting disorder that results from the lack of expression of paternal genes located in the chromosome 15q11-q13 region, and affects approximately one in 10,000 to 30,000 individuals.[16] Infants with PWS have significant hypotonia and feeding disorders. As a result, PWS may initially present as poor weight gain and failure to thrive during the first 2 years of life; the

characteristic hyperphagia and associated severe weight gain typically emerge in later childhood.[16] Clinical features of PWS to look for include

- Significant hypotonia and feeding disorders at birth
- Poor weight gain and failure to thrive during the first 2 years of life
- Developmental delay and short stature and/or decreased growth velocity
- Almond-shaped eyes, a thin upper lip, and small hands and feet (Figure 11.5)

Children with PWS typically experience hypogonadotropic hypogonadism and growth hormone deficiency. Recombinant human growth hormone (hGH) administration in youth with PWS results in increased height, improved body composition and physical strength, and beneficial cognitive effects.[17] As a result, the early initiation of hGH therapy is recommend in infant and children with PWS, and evidence suggests ongoing benefits of hGH in adults with PWS.[17] Consequently, HCPs caring for youth (and adults)

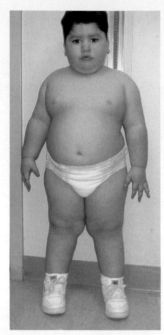

FIGURE 11.5 Typical physical features of child with Prader-Willi syndrome. Physical features associated with Prader-Willi syndrome (PWS) include severe obesity, short stature, almond-shaped eyes, a thin upper lip with a down-turned mouth, small hands and feet, and straight borders of the inner legs. (Reprinted from Angulo MA, Butler MG, Cataletto ME. Prader-Willi syndrome: a review of clinical, genetic, and endocrine findings. *J Endocrinol Invest.* 2015;38(12):1249-1263.)

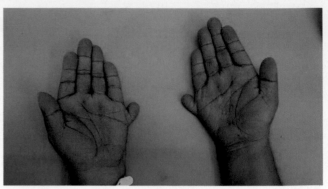

FIGURE 11.6 Brachydactyly and polydactyly in Bardet-Biedl syndrome. Individuals with Bardet-Biedl syndrome (BBS) may have dysmorphic hands and feet, including extra (polydactyly) or short (brachydactyly) digits. (Reprinted from Madireddi J, Acharya V, Suryanarayana J, Hande HM, Shetty R. Bardet-Biedl syndrome: multiple fingers with multiple defects. *BMJ Case Rep.* 2015;2015:bcr2015211776.)

with PWS should collaborate with a pediatric or adult endocrinologists as well as other specialists to ensure comprehensive care.

Bardet-Biedl Syndrome

The second most common syndromic etiology of obesity is Bardet-Biedl syndrome (BBS), a homozygous recessive multisystem disorder that affects an estimated one in 125,000 to 175,000 lives births.[18] In addition to severe, early-onset obesity, other clinical features of BBS to look for include

- Progressive visual loss as a result of a retinal disorder known as rod-cone dystrophy
- Dysmorphic extremities including polydactyly, syndactyly, and brachydactyly (Figure 11.6)
- Renal tract abnormalities including polycystic kidney disease
- Learning disabilities, developmental delay, or intellectual disability

However, the clinical presentation of BBS is variable and may also include more severe developmental delay/intellectual disability, dysmorphic facial features including a prominent forehead or hypertelorism with deep-set eyes, dental abnormalities, hearing loss, hypogonadism (particularly among males), and ataxia with impaired coordination.[18] With the exception of polydactyly, many of the signs and symptoms of BBS may not be readily apparent at birth, but begin to emerge during childhood or early adolescence. The variability in clinical phenotype in patients with BBS likely results from the fact that over 20 disease-causing genes have been identified, each encoding for proteins essential for the primary cilium/basal body complex.[19] The primary focus of treatment in BBS is clinical and supportive management of syndrome-associated comorbidities including eye disease, kidney disease and obesity.[19] Patients with BBS are also at increased risk of T2D, hypertension, and metabolic syndrome and should be screened and treated appropriately to mitigate accelerated decline in vision and kidney function. As with PWS, HCPs should collaborate with other specialists to ensure optimal care for individuals with BBS.

Monogenetic Obesity

Melanocortin 4 Receptor Deficiency

The most common monogenic cause of early-onset obesity is a heterozygous mutation in the gene encoding for the melanocortin 4 receptor (MC4R), a critical regulator of appetite and energy metabolism, affecting approximately 4% to 6% of patients with severe obesity.[15,20] In contrast to most other monogenetic or syndromic etiologies of obesity, individuals with heterozygous MC4R mutations do not demonstrate short stature, developmental delay/intellectual disability or typical phenotypic features. Although accelerated linear growth in childhood and hyperinsulinemia may be subtle features associated with MC4R mutations, youth with obesity but without MC4R mutations may also manifest similar but less prominent growth acceleration and hyperinsulinemia.[21] Given the lack of definitive characteristics besides early-onset, severe obesity, the clinical identification of individuals with MC4R mutations may be challenging without genetic testing (see below). At this time, the mainstay of treatment for patients with heterozygous MCR4 mutations is comprehensive lifestyle modification, with the potential addition of weight loss surgery.[22] The FDA recently approved setmelanotide, a selective MCR4 agonist, for the treatment of rare genetic mutations upstream of MCR4. Although treatment of MC4R mutations was not included in the initial FDA approval, the agent's role in individuals with minor MC4R defects is promising and warrants further investigation.[23]

Mutations in other single genes (e.g., leptin, leptin receptor, proopiomelanocortin [POMC] and proprotein convertase) may also result in severe, early-onset obesity, but these defects are extremely rare, typically associated with secondary endocrine dysfunction (e.g., central hypogonadism, adrenal insufficiency, or hypothyroidism), and not commonly encountered in clinical practice.[24]

When to Obtain Genetic Testing

Endocrine Society guidelines recommend consideration of genetic testing in patients with severe, early-onset obesity (before age 5 years) with clinical features of genetic syndromes and/or a family history of severe obesity.[2] The diagnosis of PWS is confirmed by DNA methylation analysis, and DNA sequencing tests for MC4R mutations are commercially available. However, genetic testing/screening for etiologies of obesity, like other conditions, should be offered in the context of high-quality genetic counseling so that families and patients are well informed of the risks, benefits, and potential implications of testing. Parental permission for genetic testing should be obtained prior to testing, as well as assent from the child, when appropriate. Thus, genetic testing is ideally conducted in collaboration with dedicated genetic counselors and clinical geneticists, and referral is recommended.

Endocrine Conditions Associated With Obesity

Endocrine disorders such as hypercortisolism, hypothyroidism, and growth hormone deficiency may also result in excess weight gain, but these conditions are rarely the primary underlying cause of obesity in children.[15] Moreover, youth with endocrine causes of obesity typically have other symptoms suggestive of the diagnosis beyond weight gain. An important clinical clue that may indicate an underlying endocrinopathy is short stature

and, even more specifically, reduced height velocity.[15] Thus, in addition to assessing trends in weight and BMI, the clinical evaluation of youth with obesity should include a careful review of the patient's height growth. Many children with overweight and obesity experience slightly accelerated growth rates (i.e., height velocities) compared with healthy-weight peers during late childhood and early adolescence, such that 10- to 12-year-old girls and 11- to 13-year-old boys with overweight and obesity are ~3 cm taller than same-sex youth with a healthy weight.[25] However, the discrepancy in height between youth according to weight status is no longer apparent in older age groups as both groups approach their genetically determined adult predicted height.[25]

The early growth spurt and advanced skeletal maturation in children with obesity is likely driven, in part, by an early onset of puberty (and associated increase in sex steroids) in youth with excess body adiposity.[26] Girls with overweight and obesity are more likely to experience earlier onset of breast and pubic hair development and menstrual periods.[27] The relation between BMI, body fat, and pubertal development in male youth is less clear, with studies suggesting that boys with overweight/obesity are more likely to experience both early and delayed pubertal development.[26,28] Elevated levels of insulin and leptin have also been implicated as contributing to the early weight-related growth acceleration in both sexes.[26]

Given the low prevalence of underlying endocrine conditions in asymptomatic youth with overweight and obesity, guidelines recommend *against* the routine laboratory evaluation for endocrine etiologies of excess weight gain (including thyroid function studies) unless the child has one of the following:[2,3]

- An attenuated height velocity (or a height that is shorter than anticipated according to genetic and familial potential).
- Clear signs or symptoms suggestive of an endocrine disorder beyond weight gain.

However, when the clinical assessment or testing suggests an underlying endocrine condition, referral to a pediatric endocrine specialist is warranted.

Hypothalamic Obesity

In light of the central role of the intricate central nervous system pathways involved in the regulation of appetite and energy metabolism, damage to these areas in the hypothalamus from tumors, surgery, radiation, trauma, or inflammatory disease may lead to marked obesity.[29] Children and adolescents with hypothalamic obesity manifest severe hyperphagia as well as metabolic changes that result in reduced energy expenditure that can contribute to ongoing weight gain even in the setting of aggressive lifestyle modification and caloric restriction.[29]

CLINICAL EVALUATION OF PEDIATRIC PATIENTS WITH OVERWEIGHT AND OBESITY

As outlined previously, an assessment of weight status and obesity risk is recommended at least annually as part of routine pediatric care. Given the substantial lifetime risk of overweight and obesity as well as the central role of dietary intake and regular physical activity in health and chronic disease prevention, it is recommended that pediatric HCPs routinely and thoughtfully assess a child's dietary and physical activity patterns, regardless of the patient's current BMI. For children and adolescents with established overweight or obesity, the initial encounter should focus on

- Establishing rapport with the patient and family.
- Identifying any underlying etiologies contributing to excess weight gain.
- Screening for the presence of weight-related comorbidities.
- Age-appropriate assessment of dietary, physical activity, sedentary behaviors, and sleep patterns.
- Collaboratively developing and implementing an age-appropriate, family-based treatment plan that accounts for the patient/family's readiness to change, unique values, and goals.

Initiating Discussions Regarding Weight and Health Behaviors During Pediatric Encounters

Tragically, many youth with overweight and obesity face significant stigmatization and discrimination at home, in school, through media, and, unfortunately, with health care.[30] Consequently, it is imperative that providers develop and refine a clinical approach and practice environment that minimizes weight-related stigma. One particular approach for establishing rapport and minimizing weight stigma is for the provider to ask permission prior to discussing weight and weight-related concerns. As with many aspects of pediatric care, providers should modify this approach to account for the developmental stage of the patient. For example, even when a parent of an older child or adolescent initiates a discussion with an HCP about weight, it is important for the provider to seek verbal assent from the patient as well.

Although pediatric guidelines recommend the use of the clinical terms of "overweight" and "obesity" for clinical documentation, experts recommend the use of different terms during clinical encounters to reduce stigma.[3] In a survey of parents of children aged 2 to 18 years regarding perceptions of different weight-related terms used by HCPs, parents indicated that more neutral words like "weight," "unhealthy weight," or "high BMI" were more desirable, motivating, and

less stigmatizing than terms like "heavy," "chubby," "obese," or "fat."[31] It may also be helpful to review concerns regarding weight in the context of reviewing the patient's growth chart: "*Your child's BMI has been increasing over the past several years and is now above the 95th percentile. What concerns, if any, do you have about his weight?*"

In addition to the thoughtful selection of terms to describe weight during encounters, providers are encouraged to use open-ended questions initially to assess both the parent and child's level of concern, followed by more direct, but still neutral, questions in order to gather additional aspects of the history. During this process, providers should consistently engage the child and adolescent as developmentally appropriate and practice reflective listening with both the patient and the caregiver.

Components of Medical History in Children With Overweight and Obesity

Weight History

The initial evaluation of a child or adolescent with overweight or obesity should include a complete medical history including details regarding the onset and pattern of abnormal weight gain. As outlined previously, severe early-onset obesity (before 5 years of age) may suggest an underlying syndromic or monogenic etiology. The sudden onset of weight gain should prompt providers to explore temporal relations to medication initiation or changes, significant changes in the social environment (e.g., change in residence, parent's divorce, family member's death), or the emergence of symptoms of disordered eating or another underlying medical problem. In addition, HCPs should inquire about previous efforts at behavior change (including who participated in the changes) as well as participation in dedicated obesity treatments including specific dietary interventions, community-based or structured weight management programs, or use of antiobesity medications.

Past Medical and Surgical History

A detailed past medical history should be obtained including the diagnosis and treatment of any weight-related comorbidities. The presence of other medical diagnoses (and associated pharmacotherapy) may not only increase the child's risk of obesity, but also significantly impact the approach to obesity treatment. Detailed information regarding current and prior medication use, including the use of over-the-counter medications and vitamin/mineral supplements, should be obtained. Children with autism spectrum disorders, Fragile X syndrome, and trisomy 21 are more likely to have overweight and obesity, and individualized treatment plans for affected youth often need to account for strong food preferences, developmental delay/

intellectual disabilities, and/or behavioral challenges. Youth with attention-deficit hyperactivity disorder (ADHD) are also at increased risk of obesity, particularly those not receiving pharmacotherapy.[32] For youth with a history of anxiety, depression, and other mood disorders, the clinical interview should also include a history of current and previous treatments and address both behavioral therapies and medication use. A complete review of systems (including snoring/sleep disturbances, headaches, abdominal pain, menstrual irregularities, hirsutism, hip/knee/leg pain, polyuria, polydipsia, depressed mood, and anxiety) should be obtained to assist HCPs in identifying any previously unidentified weight-related comorbidities and concerns.

Birth History

For younger children, details from the patient's birth history and early life may provide information regarding obesity and other cardiometabolic disease risk. A maternal history of gestational diabetes mellitus during the pregnancy, maternal tobacco use, higher birth weight, and delivery via cesarean section are associated with increased risk of obesity in the child.[33] Breastfeeding may be associated with lower risk of obesity in the child, and the introduction of solid food before 4 months of age may be associated with increased risk.[33] However, the evidence regarding both of these early dietary risk factors is inconsistent.[33]

Developmental History

Collecting a developmental history, noting any delays in early language and fine and gross motor development, is vital and may provide clues to suggest an underlying syndromic or genetic etiology of the child's weight gain. The developmental history should be expanded to include any concerns regarding attenuated growth velocity as well as a history of early or delayed pubertal development, as appropriate.

Family History

Family history should include the presence of family members with a history of overweight and obesity (as well as history of family members undergoing MBS), T2D, gestational diabetes mellitus, hypertension, dyslipidemia, and premature cardiovascular disease.

Social History

The social history should include an assessment of the child's living situation; school performance including any learning disabilities or individualized educational programs (IEPs); daycare, before- and after-school supervision, and employment; and substance use patterns. As part of the social history, it is important to identify any caregivers besides parents (e.g., grandparents, sitter) who play significant roles in the child's life who may need to be engaged in treatment plans. Given the association with childhood obesity (as well as pertinent implications to treatment plan development), an assessment of food security should be included. Although more comprehensive validated assessments are available, the inclusion of a single question (i.e., "*In the last year, did you worry that your food would run out before you got money or food stamps to buy more?*") may identify a family with food insecurity. Unfortunately, weight-based bullying is highly prevalent, both at school and at home, and should also be assessed.[30] A significant proportion of youth with obesity endorse being teased or bullied about their weight by a parent, and the clinical interview may be an opportunity for providers to model discussion using weight-neutral and nonstigmatizing language.

Assessment of Dietary and Physical Activity Patterns in Children

Other essential portions of the pediatric history include the identification of key modifiable behaviors related to energy metabolism, including an age-appropriate assessment of dietary and activity patterns.[34] HCPs may find it beneficial use a screening questionnaire (Table 11.2) to collect such information. As with all components of the pediatric encounter, the patient should be engaged in dietary and activity pattern assessments as age and developmentally appropriate, using neutral and nonjudgmental language and an interview approach that reduces stigma. In addition, as part of the assessment of dietary and physical activity patterns, providers can also begin to partner with patients and families in the identification of specific target behaviors for reducing energy intake and increasing activity.

Dietary Assessments

Traditional dietary assessment measures such as a 24-hour dietary recalls, food records, and food frequency questionnaires have been validated for use in children and are often used in research studies. However, the use of these instruments in a busy clinical practice is typically not helpful. Instead, guidelines propose that providers assess several key behaviors that significantly impact energy intake in children including: (1) consumption of sugar-sweetened beverages (SSB), (2) frequency of food consumed outside of the home, especially at fast food restaurants, (3) portion sizes, and (4) frequency, quality, and setting of meals and snacks.[34]

Assessments of SSB should extend beyond soda/soft drinks and include consumption of juice, lemonade, flavored milk, sweet tea, sports drinks, energy drinks, and coffee-based beverages. The consumption of SSB in youth has increased dramatically over the past

TABLE 11.2 Pediatric Dietary and Physical Activity Questionnaire

Please complete this from as accurately as possible. There are no right or wrong answers. This information will help us get a better picture of your child's current daily patterns.

Dietary Patterns:

How many meals does your child eat on a typical day? _____ per day

---

Does your child regularly eat:

Breakfast	Yes _____ No _____
Lunch	Yes _____ No _____
Dinner	Yes _____ No _____

How many snacks does your child eat on a typical day? _____ per day
What types of snacks does your child typically eat? _____

How many servings of fruits does your child eat on a typical day? (circle one)

None	1	2	3	4	5 or more

How many servings of vegetables does your child eat on a typical day? (circle one).

None	1	2	3	4	5 or more

Select the types of drinks your child normally consumes:

☐ Juice ☐ Lemonade ☐ Sports Drinks ☐ Sweetened Coffee

☐ Regular Soda ☐ Sweetened Tea ☐ Energy Drinks

On a typical day, how many of these types of drinks does your child consume (count them all together & enter the total here)? _____

Who normally prepares the food in the house?

☐ Mom ☐ Dad ☐ Grandparent ☐ This Child ☐ Sibling ☐ Other: _____

Who normally does the grocery shopping in the house?

☐ Mom ☐ Dad ☐ Grandparent ☐ This Child ☐ Sibling ☐ Other: _____

How many times per week do you eat together as a family? (circle one)

Never	1	2	3	4	5 or more

How many times per week does your child eat fast food? (circle one)

Never	1	2	3	4	5 or more

Concerns about your child's eating habits:

Are you satisfied with your child's eating habits?	Yes _____ No _____
Do you have concerns about your child's portion sizes?	Yes _____ No _____
Does your child ever eat in secret or sneak food?	Yes _____ No _____
Does your child ever eat to make himself/herself happy, or to feel better?	Yes _____ No _____
Does your child's weight affect how he/she feels about himself/herself?	Yes _____ No _____

Physical Activity and Screen Time:

How many times per week is your child physically active (i.e., His or her breathing gets faster)? (Circle one that best describes a typical week)

Never	1-2 days/week	3-4 days/week	5-6 days/week	Daily

What types of physical activities does your child like to participate in? _____

TABLE 11.2 Pediatric Dietary and Physical Activity Questionnaire (Continued)

How many hours does your child watch TV/movies, sit at the computer, play video games, or spend time on a phone or tablet **on a typical weekday**? _____ hours/day

How many hours does your child watch TV/movies, sit at the computer, play video games, or spend time on a phone or tablet **on a typical weekend day**? _____ hours/day

<u>**Sleep Behaviors:**</u>

Does your child have a TV or other screen device (e.g., smart phone) in the room where they sleep?

Yes _____ No _____

What time does your child typically go to bed **during the week**? _____

What time does your child typically fall asleep after going to bed **during the week**? _____

What time does your child typically wake up **during the week**? _____

What time does your child typically go to bed **during the weekend**? _____

What time does your child typically fall asleep after going to bed **during the weekend**? _____

What time does your child typically wake up **during the weekend**? _____

Which of the following habits (if any) do you feel ready to help your child and family to change? Check all that apply:

☐ Drink less soda or juice

☐ Choosing healthy snacks

☐ Eating more fruits & vegetables

☐ Eat less fast food

☐ Eat more meals as a family

☐ Plan out meals

☐ Play outside/be more active more often

☐ Spend less time watching TV & playing video games or on the computer

☐ Take the TV/Computer out of the bedroom

---

several decades, and mounting cross-sectional and longitudinal studies support a relation between SSB intake and weight gain during childhood and adolescence.[35] Moreover, pediatric intervention studies have demonstrated that the elimination of calories from SSB leads to reductions in BMI.[35] Thus, SSB intake represents a key therapeutic target when the patient and family are ready to make such changes.

The relationship between the consumption of 100% fruit juice and obesity risk in children is less clear.[34,36] However, a Policy Statement by the AAP highlights that 100% fruit juice provides no nutritional benefits for infants younger than 1 year and offers no health benefits over whole fruit in older children.[37] As such, AAP guidance recommends that 100% fruit juice should be avoided in infants younger than 12 months and limited in older infants and children: ≤4 ounces/day in toddlers 1 to 3 years of age; ≤6 ounces/day in children 4 to 6 years of age; and ≤8 ounces/day in children and adolescents 7 to 18 years of age.[37]

Low-fat milk and plain water should be recommended as the ideal beverages for children.[38] The consumption of beverages containing no- or low-calorie artificial and nonnutritive sweeteners in children is controversial, but their use may be reasonable over a limited period of time when used to support the transition between regular SSB and water.[38] However, artificially sweetened beverages offer no nutritional benefits over plain water and should ideally be limited in a child's diet.[38]

The consumption of meals at restaurants and fast-food locations outside of the home may be associated with increased energy intake as a result of increased intake of SSB and energy-dense food as well as larger portions.[38] As in adults, research demonstrates that children presented with larger food portions consume more calories.[34] One strategy that can be effective to reduce portions is to eat from a smaller sized plate, as this is associated with reductions in the amount of energy consumed at a meal. Children aged 3 to 5 years also consumed ~25% less of an entrée when they were allowed to serve themselves compared to when the entrée was served preportioned on an individual plate.[39] Educational resources regarding recommended daily caloric goals and appropriate serving sizes based on age are available at https://www.choosemyplate.gov/. Providers and caregivers may also find that referencing a child's hand can be a helpful tool in estimating appropriate serving sizes, suggesting that the child's palm, cupped hand, and fist typically reflect approximate serving sizes for meats/protein, starches/grains, and snacks, respectively, with fewer concerns related to overportioning fruits and vegetables.

Other important dietary patterns to assess in the pediatric population include the frequency, timing, quality, and setting of meals and snacks.[34,38] Reduced meal frequency, including skipping breakfast, has frequently been implicating as contributing to obesity in youth, but study results are inconsistent and causation has not been established.[34] Even though the relation between breakfast consumption and obesity has not been firmly established, the regular consumption of breakfast may still be an appropriate target for intervention for improved cognition and academic performance.[40] As children get older, skipping lunch at school may frequently be observed and can be associated with subsequent overeating when at home in the afternoon.

The frequency of snacking has increased markedly in children and adolescents over the past several decades, and accounts for greater that 25% of the daily energy intake for most youth.[41,42] Although increased frequency of snacks is associated with higher total daily energy intake, snacking frequency has not been consistently associated with BMI in youth.[41] However, as energy-dense foods and SSB represent the major sources of calories from snacks in children,[41] snacking (e.g., modifying the frequency or quality of snacks) may be an appropriate behavior change target.

Most children do not consume the recommended number of servings of fruits and vegetables per day.[43] As most fruits and vegetables are high in fiber and water content, increasing fruit and vegetable intake has been proposed as a targeted behavior to potentially promote satiety and reduce energy intake if these items displace other energy-dense foods.[34] Fruits and vegetables are essential components of a healthy diet and inadequate intake is associated with an increased lifetime risk of cardiovascular disease and certain cancers[44,45]; encouraging children and adolescents to substitute fruits and vegetables for other processed, energy-dense foods is certainly a sound nutritional recommendation. HCPs should use caution about providing guidance to simply add fruits and vegetables to children's dietary intake (in contrast to substituting them for other higher energy foods); although dietary quality might improve, this strategy would not yield a reduction in energy intake.

A vital component of the dietary assessment is determining the context in which the child consumes meals and snacks. Eating while watching screens and the frequency of family meals are two specific scenarios that are especially important to assess. Eating in front of screens can decrease attention to hunger and fullness cues and result in mindless eating. Furthermore, eating while watching television is associated with increased consumption of energy-dense foods and SSB in children and adolescents.[46] An increased frequency of eating family meals is associated with improved child and adolescent dietary quality and lower BMI, and these healthful associations appear to persist across age-groups, socioeconomic status,

meal type (i.e., breakfast, lunch or dinner), and the number of parents present.[47] Moreover, consuming family meals is associated with reduced rates of disordered eating, substance abuse, depression, and suicide; improved quality of life; and higher academic performance in children.[48] Thus, it is strongly recommended that families eat meals together, at a table, with screens off.

Disordered Eating Patterns

As part of a dietary assessment, HCPs should include a brief assessment for disordered eating patterns, with binge and loss of control eating being the most common behaviors observed in children and adolescents with overweight and obesity. Although full diagnostic criteria for binge eating disorder are rarely met, subthreshold binge and loss of control eating is observed in 22% to 31% of youth with overweight and obesity.[49] Moreover, the loss of control element is most frequently associated with greater psychopathology and distress in pediatrics. A brief four-item screener (Table 11.3) can identify adolescents who should be referred for more comprehensive evaluation and treatment by an eating disorder specialist.[50] Other subclinical dysregulated behaviors to assess include frequency of sneaking, hiding, or hoarding food. While to some extent these behaviors can be developmentally normal, they also might be associated with ineffective feeding practices (e.g., overly restrictive) and/or lack of self-regulation in children that could become a focus of treatment.

Physical Activity and Sedentary Behavior Assessment

In addition to assessing behaviors associated with energy intake, HCPs should explore behaviors related to energy expenditure in youth including (1) patterns of physical activity (PA) including exercise and lifestyle PA, (2) screen time and other sedentary behaviors, and (3) sleep duration and quality. Age is an important consideration in assessing each of these domains in pediatric patients.

TABLE 11.3 Eating Disorder Screener

1. Do you worry you have lost control over how much you eat? YES[a] NO

2. Do you ever eat in secret? YES[a] NO

3. Do you currently have or have you ever had an eating disorder? YES[a] NO

4. Do you make yourself sick when you feel uncomfortably full? YES[a] NO

For use in adolescents aged 12 to 18 years.
[a]Consider referral to eating disorder specialist for two or more affirmative responses or if YES to Question 3.
Adapted from Cotton M, Ball C, Robinson P. Four simple questions can help screen for eating disorders. J Gen Int Med. 2003;18:53-56.

High-quality evidence supports the numerous health benefits of PA across age groups, regardless of weight status.[51] To this end, guidelines recommend that all youth aged 6 to 17 years participate in at least 60 minutes of moderate to vigorous PA daily.[52] It is particularly important to highlight that the 60 minutes of PA do not need to be consecutive and briefer bouts can cumulatively contribute to these goals. To maximize health benefits, the guidelines further clarify that, throughout the week, children and adolescents should routinely participate in three different types of PA (vigorous-intensity aerobic, muscle strengthening, and bone strengthening), incorporating each type on at least 3 (but not necessarily the same) days a week.[52] In youth, the distinction between PA (i.e., any bodily movement produced by skeletal muscles that requires energy expenditure) and exercise (i.e., a specific form of PA that is planned, structured, repetitive, and performed with the goal of improving health or fitness) may be important, particularly among younger children where the majority of PA will consist of active play and not specifically exercise.[34] Thus, guidelines recommend that preschool-aged children (aged 3 to 5 years) be physically active throughout the day, participating in a variety of activity types.[52]

Of concern, most US youth do not meet these minimal daily PA recommendations.[51] In fact, levels of PA drop dramatically during adolescence, particularly among girls, racial/ethnic minorities, and youth with obesity.[53] Alarmingly, 56% of African American girls report not participating in *any* PA by the age of 16 to 17 years.[53] As part of an assessment of PA patterns, it is important to explore potential barriers to engagement in more regular PA and exercise such as access to safe environments, physical limitations (e.g., joint pain, uncontrolled asthma), reduced self-efficacy (e.g., "I am not sure what type of exercise I should do"), and concerns about stigma (e.g., "The other girls at the gym aren't overweight"). It is important to emphasize that among physically inactive youth with obesity, small increases in PA may still result in significant improvements in cardiometabolic risk factors, even when the recommended 60 minutes of PA daily are not achieved.[2] Thus, it is appropriate to collaborate with patients and families to set reasonable and achievable goals for increasing PA.

Methods for assessing levels and patterns of PA in youth that can be applied clinically include questionnaires and wearable PA monitors such as accelerometers, pedometers, and heart rate monitors.[34] Although the results of questionnaires are subject to recall bias and frequently overestimate the amount of time spent in PA, their use may still be reasonable in the clinical setting to establish baseline PA levels and patterns and assess treatment response, particularly in older children and adolescents. Children <10 years of age often cannot reliably respond to PA questionnaires, and parent estimates of their child's PA should be obtained instead.[34] Details regarding the time spent in outdoor play, recess and physical education at school, and community sports programs on a typically week may provide useful information regarding PA patterns in younger children.[34] Table 11.2 contains an example of a questionnaire that includes assessments of PA that may be applied to the primary care practice.

With the increased availability of commercially available, wearable, personal physical activity monitors, these devices may also be used to provide patients, families, and HCPs with additional data regarding PA to establish a baseline and set goal, when available.[34] However, the accuracy of such commercially available monitors are likely reduced in the pediatric population given analysis methods and the impact of body size, wear location, and PA type. Nevertheless, a pedometer count of 8,000 "steps" during a period of 60 minutes has been proposed as a reasonable estimate of 60 minutes of moderate to vigorous PA in youth aged 10 to 15 years.[54]

An assessment of time spent in sedentary behaviors is also vital in the pediatric population. Even though patterns of sedentary behaviors and PA may be related, both reduced PA and increased sedentary behaviors appear to be independent risk factors for obesity in youth, and both behaviors should be considered appropriate targets for behavioral interventions. Sedentary activity includes television viewing, video games, smart phones, tablets, and computers, and is now reflected in updated AAP guidelines.[55,56] The revised guidelines still recommend limiting media use to video-chatting only in children younger than 18 months and <1 hour of high-quality screen time in children younger than 18 months to 5 years. Recommendations for school-aged children and adolescents do not include absolute recommendations for total screen time but encourage parents to continue to set limits on screen time at every age, develop a family media use plan (https://www.healthychildren.org/English/media/), model behaviors related to media use, and create definitive media-free zones or times to avoid use during meals or at bedtime.

As in adults, mounting evidence suggests that inadequate sleep duration and reduced sleep quality during childhood are associated with increased risk of obesity.[38] In fact, a meta-analysis regarding the association between sleep and pediatric obesity risk found that, in children younger than 10 years, for each hour increase in sleep, the risk of overweight or obesity was reduced by ~9%.[57] As a result, an assessment of a child's sleep duration and patterns is essential. Potential therapeutic targets regarding sleep include removing screen media from the child's bedroom, establishing a consistent bedtime, and encouraging age-appropriate targets for sleep duration. Recommendations from the

TABLE 11.4 Recommended Healthy Sleep Durations for Infants, Children, and Adolescents

CATEGORY	AGE RANGE	RECOMMENDED SLEEP DURATION (HOURS EACH DAY)
Newborns	0-3 months	14-17
Infants	4-11 months	12-15
Toddlers	1-2 years	11-14
Preschoolers	3-5 years	10-13
School-age children	6-13 years	9-11
Teenagers	14-17 years	8-10
Adults	18-64 years	7-9

Adapted from Hirshkowitz M, Whiton K, Albert SM, et al. National Sleep Foundation's sleep time duration recommendations: methodology and results summary. Sleep Health. 2015;1(1):40-43.

National Sleep Foundation regarding appropriate sleep duration according to age-group are outlined in Table 11.4.[58]

Pediatric Physical Examination

The physical examination in infants, children and adolescents with excess weight gain should include the following six elements: (1) accurate measurement of height/weight, calculation of BMI, and determination of height/weight/BMI percentiles; (2) interpretation of the current anthropometric measurements in the context of prior growth patterns; (3) appropriate measurement and interpretation of blood pressure; (4) assessment of pubertal status (as appropriate); (5) assessment for clinical signs suggestive of a syndromic or endocrine etiology of weight gain; and (6) presence of examination findings associated with weight-related comorbidities.

Anthropometric Measurements in Children

Weight should be measured with the patient in light clothing. In practice environments providing care predominantly for children, it is vital to ensure easy access to an accurate scale that can accommodate youth with more severe obesity. As in adults, it is important that the measurement and reporting of weight be conducted by office staff in a manner that promotes privacy and reduces stigma. For example, it may be appropriate to ask a patient if he/she (or their parent) would like know what the results of the measurement instead of reflexively communicating the value.

In children ≥2 years of age who are able to stand without assistance, height should be measured (to the nearest 0.1 cm) using a stadiometer, after the patient has removed shoes and any hair braids/ornaments (as feasible). During the measurement, the child or adolescent should stand with his/her feet flat, together and against the wall; with straight legs and arms at his/her side; and looking straight ahead. In infants younger than 2 years, recumbent length (as opposed to standing height) should be determined, ideally using a dedicated measuring board. Given the challenges in the accurate measurements of height and recumbent length, it is advisable to measure height (or length) in duplicate and perform additional measurements when the first two measurements are discrepant.

Absolute BMI and age- and sex-specific percentiles for weight, height, and BMI should be determined in children ≥2 years of age using the 2000 CDC growth charts. In younger infants, a weight-to-recumbent length ratio should be calculated and age- and sex-specific percentiles determined, along with weight and length percentiles, using the 2006 WHO growth standards (https://www.cdc.gov/growthcharts/who_charts.htm).[3,5]

Assessment of Growth Patterns

It is important to evaluate the pediatric patient's current height, weight, and BMI (and associated percentiles) in the context of prior anthropometric measurements, when available, as temporal changes may provide additional pertinent information. A child or adolescent whose BMI trajectory is steadily crossing BMI percentile lines is likely to experience ongoing weight gain, even if his/her current BMI is below the 95th percentile.

As outlined, youth with obesity commonly experience their pubertal increase in height velocity slightly earlier than healthy-weight, late-childhood, and early-adolescent peers.[25] An attenuated height velocity, assessed in the context of genetic potential and pubertal stage, should prompt additional clinical or laboratory evaluation for endocrine etiologies of abnormal weight gain including hypothyroidism, hypercortisolism, or growth hormone deficiency.[2,15]

Pediatric Blood Pressure Measurement and Interpretation

The physical examination of children with overweight and obesity ≥3 years of age should include the careful measurement and interpretation of blood pressure (BP). Blood pressure readings should be obtained using an appropriately sized cuff, and values compared with normative values based on the patient's age, sex, and height.[59] In the pediatric population, BP values ≥95th percentile *or* an absolute value ≥130/80 mm Hg are consistent with hypertension (HTN), and values ≥90th percentile but <95th percentile *or* an absolute value of ≥120/80 mm Hg (if below the 90th percentile in older youth) are characterized as "elevated blood pressure." Abnormal value BP readings obtained using an automated device should be confirmed via auscultation. In addition, elevated BP readings should be confirmed on subsequent visits (and ideally ambulatory blood pressure monitoring) before diagnosing HTN.[59] A web-based tool for the age-, sex-, and height-appropriate interpretation of pediatric BP readings is available from the AAP online (https://www.mdcalc.com/aap-pediatric-hypertension-guidelines).

The prevalence of primary (i.e., essential) HTN has increased substantially in the pediatric population in conjunction with the obesity epidemic, with obesity accounting for ~85% to 90% of cases of HTN in adolescents aged 12 to 18 years.[60] Although HCPs should maintain a heightened level of suspicion for a secondary cause of HTN in all youth such as renal parenchymal disease and coarctation of the aorta, AAP guidelines recommend that children ≥6 year of age do not require an extensive evaluation for secondary causes of HTN (beyond an urinalysis and comprehensive metabolic panel) if (1) they have a positive family history of HTN *or* have overweight or obesity and (2) there is no history of physical examination findings (e.g., tachycardia, heart murmur, decreased lower extremity pulses, differential blood pressures in upper and lower extremities, edema) suggestive of a secondary cause of HTN.[59] As in adults, elevated blood pressure may also be a subtle indicator of the presence of sleep-disordered breathing and further diagnostic testing should be considered. Standard guidelines for the classification, clinical evaluation, and treatment of HTN in children and adolescents, including guidance regarding indications for referral to a pediatric HTN specialist (e.g., pediatric cardiologist or nephrologist), are available.[59]

Other Components of the Pediatric Examination

Additional examination features include assessment for the presence of acanthosis nigricans and skin tags, tonsillar hypertrophy, goiter, hepatomegaly, acne, and hirsutism. The pediatric physical examination should also include a careful evaluation of the lower extremities and gait, as children and younger adolescents with obesity may be particularly vulnerable to the development of weight-related orthopedic conditions as a result of ongoing skeletal maturation.

Tibia vara (Blount disease) results from the disruption of the medial aspect of the proximal tibial growth plate and results in unilateral or bilateral lower extremity bowing (genu varum). It is important to note that genu varum is a normal physiologic finding in infants, but typically transitions to a more neutral alignment by the age of 24 months as part of normal skeletal development.[61] Persistent, progressive, unilateral, or painful lower extremity bowing warrants further evaluation, including radiograph imaging and referral to an orthopedic specialist.[61]

Slipped capital femoral epiphysis (SCFE) refers to the displacement of the femoral head from the femoral neck through the growth plate. The condition is typically observed in early- to mid-adolescence, and obesity is a significant risk factor.[61] Adolescents with SCFE may present with (1) a limp and/or (2) acute *or* intermittent groin pain, thigh pain, or knee pain, in the absence of a history of trauma. Physical examination findings associated with SCFE include a limp with ambulation, external rotation of the foot on the affected side, and limited or painful internal rotation of the affected hip. The diagnosis is confirmed by anteroposterior and frog leg radiographs of the pelvis; imaging of both sides is recommended as 20% of cases of SCFE are bilateral, even though one side may be asymptomatic.[61] When present, SCFE requires urgent evaluation and surgery.

A funduscopic examination should be performed to assess for papilledema if the patient reports headaches; the presence of this finding may suggest pseudotumor cerebri and warrants urgent neurologic evaluation. HCPs should also remain alert to the presence of other physical examination findings (in addition to short stature and developmental delay) that could indicate the presence of a specific syndromic or genetic etiology, paying particular attention to facial features or abnormalities involving the digits, hands, or feet.

Pubertal Staging

When appropriate, the pediatric physical examination should also include an assessment of the child's pubertal development according to Sexual Maturity Rating (SMR) (i.e., Tanner Staging [Table 11.5]). Breast development (thelarche) and testicular enlargement (gonadarche) are typically the first signs of puberty in females and males, respectively; however, pubic hair development may be the initial sign of puberty (as opposed to breast development) in ~15% of girls.[62] Accurate SMR requires palpation, and it is important to differentiate glandular breast tissue from adipose tissue (adipomastia).

Precocious puberty is defined as the onset of pubertal changes in females before 8 years of age and in males before 9 years of age.[63] The lower age for the normal onset of puberty for females is debated, particularly among non-Hispanic black and Mexican American girls or girls with overweight/obesity, where the onset of breast development may be observed prior to the age of 8 years in ~12% of girls.[27] Although the onset of menses (menarche) typically occurs 2 to 2.5 years after the onset of puberty, the mean age of menarche is only slightly earlier in girls with a BMI ≥85th percentile

TABLE 11.5 Sexual Maturity Rating in Boys and Girls			
	BREAST DEVELOPMENT	**PUBIC HAIR DEVELOPMENT**	**TESTICULAR/PENILE DEVELOPMENT**
Prepubertal (Stage 1)	No breast buds	Prepubertal (may include some vellus hair)	Prepubertal
Stage 2	Subareolar breast bud	Sparse, fine, straight pubic hairs, typically at the base of penis or along labia	Enlargement of testes and scrotum, no enlargement of the penis
Stage 3	Elevation of the breast contour and enlargement of the areola	Long, dark curly pubic hairs limited to mons pubis	Enlargement of testes and scrotum, penis grows in length
Stage 4	Areola forms a secondary mound above the contour of the breast	Pubic hair is adult in quality, not yet spread to thighs	Further enlargement of testes and scrotum, penis grows in length
Stage 5	Mature female breast with dependent breast contour, recession of areola	Pubic hair has distribution of inverted triangle and spread to thighs	Mature male genitalia

Adapted from Wolf RM, Long D. Pubertal Development. Pediatr Rev. 2016;37(7):292-300.

(12.06 years of age) compared with girls with a healthy weight (12.57 years of age).[27] Although the early onset of puberty in girls before the age of 8 years may be considered normal in certain groups, girls with (1) the onset of puberty before the age of 7 years, or (2) the onset before the age of 8 years with a rapidly progressive course *or* a significant increase in growth velocity should be referred to a pediatric endocrinologist for further evaluation.

Conversely, delayed puberty is defined as the absence of breast development or testicular enlargement by the age of 13 years in females and by the age of 14 years in males.[62] Youth with obesity and delayed puberty should also be referred for endocrine evaluation. In the setting of otherwise normal pubertal development, the absence of menarche by the age of 16 years (primary amenorrhea) warrants further investigation. In particular, adolescent girls with polycystic ovary syndrome (PCOS) may present with primary amenorrhea (as opposed to irregular menstrual periods)[64]; and the diagnosis should be considered in adolescent girls with obesity (particularly those with acanthosis) if menarche has not occurred within 3 years of the onset of puberty and the patient has attained SMR Stage 4 or 5 breast development.

Recommended Comorbidity Screening and Associated Laboratory Testing in the Pediatric Population

As pediatric overweight and obesity is associated with an increased risk of the development of significant cardiometabolic comorbidities, even during childhood, it is vital to conduct appropriate screening for such conditions, many of which may be asymptomatic yet still convey significant lifetime risk. The 2007 Expert Committee Guidelines recommend conducting laboratory screening for T2D/prediabetes, dyslipidemia, and nonalcoholic fatty liver disease (NAFLD) based on severity of weight gain and other risk factors (Table 11.6).[3] Endocrine Society guidelines recommend similar screening laboratory testing in children with a BMI ≥85th percentile.[2]

Screening for undiagnosed T2D or prediabetes should be initiated in youth with a BMI ≥85th percentile at 10 years of age or the onset of puberty, whichever is earlier, and may consist of one of the following laboratory tests: measurement of a fasting serum glucose, a 2-hour oral glucose tolerance test, or HgbA1c.[65] The diagnostic criteria for impaired fasting glucose, impaired glucose tolerance, and overt diabetes mellitus in the pediatric population are the same as in adults.[65] Although the American Diabetes Association suggests that HgbA1c might still be an appropriate screening test in children and adolescents given its ease of collection,[65] Endocrine Society guidelines caution that HgbA1c may not have adequate diagnostic sensitivity in the pediatric population, underestimating the prevalence of both pre- and overt diabetes.[65] Despite the frequent presence of insulin resistance in youth with obesity, measurement of fasting insulin concentrations are not recommended given the lack of well-defined cut points to distinguish insulin-resistant and insulin-sensitive youth.[2]

Despite the clinical importance of detecting NAFLD in youth with overweight and obesity, the ideal

TABLE 11.6 Recommended Laboratory Screening for Cardiometabolic Risk Factors in Youth With Overweight and Obesity

BMI	RECOMMENDED TESTS
>85th-94th percentile, with no risk factors	Fasting lipid profile
>85th-94th percentile, with risk factors[a]	Fasting lipid profile Screening for glucose intolerance[b] AST and ALT levels
≥95th percentile	Fasting lipid profile Screening for glucose intolerance[b] AST and ALT levels

ALT, alanine aminotransferase; AST, aspartate aminotransferase; BMI, body mass index.
[a]Risk factors include family history of obesity-related diseases such as type 2 diabetes mellitus (T2D); elevated blood pressure; elevated lipid levels; or tobacco use.
[b]Screening for glucose intolerance via one of the following tests: fasting plasma glucose, oral glucose tolerance test, or HgbA1c.
Adapted from Krebs NF, Himes JH, Jacobson D, Nicklas TA, Guilday P, Styne D. Assessment of Child and Adolescent Overweight and Obesity. Pediatrics. 2007;120(suppl 4):S193-S228 and Styne DM, Arslanian SA, Connor EL, et al. Pediatric obesity-assessment, treatment, and prevention: an endocrine society clinical practice guideline. J Clin Endocrinol Metab. 2017;102(3):709-757.

approach to screening for the disorder in the pediatric population has not been established. Both the Barlow Expert Panel and Endocrine Society guidelines recommend obtaining serum aspartate aminotransferase (AST) and alanine aminotransferase (ALT) to screen for NAFLD.[3,34] These recommendations are consistent with those of the North American Society for Pediatric Gastroenterology, Hepatology, and Nutrition which proposes using a sex-specific upper limit of normal for ALT of 22 U/L in females and 26 U/L in males. The routine use of abdominal ultrasound to screen for NAFLD in the pediatric population is not recommended.[66] The diagnosis and severity of NAFLD is definitively established via liver biopsy in pediatric-aged patients as the validity of noninvasive assessment methods such as transient elastography in this population has yet to be confirmed.[66]

Although estimates of the prevalence of sleep-disordered breathing (i.e., obstructive sleep apnea [OSA]) among youth with obesity vary considerably (ranging between ~5% to 35%), routine screening for its presence is not recommended.[5] However, HCPs should maintain a high level of suspicion and consider referral for polysomnography if there is a history of elevated blood pressure, snoring, observed interruptions in breathing while asleep, secondary enuresis, daytime somnolence, or deteriorations in school performance.[34]

TREATMENT OF PEDIATRIC OBESITY AND OVERWEIGHT

The cornerstone of pediatric obesity treatment is family-based lifestyle modification that includes dietary modification, regular physical activity, and behavioral support.[2,3] In addition, pediatric obesity treatment plans should be age-appropriate, culturally sensitive, and tailored according to obesity severity. To guide providers in collaboratively establishing an appropriate treatment plan, the AAP-endorsed 2007 Expert Committee Recommendations propose a systematic approach to the intensity of clinical treatment that outlines four specific stages.[3] According to this proposed algorithm, treatment should be initiated at the least intensive stage, as appropriate given the patient's age, BMI, health risks, and motivation; treatment should then be advanced through subsequent stages based on the clinical response. Table 11.7 outlines recommended weight goals and the initial treatment stage according to the child's age and BMI category.[3] Of note, for younger children with overweight or less severe obesity, the recommended weight goal may include weight maintenance or slowing weight gain as opposed to overt weight loss. It is important to acknowledge that although many components of the stages are evidence based, the staged approach itself has not been rigorously assessed.

Several key approaches are vital at all stages of pediatric obesity treatment:

- The focus of pediatric behavioral weight management is to establish healthy dietary, activity, and family patterns that are sustainable over the long term and account for the family and patient's daily schedule, living environment, available resources, and cultural values and preferences.
- The entire family should be encouraged to engage in health behavior changes, and the specific identification of the child or adolescent as the "patient" or sole target for change should be discouraged.
- HCPs should work collaboratively with pediatric patients (as age-appropriate) and their families, using motivational interviewing techniques, to identify specific behaviors that the family is ready to modify.
- Effective behavior change should be supported by guiding the family in the development of a few specific and achievable goals and collaboratively developing implementation plans to proactively identify, and develop plans to overcome, barriers and consider strategies to increase the likelihood of goal attainment (e.g., environmental changes to promote stimulus control). The construct of SMART (Specific, Measurable, Achievable and Action-oriented,

TABLE 11.7 Pediatric Weight Goals, According to Age and BMI Category		
AGE	**BMI CATEGORY**	**WEIGHT GOAL**
2-5 years	85th-94th percentile with *no* health risks	Weight velocity maintenance
	85th-94th percentile with health risks	Weight maintenance or slow weight gain
	≥95th percentile	Weight maintenance (weight loss of up to 1 lb/mo may be acceptable if BMI >21 kg/m^2)
6-11 years	85th-94th percentile with *no* health risks	Weight velocity maintenance
	85th-94th percentile with health risks	Weight maintenance
	95th-99th percentile	Gradual weight loss (1 lb/mo or 0.5 kg/mo)
	>99th percentile	Weight loss (maximum is 2 lb/wk)
12-18 years	85th-94th percentile with *no* health risks	Weight velocity maintenance; after linear growth is complete, weight maintenance
	85th-94th percentile with health risks	Weight maintenance or gradual weight loss
	95th-99th percentile	Weight loss (maximum is 2 lb/wk)
	>99th percentile	Weight loss (maximum is 2 lb/wk)[a]

BMI, body mass index; mo, month; wk, week.

[a]*More rapid weight loss may be appropriate in adolescents with severe obesity treated with pharmacotherapy or metabolic and bariatric surgery.*

Adapted from Barlow SE; Expert Committee. Expert committee recommendations regarding the prevention, assessment, and treatment of child and adolescent overweight and obesity: summary report. Pediatrics. 2007;120(suppl 4):S164-S192.

Realistic, and Time-based) goal-setting may assist in this process. Moreover, families may need to work toward larger goals (e.g., "My child will be active 1 hour a day") by breaking behaviors down to more manageable and achievable steps that can then be subsequently built upon (e.g., "My child and I will play outside for 30 minutes after I pick him up from school 2 days next week.")

- HCPs should encourage timely follow-up, as appropriate for the stage of treatment, to partner with families and patients in nonjudgmentally assessing progress toward goals and revising the treatment plan as appropriate.

Role of Parents in Pediatric Obesity Treatment

Parental engagement is an essential component of all effective pediatric obesity treatments as parents are vital in promoting healthy behaviors in children. Parents strongly influence the home food and exercise environment. Moreover, parents are important role models of eating and activity patterns, and parent and child weight are related. In fact, studies have demonstrated that among children engaged in lifestyle modification programs, parental weight loss (even when parents are not specifically targeted in the intervention) correlates with the child's treatment response.[67] As a result, behavioral interventions for youth with overweight or

obesity should be family-based and specifically involve parents in obesity treatment through strategies such as parental monitoring, limit setting, reducing barriers, managing family conflict, and modifying the home environment. It is important to reemphasize that pediatric obesity treatment should primarily focus on the family versus the child alone as the identified patient. Indeed, parent-exclusive treatment has yielded comparable (or even superior) outcomes for children aged 6 to 11 years.[68] Although there is less clarity regarding the most effective way to engage parents in their adolescents' obesity treatment, there are well-established practices that parents can use to promote the development of healthy behaviors in their children. Efforts to enhance and reinforce parenting skills are therefore important components of pediatric obesity treatment across age ranges.

Parenting Styles

HCPs should encourage parents to adopt a parenting style known as authoritative parenting which is characterized by both responsiveness (e.g., being attuned to their child's need and emotions, fostering autonomy) yet a consistent firmness (i.e., high demands) in regard to establishing limits and providing structure. Parents employing an authoritative parenting style shape their child's behavior by explaining and discussing limits and reasoning; they listen to and acknowledge their child's viewpoint, but do not necessarily accept it. It is important to distinguish the characteristics of this authorit*ative* parenting style ("loving with limits") from other styles such as authorit*arian* or permissive parenting. An authoritarian parenting style ("strict and stern") is characterized by high demands but low responsiveness (i.e., having very high expectations of children but providing little in the way of feedback and nurturance); parents who engage in an authoritarian parenting style typically impose numerous rules, which may often seem arbitrary, and may respond to the child's mistakes or "rule-breaking" harshly. On the other hand, permissive parenting is characterized by low demands but high responsiveness (i.e., emotionally warm, yet providing little guidelines or rules). Of importance, compared with these other parenting styles, an authoritative approach to parenting is associated with healthier weight outcomes in children and adolescents.[69] To this end, providers should encourage parents to set (and discuss) age-appropriate limits with their children and consistently enforce these limits with warmth and understanding.

Feeding Styles

Authoritative feeding (e.g., providing choice within parameters; avoiding excessive restriction or control) is a separate (but not necessarily related) construct that has also been associated with improved weight outcomes in children.[70,71] A major goal of parent feeding is to teach children to self-regulate their dietary intake and to eat based on hunger and fullness cues. Overly permissive feeding (e.g., no structure or guidelines around eating) does not teach children limits and is associated with higher intake of energy-dense food. Moreover, a restrictive feeding style (e.g., having strict rules around food) can teach children to eat (or not eat) in response to guilt or shame, or due to access to a food or beverage that might be forbidden food at home. Overly restrictive feeding can be associated with dysregulated eating behaviors, including sneaking, hiding or hoarding food, or overeating/binge eating when desired food is present. Neither permissive nor restrictive feeding patterns support children in self-regulating their dietary intake based on hunger and fullness cues. Resources available on https://www.ellynsatterinstitute.org/ can be helpful to promote authoritative feeding and teach parents the "division of responsibility" in feeding (i.e., the parent's responsibility is to provide healthful food options at structured meal and snack times while it is the child's responsibility to determine specifically which of the offered foods, and how much of them, are consumed). Authoritative feeding strategies help children develop healthy eating and weight patterns.

Stage 1 Treatment: Prevention Plus

Stage 1 (prevention plus) is designed to be implemented in the primary HCP's office and focuses on developing, or reinforcing, healthy eating and activity habits for the entire family. The term "prevention plus" highlights the central role of promoting healthy dietary habits, regular physical activity, reduced sedentary activity, and sufficient sleep in youth of all ages regardless of body weight; however, these behaviors are also important key therapeutic targets in addressing the imbalance in energy metabolism that contributes to pediatric overweight and obesity (Table 11.8). During this treatment stage, the child or adolescent should be allowed to self-regulate his or her dietary intake, within the limits that parents set (e.g., eating at predictable meal and snack times, avoiding screens while eating, eating at table), while avoiding overly controlling feeding behaviors (e.g., forcing a child to clean their plate, overly restricting food). The frequency of follow-up visits during Stage 1 treatment should be tailored to the clinical scenario and account for the patient's/family's specific goals and motivation. If the desired and age-appropriate clinical response (Table 11.7) has not been achieved after 3 to 6 months, the AAP treatment algorithm recommends that the treatment approach be intensified to Stage 2 care.

Stage 2 Treatment: Structured Weight Management

Stage 2 care is also designed to be implemented in the primary care setting and is primarily distinguished from Stage 1 by an enhanced level of support and structure to assist families in implementing sustained behavior changes. To this end, recommendations for Stage 2 care includes the development of a specific eating plan designed to reduce energy intake, in collaboration with

---

TABLE 11.8 Key Behavioral Targets for Treatment of Pediatric Overweight and Obesity

- Minimize or eliminate sugar-sweetened beverage intake
- Consume ≥5 serving of fruits and vegetables every day
- Eat a healthy breakfast every day
- Set age-appropriate limits on screen time, including the establishment of screen-free zones (e.g., bedrooms at night) and times (e.g., during meals)
- Be physically active a total of ≥60 minutes each day
- Prepare more meals at home
- Eat family meals at a table five or six times a week
- Establish a regular sleeping schedule according to age-specific recommendations

Adapted from Barlow SE; Expert Committee. Expert committee recommendations regarding the prevention, assessment, and treatment of child and adolescent overweight and obesity: summary report. Pediatrics. 2007;120(suppl 4):S164-S192.

a registered dietitian nutritionist (RDN); encouraging the family (and youth as developmentally appropriate) to monitor targeted dietary and activity behaviors through the use of logging; and an increased frequency of follow-up visits (typically at least once a month).[3] In addition to the development and implementation of a specific eating plan, increasing physical activity and reducing sedentary activities remain key therapeutic targets during Stage 2 as regular engagement in PA is a significant predictor of weight loss maintenance, even in the pediatric population. A meta-analysis of the impact of pediatric weight management interventions implemented in primary care settings demonstrated that such interventions result in small but significant reductions in BMI across age groups, with greater BMI reductions observed with longer treatment duration and more frequent contact with the care team.[72]

Pediatric Dietary Interventions

A core component of Stage 2 pediatric obesity treatment is the development of a specific eating plan, which should be designed and implemented in collaboration with an RDN or by an HCP who has received additional training in the use of such plans.[3] As a result, HCPs who treat youth with overweight and obesity should seek to identify an RDN in their local community who can skillfully work with families to establish a structured eating plan. Instead of instituting a specific "diet," the Stage 2 dietary plan should focus on the consumption of macronutrient-balanced meals (breakfast, lunch, and dinner), with one to two scheduled snacks, with emphases on portion control, consumption of foods low in energy density such as fruits or vegetables, and reduced intake of processed foods (or beverages) high in added sugar, saturated fat, and sodium.[3]

As in adults, the ability to sustain adherence to a particular dietary approach that results in an energy deficit appears to overshadow any particular focus on macronutrient composition in the pediatric population. Improved dietary quality (e.g., increased consumption of complex carbohydrates and lean protein) can assist with adherence to an energy-restricted diet via enhancing satiety; intake of these foods also plays a key role in improved health and reduced disease risk. However, a focus on diet quality will only yield weight loss if it also creates an energy deficit. To this end, it may be appropriate to discuss recommended age- and sex-appropriate estimated daily calorie needs (Table 11.9) with parents and adolescent patients to provide guidance related to meal planning and adjusting dietary intake to achieve targets, even if formal calorie tracking is not being implemented. Yet, for adolescents, it may be appropriate to discuss tracking caloric intake, with parent support, to help patients learn how to make dietary choices that keep intake within their recommended calorie targets. To date, there is no evidence that monitoring energy intake, in the context

TABLE 11.9 Estimated Pediatric Daily Caloric Needs (Kcal/day) by Age and Sex[a]

AGE (YEARS)	MALES	FEMALES[b]
2	1,000	1,000
3	1,000-1,400	1,000-1,200
4	1,200-1,400	1,200-1,400
5	1,200-1,400	1,200-1,400
6	1,400-1,600	1,200-1,400
7	1,400-1,600	1,200-1,600
8	1,400-1,600	1,400-1,600
9	1,600-1,800	1,400-1,600
10	1,600-1,800	1,400-1,800
11	1,800-2,000	1,600-1,800
12	1,800-2,200	1,600-2,000
13	2,000-2,200	1,600-2,000
14	2,000-2,400	1,800-2,000
15	2,200-2,600	1,800-2,000
16-18	2,400-2,800	1,800-2,000

Adapted from U.S. Department of Health and Human Services and U.S. Department of Agriculture. 2015-2020 Dietary Guidelines for Americans. 8th ed. December 2015. https://health.gov/our-work/food-nutrition/2015-2020-dietary-guidelines/guidelines/appendix-2
[a]Range based on a sedentary to moderate physical activity level; higher caloric needs may be appropriate for more active children. Lower daily caloric targets may be necessary to induce a negative energy balance necessary for weight loss.
[b]Estimates for females do not include women who are pregnant or breastfeeding.

of a weight loss program, is associated with an increased risk of disordered eating behaviors[73]; in contrast, given that calorie labeling is ubiquitous, teaching adolescents and parents how to appropriately use this information to make choices that are consistent with their goals can empower them to more effectively engage in their weight management. Nonetheless, calorie monitoring is time intensive and may not be appropriate in all adolescent or younger patients. An alternative strategy that can more readily be applied across all age groups, and adopted by families, is to use the MyPlate meal planning guide (e.g., ½ the plate with fruits and vegetables, ¼ lean protein, ¼ whole grain) to assist in improving dietary quality and induce an energy deficit via controlling portions.

Behavioral Self-Monitoring

An additional component of Stage 2 pediatric obesity treatment is the implementation of self-monitoring techniques to assess engagement with targeted dietary, activity, or parenting behaviors. Although such self-monitoring need not necessarily include the completion of detailed dietary logs or tracking calorie intake (unless parents or older youth are motivated to engage in these specific approaches), self-monitoring is a key therapeutic approach that assists families in assessing and adjusting progress toward their selected behavioral goals and should be promoted. Approaches and targets for self-monitoring may take many forms (e.g., meal planning; monitoring SSB or fruit/vegetable intake; tracking frequency of breakfast consumption or family meals via a calendar; using physical activity monitors or sleep logs; or tracking weight) based on individual goals, the patient's age, family preference, and available resources (e.g., access to smartphone apps or physical activities monitors for tracking).

Stage 3 Treatment: Comprehensive Multidisciplinary Intervention

For patients who have not experienced a significant clinical response (Table 11.7) with Stage 2 treatment, care should be intensified to Stage 3 treatment which consists of a comprehensive multidisciplinary intervention that includes a structured behavioral modification program with frequent (ideally weekly) follow-up and is delivered by an integrated care team that includes an RDN, behavioral specialist (e.g., psychologist, social worker or other mental HCP), and exercise specialist (e.g., physical therapist or exercise physiologist). The team structure and suggested weekly contact frequency required for Stage 3 treatment interventions may exceed the capacity and resources available in many primary care offices. Although Stage 3 programs are frequently available at specialized pediatric obesity treatment centers, HCPs should familiarize themselves with what specific resources are available to families within their local practice areas.

A targeted systematic review conducted by the US Preventive Services Task Force (USPSTF) regarding the effectiveness of weight management interventions in children provides support for the efficacy of moderate- to high-intensity comprehensive multidisciplinary interventions in youth aged 4 to 18 years, with a 1.9 to 3.3 kg/m² difference in BMI reduction at 12 months compared with control interventions.[74] Importantly, multidisciplinary interventions appear to be more effective in younger children (6 to 9 years of age) and youth with less severe obesity.[75]

Stage 4 Treatment: Tertiary Care Intervention

Youth with more severe obesity, including those with underlying genetic or syndromic etiologies of obesity or multiple weight-related comorbidities, who have not experienced adequate weight loss or maintenance in response to intensive lifestyle modification (Stage 3) alone, may benefit from more specialized, evidence-based treatments including the use of antiobesity pharmacotherapy or MBS. Data regarding the use of other additional adjuvant approaches in the pediatric population including very-low-calorie diets or residential treatment programs are limited and demonstrate variable success. It is important to emphasize that intensive, family-based, lifestyle modification remains an essential foundation for effective and durable Stage 4 treatment. According to guideline recommendations, Stage 4 treatment, especially MBS, should be conducted in coordination with specialized care teams at dedicated pediatric obesity centers.[2,3]

Pharmacotherapy in Adolescents With Severe Obesity

Pediatric clinical guidelines and opinion statements propose a potential role for antiobesity pharmacotherapy in adolescents with obesity, when used in conjunction with ongoing lifestyle modification.[2,3,76] However, although adult criteria support the use of antiobesity pharmacotherapy based on BMI thresholds, the ideal criteria for the use pharmacologic therapy in the pediatric population remain unclear. At least two expert panels recommend that antiobesity pharmacotherapy in patients <18 years of age should be reserved for youth with at least Class 1 obesity (BMI ≥30 kg/m² or ≥95th percentile) and should only be prescribed by clinicians with experience in the use of such agents in this population and in conjunction with intensive multidisciplinary lifestyle modification (i.e., Stage 3 intervention).[2,76] Lastly, as in adults, treatment response should be monitored closely and medications should only be continued beyond 12 weeks in pediatric patients who experience a >4% to 5% reduction in BMI.[2] Moreover, only two antiobesity medications are currently approved by the Federal Drug Administration (FDA) for use in children and adolescents <18 years of age with obesity: orlistat and phentermine (see Chapter 8 on Pharmacotherapy).

Orlistat, a lipase inhibitor that blocks fat absorption, is FDA approved for the treatment of obesity in children ≥12 years of age at the same dose used in the adult population (i.e., 120 mg orally three times a day). In clinical trials involving youth with obesity, the addition of orlistat to lifestyle modification results in BMI reductions of -0.94 to -0.50 kg/m² over 6 to 12 months compared with placebo.[77] The adverse gastrointestinal side effects commonly associated with orlistat may be particularly troubling to youth and limit the medication's tolerability in this population. In light of the risk of malabsorption of fat-soluble vitamins and minerals with orlistat, youth on the medication should also take a multivitamin daily.

Phentermine, a norepinephrine reuptake inhibitor, has been FDA approved for the short-term treatment of obesity in individuals ≥16 years of age since 1959, yet few studies have specifically evaluated its use in adolescents.[76] In a small retrospective study comparing 6 months of phentermine 15 mg once daily plus lifestyle modification with lifestyle modification alone in adolescents with obesity, phentermine was associated with mean reductions in weight and BMI of -3.23 kg (95% confidence interval [CI], -5.95 to -0.52) and -1.57 kg/m[2] (95% CI, -2.78 to -0.36), respectively.[78] Although phentermine use was not associated with significant changes in systolic or diastolic blood pressure, mild (but persistent) elevations in heart rate from baseline were noted in the phentermine group over the 6-month study period. Phentermine is a class of amphetamines and a Class IV controlled substance that includes safety concerns regarding abuse; state bylaws and statues regarding its use should be followed. As a result, some expert panels have recommended against its use for the treatment of obesity in children and adolescents.[2]

Liraglutide (up to a dose of 1.8 mg daily) is FDA approved for use in children and adolescents aged 10 years or older with T2D[79]; the 3.0 mg dose was recently approved as a weight loss medication for youth with obesity (without T2DM) aged 12 years or older. A randomized, double-blind, placebo-controlled trial enrolling adolescent aged 12 to 17 years with obesity involving liraglutide 3.0 mg daily versus placebo, combined with intensive lifestyle modification, demonstrated modest but significant reductions in body weight (estimated difference, -4.50 kg) after 56 weeks of treatment.[80] Similar to adults, gastrointestinal symptoms including nausea, vomiting, and diarrhea were more commonly reported in youth treated with liraglutide compared with placebo. It is unclear how the gastrointestinal side effects and the subcutaneous route of administration of liraglutide will impact the clinical acceptability of the medication in the pediatric population.

Metformin, a biguanide that improves insulin sensitivity and reduces hepatic glucose production, is FDA-approved for the treatment of T2D in children ≥10 years of age, but it does not have an approved indication for obesity treatment in either the adult or pediatric populations. However, given metformin's potential suppressive effects on appetite, favorable safety profile and extensive experience in the pediatric population, the medication's mild impact on weight has been more extensively studied in youth compared with other approved pharmacologic agents for obesity. In a meta-analysis, metformin use was associated with a small but significant reduction in BMI (-0.86 kg/m[2]; 95% CI, -1.44 to -0.28) at 6 to 12 months in studies of children and adolescents.[77] Importantly, 80% of the pediatric metformin studies required that participating youth have evidence of hyperinsulinemia, insulin resistance, or glucose intolerance.[77] As such, metformin may be a component of a comprehensive treatment plan that includes lifestyle modification in adolescents with overweight and obesity who are at increased risk for the development of T2D such as youth with prediabetes, the metabolic syndrome, and PCOS. Metformin may also have a potential role in mitigating the weight gain associated with atypical antipsychotic use in the pediatric population.[34]

Pediatric MBS

In contrast to the unclear role of antiobesity pharmacotherapy in the pediatric population, mounting robust evidence supports the role of MBS as part of a comprehensive treatment plan in youth with severe obesity.[2,6,81] Roux-en-Y gastric bypass (RYGB) and vertical sleeve gastrectomy (VSG) are the two most common MBS procedures conducted in adolescents. Although RYGB was previously considered the gold-standard procedure in this population, VSG is increasingly performed in youth with severe obesity. Despite initial interest in the role of the laparoscopic adjustable gastric band in the adolescent population, it is not approved by the FDA for use in people younger than 18 years and is not used any more.

Several longitudinal cohort studies have demonstrated the impact of MBS on weight loss and weight-related comorbidities in adolescents with severe obesity, demonstrating significant (~26% weight change) and sustained (≥5 years) reductions in weight and BMI among youth undergoing MBS.[81,82] These clinical responses are similar in magnitude to MBS outcomes in adults. Moreover, youth with severe obesity may experience significant improvements in weight-related comorbidities (including T2D, HTN, OSA and NAFLD) and quality of life following MBS.[6] A recent study published by the Teen-Longitudinal Assessment of Bariatric Surgery (Teen-LABS) consortium highlighted ongoing remission rates of T2DM and HTN in adolescents of 86% and 68%, respectively, 5 years after MBS, rates that were substantially higher than those observed in adults undergoing MBS.[82]

Based on this growing body of data, the American Society for Metabolic and Bariatric Surgery (ASMBS) released revised best practice guidelines for the pediatric population in 2018, recommending consideration of MBS in youth with Class 2 obesity (BMI ≥35 kg/m[2] or a BMI ≥120% of the age- and sex-appropriate 95th percentile) with significant weight-related comorbidities or Class 3 obesity (BMI ≥40 kg/m[2] or a BMI ≥140% of the age- and sex-appropriate 95th percentile) without comorbidities, who have not experienced sufficient weight loss with intensive lifestyle modification.[6] Contraindications in the pediatric population include a medically correctable cause of obesity, uncontrolled substance abuse, uncontrolled eating or mood disorder, and difficulty adhering to lifestyle modification or follow-up. According to the most recent ASMBS guidelines, age or physical/sexual maturity is no longer proposed as a specific eligibility requirement for youth undergoing weight loss surgery. Guidelines consistently and strongly recommend that pediatric MBS should only be conducted at specialized centers with comprehensive care teams that specifically include a pediatric obesity specialist and behavioral specialist.[6,81] The Metabolic and Bariatric Surgery Accreditation and Quality Improvement Program (MBSAQIP) includes a pediatric-specific designation to assist HCPs in identifying such programs.

Surgical complications are infrequent in youth undergoing BMS and, when they do occur, are typically minor and occur early in the postoperative period (e.g., nausea and dehydration).[6,81] Extant evidence does not suggest that MBS results in significant growth impairment when conducted in the pediatric population.[81] However, as in adults, micronutrient deficiencies, especially iron deficiency, are common in youth after both RYGB and VSG. Thus, youth considering MBS should be counseled (and demonstrate understanding) regarding the need for lifelong adherence with routine vitamin and mineral supplements, as well as the recommendations for ongoing medical follow-up.[6]

Although the number of surgical procedures performed in individuals younger than 18 years have increased significantly, only a small fraction of youth who meet criteria and may benefit from the MBS undergo surgery.[81] Consequently, the AAP Policy Statement regarding Pediatric MBS strongly encourages HCPs to understand the potential role of MBS in the comprehensive treatment of youth with severe obesity and discuss options for referral to MBSAQIP-designated pediatric programs in youth who meet surgical indications; the Policy Statement authors also strongly recommend that public and private insurers cover MBS for pediatric patients who meet established, and increasingly evidence-based, indications.[81]

SUMMARY

Given the high prevalence of pediatric overweight and obesity, the substantial impact of obesity on a child's current and future health, and the importance of the identification and treatment of at-risk youth, an assessment of adiposity (via determination of BMI and age- and sex-appropriate BMI percentiles) should be routinely performed by HCPs as part of routine pediatric care. In youth with elevated BMIs, HCPs should conduct a careful history and physical examination

with the goals of identifying any underlying conditions that may directly contribute to the child's weight gain as well as any health conditions resulting from obesity. Although rare, genetic and syndromic etiologies of abnormal weight gain should be considered when there is a history of early-onset severe obesity; attenuated growth velocity may indicate an underlying endocrine etiology of abnormal weight gain. Screening for potential weight-related comorbidities should be conducted based on clinical suspicion and established guidelines considering age- and sex-appropriate cut-offs where appropriate. Lifestyle modification designed to induce a negative energy balance is the cornerstone of all pediatric obesity treatments (with relatively greater emphasis on reduction of energy intake compared with increased energy expenditure, to yield weight losses), and parental involvement to promote family-based change and empirically supported parenting skills are essential components of pediatric behavioral weight management. The impact of lifestyle modification on BMI in children and adolescence is the most robust when interventions are initiated earlier in life before more severe obesity is established. In addition to intensive lifestyle modification, the comprehensive treatment of severe obesity in older children and adolescents may include the use of pharmacotherapy or MBS when conducted by multidisciplinary teams with expertise in the application of these modalities in the pediatric population.

CLINICAL HIGHLIGHTS

- Approximately one in five and one in three youth in the United States have obesity and overweight, respectively.
- Screening for excess adiposity in children and adolescents should include calculation of BMI and determination of age- and sex-specific BMI percentiles according to the 2000 CDC growth charts: a BMI ≥85th but <95th is consistent with overweight; a BMI ≥95th percentile (*or* an absolute BMI ≥30 kg/m²) is consistent with obesity.
- The initial clinical assessment should consist of (1) a detailed history; (2) an age-appropriate assessment of dietary, physical activity, sedentary behaviors, and sleep patterns; (3) a careful review of previous growth patterns; and (4) a detailed physical examination to assess pubertal development (as appropriate), identify dysmorphic features, and screen for weight-related orthopedic conditions such as tibia vara (Blount disease) and SCFE.
- Blood pressure measurements in children should be interpreted in comparison to normative values based on the patient's age, sex, and height. Values ≥90th

percentile or 120/80 mm Hg are considered elevated, and persistent values ≥95th percentile or 130/80 mm Hg are consistent with HTN.

- The majority of youth with obesity do not have an underlying identifiable genetic defect responsible for their weight gain. However, a history of severe early-onset obesity and hyperphagia, in the setting of neurodevelopmental delay, dysmorphic features, or endocrinopathies such as hypogonadism should alert the HCP to the possibility of a specific genetic syndrome, which warrants further evaluation.

- A reduced height velocity in a child with obesity should alert the HCP to the possibility of an underlying endocrine condition responsible for abnormal weight gain.

- Many weight-related comorbidities first appear during childhood, and youth with a BMI ≥85th percentile should undergo routine laboratory screening for common cardiometabolic disorders including glucose intolerance ("prediabetes") and T2D, dyslipidemia, and NAFLD.

- The cornerstone of pediatric obesity treatment is family-based lifestyle modification that includes dietary modification, regular physical activity, and behavior support that involves the entire family.

- Parental engagement is an essential component of effective treatments, and HCPs should support parents in modifying the home environment, role modeling desired health behaviors, and implementing authoritative parenting and feeding.

- Successful pediatric behavioral weight loss strategies should involve dietary changes designed to induce a negative energy balance. High-yield dietary behaviors may include reducing SSB intake, portions sizes, snacking, and frequency of eating meals outside of the home as well as establishing family meals that are free of distractions.

- Regular physical activity is associated with obesity and comorbidity prevention as well as weight maintenance. HCPs should support families in being active together and setting goals to increase the level of activity toward recommended 60 minutes daily.

- Pediatric lifestyle modification interventions are most effective in reducing BMI trajectory when initiated early in life, before more severe obesity is established. Recommended weight goals should be determined based on the child's age and BMI category.

- If initial weight goals are not achieved, HCPs should consider resources in their community for implementing a more structured treatment approach and enhanced support for families such as the development of structured eating plan in collaboration with a registered dietitian nutritionist or referral to comprehensive multidisciplinary lifestyle intervention.

- HCPs may consider the off-label addition of metformin to lifestyle modification in older children at high risk of insulin resistance-related comorbidities such as T2D and PCOS. Few antiobesity agents are currently approved for youth and should be limited to HCPs with experience in their use in the pediatric population.

- Increasing evidence supports the long-term safety and efficacy of MBS in the treatment of severe obesity and weight-related comorbidities in older children and adolescents. Although adolescent MBS should only be conducted by specialized centers with comprehensive pediatric care teams, HCPs should discuss referral to such programs with interested youth who meet surgical indications.

WHEN TO REFER?

- Child with severe, early-onset obesity before the age of 5 years and hyperphagia, particularly if neurodevelopmental abnormalities or dysmorphic physical features are present. Refer to genetics or pediatric obesity medicine specialist.

- Child with impaired height velocity, early puberty (onset before 7 to 8 years of age in girls or 9 years of age in boys), or delayed puberty (absence of breast development by the age of 13 years [or menarche by the age of 16 years] in girls or absence of testicular enlargement by the age of 14 years in boys). Refer to a pediatric endocrinologist.

- Child with persistent, progressive, unilateral, or painful lower extremity bowing. Refer for radiograph imaging and to orthopedic specialist.

- Child with a limp and/or acute or intermittent groin, thigh, or knee pain, in the absence of a history of trauma. Refer for radiographs of the pelvis. Refer urgently to orthopedic specialist if imaging is suggestive of SCFE.

- Child with confirmed and repeated blood pressure measurements ≥95th percentile for age, sex, and height *or* ≥130/80 mm Hg. Consider referral to pediatric hypertension specialist (e.g., cardiology or nephrology).

- Child has not achieved recommended weight goals using a treatment approach implemented in the primary care setting but family is interested in intensifying treatment. Refer to a registered dietitian nutritionist or a comprehensive multidisciplinary lifestyle program.

- Child has disordered patterns of eating such as binge or loss of control eating or compensatory behaviors such as purging. Refer to an eating disorder specialist.

- Older child or adolescent with Class 2 obesity (BMI ≥35 kg/m^2 or a BMI ≥120% of the age- and sex-appropriate 95th percentile) with significant weight-related comorbidities or Class 3 obesity (BMI ≥40 kg/m^2 or a BMI ≥140% of the age- and sex-appropriate 95th percentile) without comorbidities, who have not experienced sufficient weight loss with intensive lifestyle modification. Refer to specialized pediatric obesity center with dedicated MBS program.

CASE STUDY

Discussion

In the pediatric population, BMI values should be evaluated in the context of age- and sex-specific percentiles according to the 2000 CDC growth charts. Although this girl's absolute BMI is <25 kg/m² (i.e., the adult cutpoint for defining overweight), it is >95th percentile for 10-year-old girls (corresponding BMI of 22.9 kg/m²) and would be consistent with obesity. Moreover, this girl's BMI is ~108% of the 95th percentile BMI (24.8/22.9 × 100 = 108) and which would be consistent with Class 1 obesity (BMI ≥95th percentile but <120% of the 95th percentile BMI). As part of the initial conversation, you support the mother's concerns about her daughter's weight but also engage the daughter in the discussion.

Provider: *"It sounds like your mother has some concerns about your health and how your weight may be impacting that. What concerns do you have about your health or weight?"*

Patient: *"I think that I am pretty healthy, but would like to lose some weight so that kids at school would stop teasing me."*

Provider: *"I am sorry that you have experienced that. I appreciate that topics like weight can be very personal topics for people. Is it OK if we continue to discuss these things?"*

During the ongoing discussion that engages both the patient and her mother, you confirm that the patient was the product of a full-term gestation, during which her mother had gestational diabetes mellitus, and was born by cesarean section. There were no complications for the child after delivery. Her mother notes that she first started to become concerned about her daughter weight when she was about 4 years old. The mother notes that the weight gain started to occur after the patient was treated with prednisone on several occasions for her asthma. Even though the patient has not received additional steroids over the past several years, the patient has experienced ongoing steady weight gain. You confirm that the girl met her developmental milestones appropriately and there have not been any concerns about learning problems or disabilities. You confirm that there have never been any concerns that the patient was not growing from a height standpoint. The mother denies any concerns about early puberty, and the patient has not yet had menarche.

After confirming the medical portion of the history, you transition to obtaining a focused dietary, activity, and sleep history. To continue to build rapport and minimize stigma, you offer the following:

Provider: *"I'd like to get more information about some of your and your family's eating and activity habits. There are not any right or wrong answers to these questions. The information will be useful in helping us determine the next steps to improve your health together. Can you share with me what a typical day looks like for you including what time you wake up and go to bed, when and what you usually like to eat, and how you like to spend your time?"*

Patient: *"Ok, my days look pretty different based on whether it is a school day or the weekend."*

Provider: *"That makes sense. Let's start with a school day and you can then share what is different on the weekends."*

After completing the history, you review other clinical data from the examination. You review the BP measurement of 119/78 mm Hg obtained by clinic staff by comparing it to normative values for a 10-year-old girl whose height is at the 90th percentile (based on height of 147 cm). This value is >90th percentile but below the 95th percentile and is consistent with "elevated blood pressure." You make a note to reassess the value at follow-up. You review the patient's prior growth chart obtained from her previous provider and confirm her height has steadily tracked along the 90th percentile in the past. A review of her BMI shows that she experienced adiposity rebound at about the age of 4 years. You previously did not identify any dysmorphic-appearing facial features or abnormalities with the patient's hands or feet on examination.

Based on the patient's normal developmental history, growth velocity, and lack of concern in examination findings, you decide that additional testing for a syndromic or endocrine etiology (including thyroid function testing) for the patient's weight gain is not warranted and communicate these recommendations to the family. However, you do discuss recommendations regarding laboratory screening for weight-related comorbidities. As the patient is 10 years of age, has started puberty, and has a BMI ≥95th percentile, you recommend obtaining a fasting glucose, lipid panel, AST, and ALT.

Lastly, you initiate a discussion about treatment goals highlighting the importance of family-based changes. After highlighting the numerous benefits of regular PA and reflecting the family's frustration that the patient's weight has not decreased despite regular exercise, you review that exercise alone is typically not sufficient to induce a negative energy balance that results in weight loss and you would like to help the family identify some changes to eating patterns that they would like to focus on to improve health:

Provider: *"We spent some time discussing your family's normal routines and eating patterns. After that discussion, are there any specific changes that you think would help improve your health and weight that you feel ready to change?"*

Mother: *"Yes, I think we should eat out less."*

Provider: *"Eating out less sounds like a great change; let's see if we can be more specific with your goal and plan (so that you know what 'less' means)."*

Mother: *"Ok, I think we should just cut it out completely."*

Provider: *"That certainly could be a great goal and it would be healthy for you and your family to eat more meals at home together. Although, let's just consider if completely cutting out eating out is realistic… or would maybe reducing the number of meals you eat out be more realistic to start? I know for some other busy families who eat out often, a great first step might be trying first try to limit the number of times you eat out each week. You know yourself best, though what do you think would be realistic for you?"*

You work with the patient and her family to identify two SMART-style goals regarding dietary changes: (1)

"We will reduce the number of times we eat out during the next month to one time per week," and (2) "We will preportion snacks into small bags after we return from the grocery store and the kids can select one snack-bag to enjoy each day (with screens off) when they get home from school." To end the encounter, you provide the patient and her mother written copies of their goals, express confidence in their ability to reach these goals, and ask them if they would like to return to the clinic in a month to check on their progress.

QUIZ QUESTIONS

1. You are evaluating a 13-year-old boy with obesity. The patient's current BMI is 31.8 kg/m². The BMI value that corresponds to the 2000 CDC 95th percentile for 13-year-old males is 25.1 kg/m².

   Which of the following would be the most appropriate classification regarding the severity of the child's obesity according to pediatric definitions?

   A. Class 1 obesity
   B. Class 2 obesity
   C. Class 3 obesity
   D. Morbid obesity

   Answer: B. *In children and younger adolescents, the classification of weight status, including obesity severity, cannot always be determined by absolute BMI values alone. Although this child's absolute BMI value falls in the range for Class 1 obesity according to adult criteria (i.e., 30 to <35 kg/m²), a BMI of 31.8 kg/m² is ~ 127% of the 95th percentile for 13-year-old males (i.e., 31.8/25.1 × 100 = 127) which is consistent with Class 2 obesity in children (defined by a BMI between the 120% to 140% of the 95th percentile). For a 13-year-old boy, a BMI >35.1 kg/m² (140% of 25.1 kg/m² [i.e., 25.1 ×1.4]) would be consistent with Class 3 obesity. The term morbid obesity should typically be avoided in both adult and pediatric populations.*

2. A 10-year-old girl returns for follow-up of obesity. She is accompanied by her mother. At a previous visit, the patient and her mother identified reducing the consumption of energy-dense desserts as one dietary goal in their family-based lifestyle modification plan. When you assess the family's progress, the mother indicates that there has been significant conflict among members of the family regarding the best strategies to achieve the goal. As part of treatment, you have supported the mother in adopting a more authoritative parenting and feeding style.

   Which of the following responses from the mother would be most consistent with this approach?

   A. "We need to make some changes, and everyone in the family is going to cut out dessert completely."
   B. "Whoever eats all their vegetables at dinner can have dessert."
   C. "We have decided to limit dessert to one night per week. What night would we like to enjoy it this week?"
   D. "This isn't going to work. We should pick a different goal."

   Answer: C. *An authoritative parenting style is associated with reduced rates of pediatric obesity and should be supported as part of family-based behavior change. Authoritative parenting (as in response C) is characterized by both high responsiveness and high demands ("loving with limits"). Although response "A" alludes to family-based change, it is likely more consistent with an overly restrictive or authoritarian style. Use of food as a reward or encouraging that the child only receives dessert after eating certain other foods or "cleaning" her plate should be avoided (response B). Although families should decide what specific goals they are ready pursue, response D suggests a more permissive parenting style.*

REFERENCES

1. Skinner AC, Ravanbakht SN, Skelton JA, Perrin EM, Armstrong SC. Prevalence of obesity and severe obesity in US children, 1999-2016. *Pediatrics.* 2018;141(3):e20173459. PubMed PMID: 29483202; PMCID: PMC6109602.

2. Styne DM, Arslanian SA, Connor EL, et al. Pediatric obesity-assessment, treatment, and prevention: an endocrine society clinical practice guideline. *J Clin Endocrinol Metab.* 2017;102(3):709-757. PubMed PMID: 28359099; PMCID: PMC6283429.

3. Barlow SE; Expert Committee. Expert committee recommendations regarding the prevention, assessment, and treatment of child and adolescent overweight and obesity: summary report. *Pediatrics.* 2007;120(suppl 4):S164-S192. PubMed PMID: 18055651.

4. Whitaker RC, Pepe MS, Wright JA, Seidel KD, Dietz WH. Early adiposity rebound and the risk of adult obesity. *Pediatrics.* 1998;101(3):E5. PubMed PMID: 9481024.

5. Kelly AS, Barlow SE, Rao G, et al; on behalf of the American Heart Association Atherosclerosis Hypertension, and Obesity in the Young Committee of the Council on Cardiovascular Disease in the Young, Council on Nutrition, Physical Activity, and Metabolism, and Council on Clinical Cardiology. Severe obesity in children and adolescents: identification, associated health risks, and treatment approaches. A scientific statement from the American Heart Association. *Circulation.* 2013;128(15):1689-1712. PubMed PMID: 24016455.

6. Pratt JSA, Browne A, Browne NT, et al. ASMBS pediatric metabolic and bariatric surgery guidelines, 2018. *Surg Obes Relat Dis.* 2018;14(7):882-901. PubMed PMID: 30077361; PMCID: PMC6097871.

7. *WHO Growth Standards Are Recommended for Use With Children Younger Than Aged 2 Years in the United States.* Division of Nutrition, Physical Activity, and Obesity, National Center for Chronic Disease Prevention and Health Promotion; 2015. Updated April 15, 2015. Accessed January 30, 2020. https://www.cdc.gov/nccdphp/dnpao/growthcharts/who/recommendations/index.htm

8. Hales CM, Carroll MD, Fryar CD, Ogden CL. Prevalence of obesity among adults and youth: United States, 2015-2016. *NCHS Data Brief.* 2017;288:1-8. PubMed PMID: 29155689.

9. Ward ZJ, Long MW, Resch SC, Giles CM, Cradock AL, Gortmaker SL. Simulation of growth trajectories of childhood obesity into adulthood. *N Engl J Med.* 2017;377(22):2145-2153. PubMed PMID: 29171811.

10. Franks PW, Hanson RL, Knowler WC, Sievers ML, Bennett PH, Looker HC. Childhood obesity, other cardiovascular risk factors, and premature death. *N Engl J Med.* 2010;362(6):485-493. PubMed PMID: 20147714; PMCID: PMC2958822.

11. Schwimmer JB, Burwinkle TM, Varni JW. Health-related quality of life of severely obese children and adolescents. *J Am Med Assoc.* 2003;289(14):1813-1819. PubMed PMID: 12684360.

12. Olshansky SJ, Passaro DJ, Hershow RC, et al. A potential decline in life expectancy in the United States in the 21st century. *N Engl J Med.* 2005;352(11):1138-1145. PubMed PMID: 15784668.

13. Whitaker KL, Jarvis MJ, Beeken RJ, Boniface D, Wardle J. Comparing maternal and paternal intergenerational transmission of obesity risk in a large population-based sample. *Am J Clin Nutr.* 2010;91(6):1560-1567. PubMed PMID: 20375189.

14. Rohde K, Keller M, la Cour Poulsen L, Bluher M, Kovacs P, Bottcher Y. Genetics and epigenetics in obesity. *Metabolism.* 2019;92:37-50. PubMed PMID: 30399374.

15. Reinehr T, Hinney A, de Sousa G, Austrup F, Hebebrand J, Andler W. Definable somatic disorders in overweight children and adolescents. *J Pediatr.* 2007;150(6):618-622.e5. PubMed PMID: 17517246.

16. Angulo MA, Butler MG, Cataletto ME. Prader-Willi syndrome: a review of clinical, genetic, and endocrine findings. *J Endocrinol Invest.* 2015;38(12):1249-1263. PubMed PMID: 26062517; PMCID: PMC4630255.

17. Deal CL, Tony M, Hoybye C, et al; the 2011 Growth Hormone in Prader-Willi Syndrome Clinical Care Guidelines Workshop Participants. Growth Hormone Research Society workshop summary: consensus guidelines for recombinant human growth hormone therapy in Prader-Willi syndrome. *J Clin Endocrinol Metab.* 2013;98(6):E1072-E1087. PubMed PMID: 23543664; PMCID: PMC3789886.

18. Castro-Sanchez S, Alvarez-Satta M, Valverde D. Bardet-Biedl syndrome: a rare genetic disease. *J Pediatr Genet.* 2013;2(2):77-83. PubMed PMID: 27625843; PMCID: PMC5020962.

19. Forsythe E, Kenny J, Bacchelli C, Beales PL. Managing Bardet-Biedl syndrome-now and in the future. *Front Pediatr.* 2018;6:23. PubMed PMID: 29487844; PMCID: PMC5816783.

20. Vaisse C, Clement K, Durand E, Hercberg S, Guy-Grand B, Froguel P. Melanocortin-4 receptor mutations are a frequent and heterogeneous cause of morbid obesity. *J Clin Invest.* 2000;106(2):253-262. PubMed PMID: 10903341; PMCID: PMC314306.

21. Martinelli CE, Keogh JM, Greenfield JR, et al. Obesity due to melanocortin 4 receptor (MC4R) deficiency is associated with increased linear growth and final height, fasting hyperinsulinemia, and incompletely suppressed growth hormone secretion. *J Clin Endocrinol Metab.* 2011;96(1):E181-E188. PubMed PMID: 21047921.

22. Censani M, Conroy R, Deng L, et al. Weight loss after bariatric surgery in morbidly obese adolescents with MC4R mutations. *Obesity (Silver Spring).* 2014;22(1):225-231. PubMed PMID: 23740648; PMCID: PMC3880391.

23. Collet TH, Dubern B, Mokrosinski J, et al. Evaluation of a melanocortin-4 receptor (MC4R) agonist (Setmelanotide) in MC4R deficiency. *Mol Metab.* 2017;6(10):1321-1329. PubMed PMID: 29031731; PMCID: PMC5641599.

24. Huvenne H, Dubern B, Clement K, Poitou C. Rare genetic forms of obesity: clinical approach and current treatments in 2016. *Obes Facts.* 2016;9(3):158-173. PubMed PMID: 27241181; PMCID: PMC5644891.

25. Johnson W, Stovitz SD, Choh AC, Czerwinski SA, Towne B, Demerath EW. Patterns of linear growth and skeletal maturation from birth to 18 years of age in overweight young adults. *Int J Obes.* 2012;36(4):535-541. PubMed PMID: 22124455; PMCID: PMC3312969.

26. Shalitin S, Kiess W. Putative effects of obesity on linear growth and puberty. *Horm Res Paediatr.* 2017;88(1):101-110. PubMed PMID: 28183093.

27. Rosenfield RL, Lipton RB, Drum ML. Thelarche, pubarche, and menarche attainment in children with normal and elevated body mass index. *Pediatrics.* 2009;123(1):84-88. PubMed PMID: 19117864.

28. Crocker MK, Stern EA, Sedaka NM, et al. Sexual dimorphisms in the associations of BMI and body fat with indices of pubertal development in girls and boys. *J Clin Endocrinol Metab*. 2014;99(8):E1519-E1529. PubMed PMID: 24780051; PMCID: PMC4121027.

29. Lustig RH. Hypothalamic obesity: causes, consequences, treatment. *Pediatr Endocrinol Rev*. 2008;6(2):220-227. PubMed PMID: 19202508.

30. Pont SJ, Puhl R, Cook SR, Slusser W, Section on Obesity and the Obesity Society. Stigma experienced by children and adolescents with obesity. *Pediatrics*. 2017;140(6):e20173034. PubMed PMID: 29158228.

31. Puhl RM, Peterson JL, Luedicke J. Parental perceptions of weight terminology that providers use with youth. *Pediatrics*. 2011;128(4):e786-e793. PubMed PMID: 21949145.

32. Cortese S, Tessari L. Attention-deficit/hyperactivity disorder (ADHD) and obesity: update 2016. *Curr Psychiatr Rep*. 2017;19(1):4. PubMed PMID: 28102515; PMCID: PMC5247534.

33. Woo Baidal JA, Locks LM, Cheng ER, Blake-Lamb TL, Perkins ME, Taveras EM. Risk factors for childhood obesity in the first 1,000 days: a systematic review. *Am J Prev Med*. 2016;50(6):761-779. PubMed PMID: 26916261.

34. Krebs NF, Himes JH, Jacobson D, Nicklas TA, Guilday P, Styne D. Assessment of child and adolescent overweight and obesity. *Pediatrics*. 2007;120(suppl 4):S193-S228. PubMed PMID: 18055652.

35. Scharf RJ, DeBoer MD. Sugar-sweetened beverages and children's health. *Annu Rev Public Health*. 2016;37:273-293. PubMed PMID: 26989829.

36. Crowe-White K, O'Neil CE, Parrott JS, et al. Impact of 100% fruit juice consumption on diet and weight status of children: an evidence-based review. *Crit Rev Food Sci Nutr*. 2016;56(5):871-884. PubMed PMID: 26091353.

37. Heyman MB, Abrams SA; Section on Gastroenterology, Hepatology, and Nutrition, and Committee on Nutrition. Fruit juice in infants, children, and adolescents: current recommendations. *Pediatrics*. 2017;139(6):e20170967. PubMed PMID: 28562300.

38. Daniels SR, Hassink SG; Committee on Nutrition. The role of the pediatrician in primary prevention of obesity. *Pediatrics*. 2015;136(1):e275-e292. PubMed PMID: 26122812.

39. Orlet Fisher J, Rolls BJ, Birch LL. Children's bite size and intake of an entree are greater with large portions than with age-appropriate or self-selected portions. *Am J Clin Nutr*. 2003;77(5):1164-1170. PubMed PMID: 12716667; PMCID: PMC2530925.

40. Hoyland A, Dye L, Lawton CL. A systematic review of the effect of breakfast on the cognitive performance of children and adolescents. *Nutr Res Rev*. 2009;22(2):220-243. PubMed PMID: 19930787.

41. Piernas C, Popkin BM. Trends in snacking among U.S. children. *Health Aff (Millwood)*. 2010;29(3):398-404. PubMed PMID: 20194979; PMCID: PMC2837536.

42. Sebastian R, Goldman J, Wilkinson Enns C. *Snacking Patterns of U.S. Adolescents: What We Eat in America, NHANES 2005-2006*. US Department of Agriculture, Food Surveys Research Group; 2010.

43. Kim SA, Moore LV, Galuska D, et al; Centers for Disease Control and Prevention. Vital signs: fruit and vegetable intake among children - United States, 2003-2010. *MMWR Morb Mortal Wkly Rep*. 2014;63(31):671-676.

44. He FJ, Nowson CA, MacGregor GA. Fruit and vegetable consumption and stroke: meta-analysis of cohort studies. *Lancet*. 2006;367(9507):320-326. PubMed PMID: 16443039.

45. Riboli E, Norat T. Epidemiologic evidence of the protective effect of fruit and vegetables on cancer risk. *Am J Clin Nutr*. 2003;78(suppl 3):559S-569S. PubMed PMID: 12936950.

46. Avery A, Anderson C, McCullough F. Associations between children's diet quality and watching television during meal or snack consumption: a systematic review. *Matern Child Nutr*. 2017;13(4):e12428. PubMed PMID: 28211230.

47. Dallacker M, Hertwig R, Mata J. The frequency of family meals and nutritional health in children: a meta-analysis. *Obes Rev*. 2018;19(5):638-653. PubMed PMID: 29334693.

48. Harrison ME, Norris ML, Obeid N, Fu M, Weinstangel H, Sampson M. Systematic review of the effects of family meal frequency on psychosocial outcomes in youth. *Can Fam Physician*. 2015;61(2):e96-e106. PubMed PMID: 25676655; PMCID: PMC4325878.

49. He J, Cai Z, Fan X. Prevalence of binge and loss of control eating among children and adolescents with overweight and obesity: an exploratory meta-analysis. *Int J Eat Disord*. 2017;50(2):91-103. PubMed PMID: 28039879.

50. Cotton MA, Ball C, Robinson P. Four simple questions can help screen for eating disorders. *J Gen Intern Med*. 2003;18(1):53-56. PubMed PMID: 12534764; PMCID: PMC1494802.

51. Physical Activity Guidelines Advisory Committee. *2018 Physical Activity Guidelines Advisory Committee Scientific Report*. US Department of Health and Human Services; 2018.

52. US Department of Health and Human Services. *Physical Activity of Guidelines for Americans*. 2nd ed. US Department of Health and Human Services; 2018.

53. Kimm SY, Glynn NW, Kriska AM, et al. Decline in physical activity in black girls and white girls during adolescence. *N Engl J Med*. 2002;347(10):709-715. PubMed PMID: 12213941.

54. Jago R, Watson K, Baranowski T, et al. Pedometer reliability, validity and daily activity targets among 10- to 15-year-old boys. *J Sports Sci*. 2006;24(3):241-251. PubMed PMID: 16368634.

55. Council on Communications and Media. Media and young minds. *Pediatrics*. 2016;138(5):e20162591. PubMed PMID: 27940793.

56. Council on Communications and Media. Media use in school-aged children and adolescents. *Pediatrics*. 2016;138(5):e20162592. PubMed PMID: 27940794.

57. Chen X, Beydoun MA, Wang Y. Is sleep duration associated with childhood obesity? A systematic review and meta-analysis. *Obesity (Silver Spring)*. 2008;16(2):265-274. PubMed PMID: 18239632.

58. Hirshkowitz M, Whiton K, Albert SM, et al. National Sleep Foundation's sleep time duration recommendations: methodology and results summary. *Sleep Health*. 2015;1(1):40-43. PubMed PMID: 29073412.

59. Flynn JT, Kaelber DC, Baker-Smith CM, et al; Subcommittee on Screening and Management of High Blood Pressure in Children and Adolescents. Clinical practice guideline for screening and management of high blood pressure in children and adolescents. *Pediatrics*. 2017;140(3):e20171904. PubMed PMID: 28827377.

60. Viera AJ, Neutze DM. Diagnosis of secondary hypertension: an age-based approach. *Am Fam Physician.* 2010;82(12):1471-1478. PubMed PMID: 21166367.

61. Scherl SA. Common lower extremity problems in children. *Pediatr Rev.* 2004;25(2):52-62. PubMed PMID: 14754927.

62. Wolf RM, Long D. Pubertal development. *Pediatr Rev.* 2016;37(7):292-300. PubMed PMID: 27368360.

63. Long D. Precocious puberty. *Pediatr Rev.* 2015;36(7):319-321. PubMed PMID: 26133309.

64. Rachmiel M, Kives S, Atenafu E, Hamilton J. Primary amenorrhea as a manifestation of polycystic ovarian syndrome in adolescents: a unique subgroup? *Arch Pediatr Adolesc Med.* 2008;162(6):521-525. PubMed PMID: 18524741.

65. American Diabetes Association. 2. Classification and diagnosis of diabetes: standards of medical care in diabetes-2020. *Diabetes Care.* 2020;43(suppl 1):S14-S31. PubMed PMID: 31862745.

66. Shah J, Okubote T, Alkhouri N. Overview of updated practice guidelines for pediatric nonalcoholic fatty liver disease. *Gastroenterol Hepatol (NY).* 2018;14(7):407-414. PubMed PMID: 30166956; PMCID: PMC6111502.

67. Wrotniak BH, Epstein LH, Paluch RA, Roemmich JN. Parent weight change as a predictor of child weight change in family-based behavioral obesity treatment. *Arch Pediatr Adolesc Med.* 2004;158(4):342-347. PubMed PMID: 15066873.

68. Golan M. Parents as agents of change in childhood obesity–from research to practice. *Int J Pediatr Obes.* 2006;1(2):66-76. PubMed PMID: 17907317.

69. Vollmer RL, Mobley AR. Parenting styles, feeding styles, and their influence on child obesogenic behaviors and body weight. A review. *Appetite.* 2013;71:232-241. PubMed PMID: 24001395.

70. Kitzmann KM, Dalton WT III, Stanley CM, et al. Lifestyle interventions for youth who are overweight: a meta-analytic review. *Health Psychol.* 2010;29(1):91-101. PubMed PMID: 20063940.

71. Rhee KE, Jelalian E, Boutelle K, Dickstein S, Seifer R, Wing R. Warm parenting associated with decreasing or stable child BMI during treatment. *Child Obes.* 2016;12(2):94-102. PubMed PMID: 26895374; PMCID: PMC4817557.

72. Mitchell TB, Amaro CM, Steele RG. Pediatric weight management interventions in primary care settings: a meta-analysis. *Health Psychol.* 2016;35(7):704-713. PubMed PMID: 27089458.

73. Hayes JF, Fitzsimmons-Craft EE, Karam AM, Jakubiak J, Brown ML, Wilfley DE. Disordered eating attitudes and behaviors in youth with overweight and obesity: implications for treatment. *Curr Obes Rep.* 2018;7(3):235-246. PubMed PMID: 30069717; PMCID: PMC6098715.

74. Whitlock EP, O'Connor EA, Williams SB, Beil TL, Lutz KW. Effectiveness of weight management interventions in children: a targeted systematic review for the USPSTF. *Pediatrics.* 2010;125(2):e396-e418. PubMed PMID: 20083531.

75. Danielsson P, Kowalski J, Ekblom O, Marcus C. Response of severely obese children and adolescents to behavioral treatment. *Arch Pediatr Adolesc Med.* 2012;166(12):1103-1108. PubMed PMID: 23108856.

76. Srivastava G, Fox CK, Kelly AS, et al. Clinical considerations regarding the use of obesity pharmacotherapy in adolescents with obesity. *Obesity.* 2019;27(2):190-204. PubMed PMID: 30677262; PMCID: PMC6449849.

77. O'Connor EA, Evans CV, Burda BU, Walsh ES, Eder M, Lozano P. Screening for obesity and intervention for weight management in children and adolescents: evidence report and systematic review for the US preventive Services Task Force. *J Am Med Assoc.* 2017;317(23):2427-2444. PubMed PMID: 28632873.

78. Ryder JR, Kaizer A, Rudser KD, Gross A, Kelly AS, Fox CK. Effect of phentermine on weight reduction in a pediatric weight management clinic. *Int J Obes.* 2017;41(1):90-93. PubMed PMID: 27773937; PMCID: PMC5891125.

79. Tamborlane WV, Barrientos-Perez M, Fainberg U, et al; for the Ellipse Trial Investigators. Liraglutide in children and adolescents with type 2 diabetes. *N Engl J Med.* 2019;381(7):637-646. PubMed PMID: 31034184.

80. Kelly AS, Auerbach P, Barrientos-Perez M, et al; for the NN8022-4180 Trial Investigators. A randomized, controlled trial of liraglutide for adolescents with obesity. *N Engl J Med.* 2020;382(22):2117-2128. PubMed PMID: 32233338.

81. Armstrong SC, Bolling CF, Michalsky MP, Reichard KW; Section on Obesity, Section on Surgery. Pediatric metabolic and bariatric surgery: evidence, barriers, and best practices. *Pediatrics.* 2019;144(6):e20193223. PubMed PMID: 31656225.

82. Inge TH, Courcoulas AP, Jenkins TM, et al. Five-year outcomes of gastric bypass in adolescents as compared with adults. *N Engl J Med.* 2019;380(22):2136-2145. PubMed PMID: 31116917.

12

PRACTICE MANAGEMENT

Ethan A. Lazarus, Adam H. Gilden

CASE STUDY

A 62-year-old male patient with hypertension and obesity has recently retired. He wants to enjoy a better quality of life, but knee osteoarthritis limits his movement. He has struggled with his weight for decades and knows that weight loss would improve his overall health and daily function. Medications include losartan/hydrochlorothiazide 50/12.5 mg and ibuprofen prn. He has a supportive wife who is ready to help. He is not interested in joining a group but would be willing to take a medication if it would help with weight loss. His insurance plan does not include any coverage for weight loss medications. He does not want to have bariatric surgery.

On examination, height is 68 inches, weight 109 kg (240 lb), blood pressure 128/86, heart rate 88, and body mass index (BMI) 37.0 kg/m². Electrocardiogram (ECG) is normal. The remainder of the physical examination and laboratory tests are unremarkable.

CLINICAL SIGNIFICANCE

Treating obesity in clinical practice requires a multidisciplinary approach to achieve clinically significant patient outcomes. However, since primary care physicians have limited time during office visits, and because the treatments used for obesity have variable reimbursement, healthcare professionals (HCPs) who want to provide competent and compassionate obesity care face multiple office-based challenges. This chapter will discuss issues of staffing, office infrastructure, clinical protocols, billing and health insurance, weight bias, and the ethics of incorporating obesity into clinical practice.

STAFFING, EQUIPMENT, AND EDUCATIONAL CONSIDERATIONS TO PROVIDE COMPETENT OBESITY CARE

Professional staff from multiple disciplines are involved directly or indirectly in the treatment of obesity. This includes front office registration staff who provide check-in and check-out services; medical assistants who obtain vital signs (including measurement of weight and height); HCPs (physician, physician assistant, and nurse practitioner) who conduct the medical encounter; other team members (registered dietitian nutritionist [RDN], exercise specialist, social worker, health psychologist) who provide counseling; and "back office" staff who support billing and other office-based business activities. While many HCPs will not have *all* of these personnel within the office, most will have at least *some*. These individuals constitute a healthcare team.

Obesity is a complex, multifactorial disease, and as such, treatment is best accomplished by incorporation of a multidisciplinary team. This is consistent with the management of other chronic diseases such as diabetes, depression, and low back pain where certified diabetes educators, mental health counselors, and physical therapists, respectively, are routinely employed. The team approach to obesity care is further discussed in Chapter 13.

For decades, research has shown that multidisciplinary care is more effective than treatment rendered by a single provider. For example, a 12-month randomized trial demonstrated greater weight loss with the combination of intensive lifestyle intervention (ILI), pharmacotherapy, and meal replacements (16.5% loss of initial body weight), compared with medication alone (4.1%) or medication plus ILI (10.8%).[1] Another study found that ILI with a multidisciplinary team resulted in more weight loss than usual care for patients with type 2 diabetes (8.6% vs. 0.7% after 1 year), and that this weight loss continued to be significant after 8 years.[2] The value of an interprofessional team lies in its ability to provide expert assistance in multiple aspects of patient care. For example, if the medical assistant is properly trained to obtain anthropometric measurements, i.e., height, weight, waist circumference, and take vital signs, and an RDN is available to provide counseling on the implementation of lifestyle changes, this leaves more time for HCPs to focus on the medical aspects of obesity care.

Provision of care for obesity should ideally include a full array of professional resources. Although primary care practices are not likely to have all team members in the office, they should have a referral process in place to assist in comprehensive care of the patient with obesity. Team members may include:

- Medical provider (physician, physician assistant, nurse practitioner)
- Metabolic and bariatric surgeon
- RDN
- Office support staff
- Psychologist or other mental health professional (e.g., licensed professional counselor [LPC])
- Exercise physiologist/physical therapist

The roles and responsibilities of the team members are displayed in Table 12.1.

Team Members

Medical Provider

Since obesity is recognized as a chronic disease, it is important that a properly trained HCP directs patient care. Most often, this will be a physician. While all providers are *able* to treat obesity, unfortunately many often feel that they have inadequate *training* to do so. A recent study found that many providers make recommendations that are not consistent with current medical evidence.[3] While there are multiple opportunities to obtain updates and practice tips on obesity care through continued medical education conferences, online training, and journal article reviews, studies show that education around obesity and nutrition continues to be limited.[4,5] The role of the HCP is to have a fundamental understanding of all the aspects of obesity care (e.g., how to take an obesity history, evaluate for comorbid conditions, conduct an obesity-focused physical examination, and discuss treatment options including lifestyle management, pharmacotherapy, and bariatric surgery) and then to direct the patient to the resources most needed. The HCP is also responsible for setting the overall philosophy and direction of the practice. As a specific example of philosophy/direction, some HCPs may personally favor a specific eating plan (e.g., plant-based, low-carbohydrate, Mediterranean)

TABLE 12.1 Clinicians Involved in Treatment of Obesity

STAFF	SERVICE
HCP	Prescribe pharmacotherapy Manage comorbidities Refer to other services—RDN, exercise, behavior, psychologist, surgeon Provide perioperative care for patients who undergo bariatric surgery Arrange follow-up
RDN	Within practice or by referral Perform dietary assessment Review food journals Provide individualized structured food planning, intensive lifestyle intervention Provide dietary and nutritional education
Exercise physiologist/ trainer	Typically by referral Assess physical limitations and abilities Develop individualized physical activity program
Psychologist/ therapist	Typically by referral Assess psychological stressors and barriers Perform motivational interviewing Provide cognitive behavioral therapy
Bariatric surgeon	Typically by referral Assess patient appropriateness for bariatric procedures Perform procedures and arrange follow-up

HCP, healthcare professional; RDN, registered dietitian nutritionist

for weight management. However, HCPs who can counsel patients on a wide variety of evidence-based eating plans are more likely to have success in treating obesity.

Metabolic and Bariatric Surgeon

For some patients, particularly those with a BMI $\geq$40 kg/m^2 (or $\geq$35 kg/m^2 with a comorbidity such as type 2 diabetes) who have been unsuccessful at achieving and maintaining medically meaningful weight loss through noninvasive means, referral to a properly trained metabolic and bariatric surgeon is indicated. Surgery can improve lifespan, reduce the burden of medical comorbidities, and improve quality of life. Surgery has been proven to be a powerful tool for obesity treatment. (*Like all fields of medicine, these guidelines are constantly changing. Newer surgical guidelines may lower these BMI reference ranges. Often, insurance coverage for treatment lags behind any changes in guidelines.*)

Although some general surgeons perform bariatric surgery, many choose to specialize in bariatric surgery. In general, it is preferable for the HCP to refer to a surgeon who does only (or at least primarily) bariatric surgery. Many of these surgeons have completed fellowship training in performing bariatric procedures. Ideally, the surgeon should practice in a bariatric "center of excellence," accredited by the MBSAQIP (Metabolic and Bariatric Surgery Accreditation and Quality Improvement Program). Patients or HCPs can search the website of the American Society of Metabolic and Bariatric Surgeons to find a provider in their area.[6] For more information on bariatric surgery, please refer to Chapter 9.

Registered Dietitian Nutritionist

RDNs are certified by the Academy of Nutrition and Dietetics. RDNs must complete a bachelor's degree at a US regionally accredited university or college and a course work accredited by the Accreditation Council for Education in Nutrition and Dietetics (ACEND) of the Academy of Nutrition and Dietetics. They must further complete an ACEND-accredited supervised practice program consisting of a minimum of 1,200 hours of supervised practice and pass a national examination administered by the Commission on Dietetic Registration (CDR). Once credentials for RDN have been met, the RDN must maintain 75 hours of continuing medical education every 5 years. Where there are legal standards for RDNs, the term "nutritionist" is less standardized and less regulated. A nutritionist can have nutrition training or no nutrition training. Thus, if the HCP is referring a patient for dietary/ behavioral treatment, it is preferable to collaborate with an RDN.

RDNs play an important role in assessment and treatment of the patient with obesity. They excel at implementing specific, individualized dietary strategies. The CDR also offers a certificate of training in adult weight management and an Interdisciplinary Specialist Certification in Obesity and Weight Management. The RDN can be helpful in the initial assessment of the patient with obesity by performing a comprehensive nutrition history using a variety of tools that may include a Food Frequency Questionnaire, Diet History Questionnaire, 24-hour dietary recall, or a typical sample food intake day. They can then implement a nutritional intervention that is appropriate for the patient (see Chapter 5).

RDNs also excel at ILI. In a high-intensity weight management program, patients are typically seen every week or every other week. Many of these visits are performed by the RDN. In addition to supervising the food plan, the RDN can work with the patient on specific behavior changes. This can be accomplished during one-on-one visits or in group settings. (In a randomized trial, group intervention has been shown to be at least as effective as one-on-one visits, even when participants expressed a preference for individual treatment.) RDNs can cover topics related to behavior modification (see Chapter 7).

Losing weight and sustaining weight loss is challenging. It is often difficult for patients to remain motivated, engaged, and committed to change. RDNs can help patients maintain a high level of motivation and improve treatment outcomes. The 2013 AHA/ACC/TOS guideline on obesity treatment recommends at least monthly contact to help maintain weight loss; RDNs are well suited to support long-term treatment.

Office Support Staff

As with other chronic diseases, a well-functioning office staff will help improve patient satisfaction and health outcomes. Key personnel include:

- Front office staff: check-in, check-out, scheduling, phone calls, billing
- Medical assistants and nurses: assess vital signs, weight, blood draws, ECGs. Specific testing for obesity may include body composition or resting metabolic rate (RMR) testing
- Administrative staff/office manager: insurance billing, prior authorizations
- Patient advocate/case manager

Support staff must ensure a positive patient experience. They should be trained on the topic of weight bias (see Weight Bias section). Patient confidentiality must always be respected. Weight should be checked privately, and staff should be trained to provide encouragement.

Psychologist or Therapist

There are several types of training in psychology. The traditional PhD in psychology is qualified to work in clinical or counseling psychology. They may also choose to teach at the university level, practice at mental health clinics and hospitals, or have a private practice. It takes the typical candidate 4 to 8 years to obtain a PhD in psychology. The PsyD is a more practice-based degree. As a result, this degree requires fewer research and statistics courses and thus takes less time, typically 4 to 6 years. Finally, LPCs must have a master's degree in a counseling or related field and must have 2 years of supervised clinical experience before becoming credentialed to provide psychotherapy on their own. Thus, LPCs may include clinical social workers. All of these types of clinicians (PhD, PsyD, LPC) are qualified to treat patients with overlapping weight and mental health concerns, although not all have interest or expertise in this patient population.

Many patients with obesity have coexistent mental health concerns and/or psychosocial treatment barriers. They may have inadequate social support and/or saboteurs, which increases the difficulty of implementing treatment recommendations. There may be a history of verbal, physical, or sexual abuse. Patients may suffer from clinical depression, anxiety disorders, eating disorders including binge eating disorder, or other issues contributing to their obesity. For patients suffering from obesity and coexistent mental health problems, treatment by a psychologist with the proper evidence-based tools will enable improved outcomes. In addition, a psychologist can participate in ILI and address many of the psychological issues common with obesity, including stress management, building support, and increasing assertiveness. Finally, a psychological assessment is typically required before embarking on bariatric surgery (see Chapter 9 for more details).

Exercise Physiologist/Physical Therapist

Reduced calorie diets have been shown to be the most effective approach to achieve initial weight loss. Regular physical activity is key to keeping weight off and to improve fitness and overall health. Many patients with obesity have significant physical limitations. Thus, general recommendations to simply "move more" or begin a vigorous exercise program may lead to injury or further resistance to incorporate physical activity into their daily routine. Rather, the goal is to develop an individualized structured physical activity program, accounting for the patient's likes, dislikes, and physical limitations.

An exercise physiologist is properly trained to assess a patient's ability to engage in physical activity. A clinical exercise physiologist is certified by the American College of Sports Medicine (ASCM-CEP) and has either (1) a bachelor's degree in exercise science or equivalent and 1,200 hours of clinical hands-on experience or (2) a master's degree in clinical exercise physiology and 600 hours of hands-on clinical experience. The ASCM-CEP can perform body composition analysis, RMR and exercise testing, muscle strength and flexibility testing, and even gait analysis. Working one-on-one with the patient, the exercise physiologist can develop an individualized physical activity program for the patient, including specific goals and metrics. A licensed physical therapist can help carry out the exercise plan developed by the exercise physiologist (or the HCP) (see Chapter 6 for more details).

Office Equipment

Patients with obesity should be able to feel physically and psychologically comfortable in the HCP office. For example, office and examination room chairs should be armless or extra wide (28 inches) to accommodate patients who weigh 300 lb or more. If the office has sofas, they should ideally have firm seats at a higher height to allow patients to get on and off easily. Recommendations for the waiting room include having several sturdy armless chairs (again, to support patients weighing 300 lb or more) with at least 6 to 8 inches of space between them and firm high sofas if possible. Magazines could include those from organizations such as the Obesity Action Coalition (OAC) (obesityaction.org), a national advocacy organization that promotes improved healthcare for persons with obesity. Magazines should not include photographs that depict unrealistic body shape (e.g., supermodels). Measurement of an accurate height and weight is vital to treating patients with obesity. Office scales should be able to accommodate patients with weight up to 600 lb, ideally with a wide base and a handlebar for support, if necessary. A wall-mounted stadiometer is most accurate for measuring height, but a height meter attached to the scale is considered adequate. Office staff should always obtain permission to weigh patients, especially for those with visibly high weight. As stated above, office staff should be trained not to make disparaging comments about patients' weights.

Examination rooms should have both regular and large gowns available to wear as well as a sturdy step stool to mount the examination tables. Some practices may consider having a bariatric examination room table that is electronically controlled. Equipment for nonobesity care should also include different sizes (e.g., specula for Pap smears). In addition to standard adult blood pressure cuffs, practices should have large adult and thigh size blood pressure cuffs to ensure that blood pressure is correctly measured on patients of all sizes (see Chapter 2 for additional details). Finally, a cloth, vinyl, or metal tape measure should be available for measurement of waist circumference.

Getting Started With Obesity Treatment

HCPs may not have access to all the professionals listed above. In some parts of the country, there may not be an exercise physiologist or a bariatric surgeon. Or, an HCP may work in a small practice and not have access to all the above support personnel. While a multidisciplinary team is ideal, any treatment (if available) is better than no treatment at all. Patients affected by obesity and their HCP can work together using shared decision-making to implement a realistic and practical treatment plan.

For example, an HCP can prescribe medication and monitor weight, BMI, and medication side effects. If the HCP has an RDN in his/her practice or in their health system, the patient can be referred for consultation. If more aggressive lifestyle treatment is indicated, the HCP can refer the patient to an intensive group program. This may include a program based at an academic medical center, the YMCA-based Diabetes Prevention Program, an evidence-based commercial program (such as WW), or a self-directed program that incorporates some of the principles of behavioral treatment (i.e., self-monitoring and feedback), such as Noom. If the patient does have the time or resources to engage in intensive treatment, the HCP can ask the patient to start by self-monitoring diet with a free smartphone application, such as Lose It! or MyFitnessPal.

With physical activity, if the HCP does not have access to an exercise physiologist, the patient could be referred to a skilled personal trainer with experience working with patients with obesity. Physical therapists are typically more accessible in clinical practice compared with exercise physiologists and can create individualized activity plans. For example, a physical therapist can do a teaching visit for patients to use Therabands or Theratubes at home, thus allowing the patient to start an exercise program without the time, cost, or weight stigma barriers of exercising at a gym. Patients can also engage in self-directed physical activities—walking, swimming, or cycling (e.g., stationary bike—easier for patients with obesity as non–weight bearing).

One treatment option for the HCP is to prescribe pharmacotherapy for obesity. As detailed in Chapter 8, patients starting medication should be assessed monthly for the first 3 months and then at least every 3 months thereafter. Patient contacts with the practice between these HCP assessments are likely to be conducted by RDNs or other clinicians. Depending on several factors including patient need, as well as HCP availability/access, assessment after the first 3 months of treatment could take different forms. The assessment may include a 1:1 visit with the HCP or, to reduce patient out-of-pocket cost, could be a nurse visit to evaluate vital signs, with data forwarded to the HCP for prescribing. The HCP must also pay attention to adjusting therapies for weight-related conditions (e.g., diabetes, hypertension), which may need a reduction in dose if patients successfully lose 5% to 10% of initial body weight.

When patients achieve clinically significant weight loss, a significant challenge remains how to help them maintain success. As mentioned above, the 2013 AHA/ACC/TOS guideline recommends at least monthly contact to help patients with weight loss maintenance. The HCP and RDN may provide any schedule of visits that works for the practice, provided that it is intensive enough for the patient to continue practicing the behaviors that led to initial weight loss. Some patients may need more intensive dietary, physical activity, or behavioral support during weight loss maintenance, and some patients may achieve 5% to 10% initial weight loss but not be satisfied with their progress. For patients in the latter category, an office visit with the HCP to determine next steps for treatment intensification may be indicated. An office-based audit for initiation of obesity care is included (Table 12.2).

WEIGHT BIAS

Obesity stigma is a major issue in our society. This type of stigma has negative effects on patients and needs to be addressed and minimized. Weight bias comprises negative attitudes, beliefs, judgments, stereotypes, and discriminatory acts aimed at individuals primarily because of their weight. It can be overt or subtle and can occur in any setting, including employment, healthcare, education, mass media, and relationships with family and friends. It also takes many forms—verbal, written, media, online, and more. For example, a subtle example of weight bias is the common use of photographs that only show the bodies of individuals with obesity (not showing their faces). Weight bias is dehumanizing and damaging; it can cause adverse physical and psychological health outcomes and promotes a social norm that marginalizes people.[7]

Perceptions that obesity is caused by a lack of self-discipline contribute to weight bias. Many people believe that obesity is not a chronic metabolic disease, but instead is caused by willful selection of poor dietary and activity choices. This leads to discriminating treatment in many areas, including work, education, and healthcare. People affected by obesity have more trouble getting hired and promoted and are paid less than their counterparts without obesity. They have lower college acceptance rates and suffer peer victimization and negative attitudes by other students and educators. Furthermore, patients with obesity are viewed by their healthcare providers as being less motivated, honest, compliant, and intelligent, compared to their normal weight counterparts. In one study, 69% of respondents reported that their physicians were a source of weight bias.[8] These biases can result in adverse health consequences including depression, anxiety, low self-esteem, poor body image, reduced quality of interpersonal relationships, unhealthy weight control practices, binge eating, diminished physical activity, and avoidance of healthcare including routine preventive care.

It is important that we work toward acceptance of people of all weights and sizes and that we advocate for fair and equal treatment. One specific way that HCPs can reduce weight bias is to use "person-first language." This term refers to describing people with diseases, rather than labeling a person by their disease. For example,

TABLE 12.2 Office Audit for Delivery of Office-based Obesity Care

AUDIT CATEGORIES

Do you routinely assess and evaluate patients for overweight and obesity?

a. measure height, weight, waist circumference, and calculate body mass index (BMI)

b. take a focused obesity history (see Chapter 2)

c. assess readiness for and barriers to weight loss

What kinds of services or programs do you routinely provide to your patients who have obesity?

a. high-intensity dietary and exercise counseling (individual or group)

b. referral to a registered dietitian nutritionist (RDN), exercise specialist, obesity medicine specialist, or bariatric surgeon

c. email correspondence

d. use of antiobesity medications or medically supervised diets

What are the services or programs recorded in the patient's chart?

a. recommended dietary and exercise behavioral changes

b. percent weight loss goal

c. correspondence to an RDN, health psychologist, or exercise specialist

d. uses and risks of antiobesity medication

What policies and procedures do you have in place for providing obesity care?

a. all patients have a height, weight, waist circumference, and BMI measured and recorded in the chart

b. the patient's readiness is assessed before initiating treatment

c. weight loss goals are established and tracked in the progress notes

d. services are in place to provide high-intensity behavioral treatment, individualized physical activity plans, and behavioral treatment

e. patients with a BMI of $\geq$30 kg/m^2 or $\geq$27 kg/m^2 with a comorbidity are assessed for antiobesity medications

f. patients with a BMI of $\geq$40 kg/m^2 or $\geq$35 kg/m^2 with a comorbidity are assessed for bariatric surgery

What forms, patient handouts, and educational materials are you using?

a. focused obesity history form

b. diet and exercise history forms

c. guidance on diet (including popular eating plans), physical activity, and behavioral change, as well as emotional and stress eating

d. food and activity logs

e. education sheets on antiobesity medications

f. education sheets on bariatric surgery

How does your office environment support or inhibit delivery of obesity care?

a. sturdy armless chairs

b. large and thigh blood pressure cuffs

c. large gowns

d. measuring of body weight in a private setting

e. a sensitive and informed office staff and including the use of person-first language for obesity

What functions do staff currently serve in the provision of obesity care?

a. office nurse or MA obtains weight, height, and BMI

b. healthcare provider (MD, NP, or PA) reviews food and activity diaries and medication side effects

c. receptionist schedules referral appointments with RDN, exercise specialist, or clinical psychologist

Adapted from Agency for Healthcare Research and Quality. 10 Steps: Implementation Guide. Put Prevention Into Practice. Adapted from The Clinicians' Handbook of Preventive Services. *2nd ed. Publication No. 98-0025. Agency for Healthcare Research and Quality; 1998.*

using the term "patient with obesity" rather than "obese patient." HCPs typically no longer refer to patients as "diabetics" or as "epileptics." However, more deliberate attention is needed to limit the use of the word "obese" as an adjective in patient care. HCPs are encouraged to take the pledge to use person-first language at www.obesityaction.org/ow2019/people-first-language. HCPs who take the pledge have access to "A guide for Health Providers Working with Individual Affected by Obesity." This guide from the OAC includes helpful topics for the HCP to reduce bias in daily practice. In addition to the OAC, other organizations have worked to educate and reduce weight bias. These include the following:

- American Medical Association (AMA): Passed policy in 2017 encouraging the use of person-first language regarding obesity, using preferred terms regarding obesity, and educating healthcare providers (Policy H-440.821).
- American Academy of Family Physicians: Passed policy in 2019 to reduce weight stigma in the office practice environment and advocate for patient-centered communication strategies to reduce weight bias in schools, communities, and the media.[9]
- The Rudd Center at the University of Connecticut (www.uconnruddcenter.org).

PROVISION OF BEHAVIORAL TREATMENT

The 2013 guidelines on evaluation and treatment of obesity state "… prescribe on site, high-intensity (i.e., ≥14 sessions in 6 months) comprehensive weight loss interventions provided in individual or group sessions by a trained interventionist." Some healthcare systems have begun weight management programs that provide these services. Although many patients would benefit from participating in such a program, they are not broadly available.

Insurance plays an important role in coverage. If a patient is participating in a "nongrandfathered plan" (i.e., a plan established since the start of the Affordable Care Act in 2014) through a health insurance exchange, then that plan is legally required to provide high-intensity behavioral treatment with zero out-of-pocket cost. For other patients, they may have an out-of-pocket cost for this service, but several options exist. The spread of the National Diabetes Prevention Program (https://www.cdc.gov/diabetes/prevention/index.html) has made this program increasingly available, especially in urban areas. Clinicians can also use the reimbursement for "IBT" (intensive behavioral therapy) for obesity that has been reimbursed by Medicare since 2011 (see Health Insurance and Obesity section for detailed description).[10]

Commercial weight loss programs also are an option for patients seeking high-intensity behavioral treatment for obesity. Although they have an out-of-pocket cost, commercial programs are endorsed in the 2013 obesity treatment guidelines as a reasonable treatment option, provided they have published evidence of efficacy in the peer-reviewed literature. Take Off Pounds Sensibly (TOPS) is a low-cost, nonprofit group weight loss program that is led by trained laypersons and offers frequent contact. Some technology-based interventions (e.g., Noom) now offer weight loss coaching, which would meet the criteria outlined in the obesity treatment guidelines (high-intensity contact with personalized feedback from a trained interventionist). Finally, some interventions may not meet the criteria outlined in the obesity treatment guidelines but provide a structure and support that patients find useful. For example, websites such as www.sparkpeople.com offer free email support and a community of individuals seeking weight loss. Patients may also use free smartphone applications, such as MyFitnessPal or Lose It! to track food intake. For HCPs working in small practices or in areas where there are no local weight loss groups, they may need to offer a regular group check-in for their patients.

POLICIES AND PROTOCOLS

The HCP should establish practice protocols for patient care that conform with published clinical guidelines. For example, physicians and other providers in a group practice should hold similar practice styles and prescribing patterns. One practical example of a protocol question that inevitably arises is the long-term use of phentermine, a drug that remains the most commonly prescribed agent for weight loss in the United States but is not FDA-approved for long-term use. Some commonly used medical websites (e.g., WebMD) suggest that the use of phentermine should be limited to 12 weeks. The 2015 Endocrine Society guideline indicates that long-term use of phentermine may be appropriate, provided that certain conditions are met (patient has lost weight and maintained weight loss; patient is being regularly monitored; patient does not develop contraindications to treatment during therapy; patient has been informed about therapies that are FDA-approved for long-term use). Given the marginal recognition of obesity as a chronic disease and the lack of reimbursement for pharmacotherapy, it seems appropriate to use phentermine as a single agent for long-term use, provided that the patient has success with this therapy. HCPs that prescribe weight loss agents should have protocols for this off-label use of phentermine. The language in the following box is an example of language that can be provided to patients (e.g., in the printed "after visit summary" after office visits).

Sample Protocol Language for Long-Term Prescribing of Phentermine

We are prescribing you phentermine for long-term use.

Phentermine is FDA-approved only for short-term use, and thus, the way we are using this medicine is "off label." Off label means that we are using the medicine in a way that is not formally approved by the FDA. There may be long-term risks of phentermine use that we do not know about, including the risk of heart disease.

We believe that the benefits of long-term phentermine use outweigh the risks, provided that:

1. the initial prescription for the medicine was done when your body mass index was 30 (or BMI was 27 with a weight-related medical condition);

2. you have lost at least 5% of your body weight since starting the medicine and you have kept off that weight; and

3. you are following up at least every 3 months, either with your primary care physician or provider or with your weight management specialist for monitoring of weight, blood pressure, and pulse.

CULTURALLY TAILORED COMMUNICATION

The high prevalence of obesity in the United States masks some of the racial and ethnic disparities that exist in weight and in weight-related comorbidities.[11] These disparities are primarily based on socioeconomic, cultural, and environmental factors. Individuals with income 350% of the federal poverty level, as well as those with college education, have a significantly lower obesity prevalence, compared with those with lower income and education levels (28% to 30% for higher SES groups, compared with about 40% for lower to middle SES groups). African Americans and Latinos in the United States have the highest prevalence of obesity (46.8% and 47%, respectively), with Caucasians intermediate (37.9%), and Asian Americans lowest (12.7%). Important differences persist within these race/ethnicity categories. For example, African American women have the highest obesity prevalence of any subgroup (54.8%) and Asian American men the lowest (10.1%).

The relationship between obesity, race/ethnicity, gender, and socioeconomic status is complex.[11] For example, obesity rates are lower in higher SES whites and higher SES African American women, compared to lower SES whites and lower SES African American woman, respectively. However, obesity rates are similar in African American men of all SES levels. The reasons for these differences are not entirely clear and may be multifactorial. For example, obesity may be somewhat more culturally acceptable among African Americans, and in general (among all ethnic groups), men feel less stigmatized by obesity compared with women.

HCPs should be aware of racial/ethnic and socioeconomic differences in perception of weight and related health risk. For example, in a study of national data in the United States, 37.2% of individuals with BMI 25 to 29.9 kg/m² and 7.8% of individuals with a BMI ≥ 30 kg/m² stated that they were "about the right weight," as opposed to "overweight." Among men, African Americans and those with less than high school education were more likely to misjudge their weight, and similarly among women, African Americans and Mexican Americans, as well as those with less than high school education, were more likely to misjudge their weight.[12]

It is important to acknowledge that there are biological differences based on race/ethnicity. African American women have a lower RMR, compared with white women, even after adjusting for body composition.[13] African American patients, compared with whites at the same BMI, have a lower rate of dyslipidemia.[14] East Asian and South Asian patients have greater diabetes risk at the same waist circumference, compared to whites.[15] Despite the international consensus on ethnic difference in weight-related health risk, North American obesity guidelines do not recommend different BMI or waist circumference cutoffs based on race or ethnicity. A unifying principle of efforts at counseling is that patients, regardless of ethnicity, should aim for a degree of weight loss that improves energy level and functioning (subjective) and that also decreases the severity of comorbid conditions (objective). For example, a patient with a starting BMI of 50 kg/m² does not need to achieve a "normal" weight on the BMI charts to achieve optimal health.

PHYSICIAN HEALTH BEHAVIORS

Since body weight is visibly notable, it is highly likely that patients will contemplate what their HCPs and staff are doing for their own self-care. The question of "self-disclosure" is a controversial and personal decision. All clinicians need to be prepared for questions that will inevitably arise from patients.

Regarding their weight status, it is important for HCPs and their staff to model healthy behaviors. The perceptions that patients hold will vary based on the BMI of the clinician. On one hand, providers with lower BMI may serve as better role models for patients who are trying to lose weight. On the other hand, practitioners who have struggled with their weight may be better able to empathize with their patients. In a national sample of 500 physicians, those with a BMI in the healthy range were more likely to initiate discussions about weight and to feel comfortable in providing counseling. In the same study, if the physician perception of the patient's weight exceeded the perception of their own weight, the physician was much more likely to initiate a discussion. Thus, physicians appear to use a comparison of weight status more than they use their own weight status.[16] Qualitative studies indicate a range of patient views on whether they prefer a physician with lower BMI ("weight discordant") versus a physician with similar weight to their own ("weight concordant").[17-19] One qualitative study suggested that male patients tended to prefer a physician role model, whereas female patients tended to prefer greater empathy.[18]

ETHICS IN CLINICAL PRACTICE

The field of obesity medicine raises several ethical issues that merit discussion. Despite evidence-based guidelines, position papers, and best practices, some private weight management clinics continue to offer treatment with non–evidence-based therapies such as vitamin B_{12} injections, HCG drops, unproven dietary supplements, or sell sprinkles that change a patient's sense of smell and taste. Herein we discuss two ethical topics that are commonly faced.

The Case of Phentermine

One practical example of ethics in obesity medicine is the choice of pharmacotherapy agents. The four drugs that are FDA-approved for long-term use in the treatment of obesity (orlistat, phentermine-topiramate, naltrexone-bupropion, and liraglutide) have all been tested in prospective, randomized trials lasting at least 1 year, with safety data on several thousand participants. In addition, all FDA-approved medications for obesity now must undergo large postmarketing safety trials, lasting several years and including thousands of patients. Comparatively, phentermine has only been studied for up to 6 months, with much smaller sample sizes, and has limited data on long-term safety and efficacy.[20,21] The costs for the newer agents range from $100 to $1,200 per month, whereas phentermine is $10 to $20 per month. Generic phentermine can be combined with generic topiramate at less cost than the brand name drug (phentermine-topiramate extended release). Weight loss in the first 6 months is approximately 6% of initial body weight with generic phentermine versus 9% to 10% with the most effective of the newer agents (including phentermine-topiramate extended release). No data have been published using the combination of generic phentermine with generic topiramate. On the other hand, both phentermine and topiramate have individual track records of safety dating back decades. Current guidelines on the use of

pharmacotherapy for treatment of obesity specify the conditions under which long-term use of phentermine is appropriate (see Policies and Protocols section).[21] Thus, the HCP is faced with the issues of beneficence (i.e., wanting to prescribe the most beneficial treatment) and of nonmaleficence (i.e., not wanting to pressure a patient into taking a costly drug that will be needed long term and may not provide the degree of weight loss that the patient is seeking).

In the context of inadequate reimbursement for medical treatment of a chronic disease, it may be appropriate to help patients save money (nonmaleficence) by using lower cost generic drugs. When HCPs prescribe the generic medications, they have a responsibility to explain the reasoning to patients to facilitate patient autonomy and shared decision-making. For example, the HCP can explain that (1) the use of generics is meant to mimic the FDA-approved compound; (2) the two component medicines are the same, but the dose and dosing regimen are not exactly the same; (3) there are no published safety and efficacy data on the generic combination; and (4) all of the same safety precautions must be taken with generic topiramate as for the branded drug (i.e., highly reliable birth control and regular pregnancy testing in women of reproductive age). It would also be reasonable for an HCP to follow FDA guidance and not prescribe the combination of generic topiramate and phentermine off label and only prescribe the brand name combination that has been tested.

The Case of Selling Commercial Products in the Office

A second example of ethics in clinical practice is the sale of medical products from the physician office. HCPs may decide, as part of their obesity treatment program, to sell meal replacement products directly from their offices. The HCP should ensure that sales of any products to patients does not place undue pressure on the patient, erode patient trust, or undermine the obligation to put patient interests first. The AMA Code of Medical Ethics has outlined guidelines under which products may be sold directly from the physician office:[22]

1. Patients must have freedom of choice. Do not require any patient to purchase products from your office.
2. Only offer products that either have published efficacy data or that are part of a strategy with published efficacy data.
3. Fully disclose that the use of the products is optional and that patients can purchase products wherever they would like to. Also, avoid exclusive distributorship arrangements with manufacturers.

4. Provide adequate informed consent regarding the use of the products.
5. Limit sales of products to those that serve immediate needs of patients.

HEALTH INSURANCE AND OBESITY

Obesity was formally recognized as a disease in the United States by the AMA in 2013.[23] However, insurance reimbursement for weight loss services remains a challenge. Health insurance often does not provide coverage for behavioral treatment of obesity. Coverage for antiobesity medications is even more limited, with many insurers categorically denying all evidence-based treatment options. For example, Medicare specifically excludes drug therapy for obesity, and only seven state Medicaid programs currently have drug coverage.

However, the situation has been improving. Before the passage of the Affordable Care Act, and before the 2013 AMA resolution, few insurers covered weight loss services including behavioral weight loss programs, antiobesity medications, or bariatric surgery. Now many insurers cover some services, medications, and/or surgical procedures. At the time of publication of this book, roughly half of the states include bariatric surgical benefits in their essential health benefits package. Also, in the past, HCPs were hesitant to code obesity as a medical diagnosis for fear that insurance would not pay for the visit. Now, most insurers require obesity and BMI to be properly coded. The transition to ICD-10 added many new codes (including specific BMI codes) to more accurately describe a patient's weight. This is expected to change again when ICD-11 is completed.

Insurance-Based Versus Cash-Based Practice Models

Because of the challenges entailed in billing medical insurance for obesity care services, many HCPs who treat obesity have operated outside of the insurance world. Because most patients affected by obesity who seek out treatment are still choosing commercial weight loss programs (which are not reimbursed by health insurance) in lieu of working with their medical provider, this model has been popular among medical providers offering weight loss programs. These so-called "cash practices" directly bill patients for services provided. Often services are bundled into program packages, which simplifies the cost of the program for patients compared to itemized medical billing. Some of these practices will provide receipts with ICD-10 and Current Procedural Technology (CPT) codes for patients to submit to their insurance companies. Conversely, some practices offer weight loss services within their scope of patient care and submit directly to insurance for reimbursement. This offers patients the convenience of having their treatment

reimbursed by their insurance company, similar to treatment for other chronic diseases. This approach requires skilled medical billing practices to ensure accuracy and proper reimbursement. There are also many different practice models used in obesity care (see Table 12.3).

Because of these issues, including poor training in obesity medicine, a lack of insurance coverage, and concerns among patients and HCPs that weight loss medications may have excessive side effects, it is estimated that only 2% of patients who are eligible for treatment with antiobesity medication receive a prescription. Additionally, despite the documented benefits of metabolic and bariatric surgery on weight loss, resolution of comorbidities, and longevity, only around 1% of individuals eligible for surgery receive this treatment approach.[24] A bill has been drafted in the US Congress for consideration called the Treat and Reduce Obesity Act (https://www.obesityaction.org/troa). At the time of writing this book, it has not passed. If passed, it would remove the Medicare part D exclusion of obesity pharmacotherapy, and it would expand the list of providers that are able to provide IBT for obesity.

ICD-10 Codes

The International Classification of Disease (ICD-10) codes are used for coding medical diagnoses.[25] The following list of obesity codes is provided in Table 12.4A and B. However, consultation with a qualified billing specialist is recommended for all clinicians engaging in

TABLE 12.3 Models of Obesity Care	
Primary care, insurance-based	Obesity is treated as a chronic disease, similar to other diseases. Insurers are billed for the treatments provided.
Specialty care, insurance-based	Comprehensive obesity management practice including medical specialist and other obesity-specific services such as intensive lifestyle modification, exercise training, structured food plans, etc.
Comprehensive care, insurance-based	Similar to above, but offering further services such as exercise therapist, psychologist, individual and group visits, and bariatric surgery.
Cash-based practice	These practices offer obesity care but opt out of insurance assignment. Patients pay practices directly in a fee-for-service model or sometimes pay for bundled services (such as a 12-week weight loss program including medical monitoring, dietitian visits, etc.)

TABLE 12.4A Obesity Codes

ICD-10 CODE	DESCRIPTION
E65	Localized adiposity Fat pad
E66	Overweight and obesity Use additional code to identify body mass index (BMI) Excludes • adiposogenital dystrophy (E23.6) • lipomatosis NOS (E88.2) • lipomatosis dolorosa (Dercum) (E88.2) • Prader-Willi syndrome (Q87.1)
E66.0	Obesity due to excess calories
E66.01	Morbid (severe) obesity due to excess calories Excludes • morbid (severe) obesity with alveolar hypoventilation (E66.2)
E66.09	Other obesity due to excess calories
E66.1	Drug-induced obesity Use additional code for adverse effect, if applicable, to identify drug (T36-T50 with fifth or sixth character 5)
E66.2	Morbid (severe) obesity with alveolar hypoventilation Pickwickian syndrome
E66.8	Other obesity
E66.9	Obesity, unspecified Obesity NOS
R60.9	Lipedema
Z86.39	Personal history of other endocrine, nutritional, and metabolic disease • includes history of obesity, adults • history of obesity BMI 95-100 percentile
Z98.84	Bariatric surgery status Gastric banding status Gastric bypass status for obesity Obesity surgery status Excludes • bariatric surgery status complicating pregnancy, childbirth, or the puerperium (O99.84) Excludes • intestinal bypass and anastomosis status (Z98.0)

billing for obesity care services. There are many other codes including pediatric weight management codes, related comorbidities, and others. These are all available as part of ICD-10 and can be found at www.cdc.gov. It is important to code both the medical diagnosis of obesity and the corresponding BMI code. For example, for a patient with obesity and a BMI of 33.4, the HCP should code E66.0 (obesity due to excess calories) and Z68.33 (BMI 33.0 to 33.9, adult).

Current Procedural Technology Codes

CPT codes are used to report medical, surgical, and diagnostic procedures and services to entities such as physicians, health insurance companies, and accreditation organizations.[26] Some of the codes that are most commonly used are listed in Table 12.5; however, it is important to review your billing practices with a medical billing specialist.

Medicare Benefit for Intensive Behavior Therapy for Obesity

Medicare beneficiaries with BMI $\geq$30 kg/m^2 may qualify for intensive behavioral counseling. This must be

TABLE 12.4B Body Mass Index (BMI) Codes

ICD-10 CODE	DESCRIPTION
Z68.3	BMI 30-39, adult
Z68.30	BMI 30.0-30.9, adult
Z68.31	BMI 31.0-31.9, adult
Z68.32	BMI 32.0-32.9, adult
Z68.33	BMI 33.0-33.9, adult
Z68.34	BMI 34.0-34.9, adult
Z68.35	BMI 35.0-35.9, adult
Z68.36	BMI 36.0-36.9, adult
Z68.37	BMI 37.0-37.9, adult
Z68.38	BMI 38.0-38.9, adult
Z68.39	BMI 39.0-39.9, adult
Z68.4	BMI 40 or greater, adult
Z68.41	BMI 40-44.9, adult
Z68.42	BMI 45.0-49.9, adult
Z68.43	BMI 50.0-59.9, adult
Z68.44	BMI 60.0-69.9, adult
Z68.45	BMI 70 or greater, adult

TABLE 12.5 Current Procedural Technology Codes

HEALTH AND BEHAVIOR ASSESSMENT CODES	NOTES	TIME
96150	Initial assessment	Billed in 15-minute increments
96151	Follow-up assessment	Billed in 15-minute increments
Health and Behavior Intervention Codes		
96152	Individual	Billed in 15-minute increments
96153	Group	Billed in 15-minute increments
96154	Family (patient present)	Billed in 15-minute increments
96155	Family (patient not present)	Billed in 15-minute increments
Preventive Visit Codes		
99381-99387	New patient	N/A
99391-99397	Established patient	N/A
Counseling/Risk Factor Reduction Codes		
99401	Preventive counseling	15 minutes
99402	Preventive counseling	30 minutes
99403	Preventive counseling	45 minutes
99404	Preventive counseling	60 minutes
Medical Nutrition Therapy Codes		
97802	Initial assessment	Billed in 15-minute increments
97803	Re-assessment	Billed in 15-minute increments
97804	Group	Billed in 15-minute increments
Test Codes		
0358T	BIA whole body composition assessment	

BIA, bioelectrical impedance analysis.

provided by the primary care provider in the primary care setting. Up to 22 visits are covered in the first 12 months. During the first month, patients can be seen every week. During months 2 to 6, patients can be seen every other week. Then, from months 7 to 12, patients can be seen once per month. For Medicare to cover the visits during months 7 to 12, patients must be assessed at month 6 and must have lost at least 3 kg.

Codes:

G0447: Individual face-to-face obesity counseling, 15 minutes.

G0473: Group face-to-face counseling, 30 minutes.

Evaluation and Management Codes (E&M Codes:)

New patient codes: 99201 to 99205
Established patient codes: 99211 to 99215

ADVOCACY AND PUBLIC HEALTH

Given the continued presence of weight bias in healthcare and in the US society, it is important for the HCP to advocate for their patients. Advocacy for improved treatment of obesity can include any of the following: (1) advocacy for appropriate clinical care; (2) education of other clinicians; and (3) education of the public, including work with obesity advocacy groups.[27]

Advocacy on behalf of patients is an important aspect of care delivery. As described above, the HCP may need to take extra steps to help their patients find the high-intensity behavioral treatment that is now recommended as a standard of care. In some cases, this could involve letters to insurance payers to document the medical necessity of such treatment. The exclusion of pharmacotherapy from most insurance formularies may also necessitate letters of appeal or of medical necessity. While it is unfortunate for HCPs to spend time on these tasks, it may be necessary to ensure that patients receive evidence-based treatment.

HCPs who treat obesity may choose to educate their colleagues regarding the concept of obesity as a chronic relapsing disease, including the need for long-term treatment. This may include formal conferences, webinars, informal lunch time talks, or academic detailing to HCPs who treat obesity should appreciate that primary care physicians often have limited knowledge about obesity, and thus, education must start with basic principles. For example, fewer than 20% of both internists and family physicians know the FDA criteria for initiating pharmacotherapy for treatment of obesity.[3] An understanding of the biological barriers to successful long-term weight loss may be a prerequisite for a more open discussion about the use of pharmacologic or surgical treatment of obesity.

Education of the public is an important aspect of advocacy for the chronic condition of obesity. Physicians or other providers may choose to participate in public events in their local area including newspaper or radio interviews or engage in social media such as twitter, Facebook, or personal blogging. Partnering with patients who have successfully lost weight can be a helpful tool for demonstrating to the public the benefits of structured obesity treatment. Finally, HCPs treating obesity can become involved with public advocacy through the advancement of legislation, specifically the Treat and Reduce Obesity Act, as described above.

CLINICAL HIGHLIGHTS

- This chapter has reviewed practical aspects of obesity treatment in the office setting, including the clinical teams and equipment needed to conduct treatment, as well as the tools available to help patients initiate behavior modification and to engage in high-intensity lifestyle programs.
- The chapter also has reviewed the important issue of weight bias and suggestions to mitigate it.
- Recommendations for treatment protocols, communication with patients of varying backgrounds, and financial and billing consideration were also covered.

WHEN TO REFER?

Registered Dietitian Nutritionist
- Patients needing basic nutrition education (calorie counting, macronutrients)
- Patients needing assistance with implementing a specific dietary intervention
- Patients needing high-intensity behavioral intervention

Exercise Physiologist/Physical therapist
- Patients needing individualized exercise plans or supervision
- Patients needing advanced assessment (metabolic rate or muscle strength testing)

Psychologist
- Patients with a high level of emotional distress about their weight
- Patients with an eating disorder including binge eating disorder, bulimia, or night eating syndrome
- Patients with a long history of multiple weight loss attempts but difficulty keeping the weight off due to stress eating/emotional factors

CASE STUDY

Discussion

The case study illustrates two aspects of practice management that are relevant for clinical care. First is the issue of offering or providing intensive behavioral support for weight loss. The 2013 AHA/ACC/TOS guideline on obesity management states that in-person, high-intensity treatment (≥14 sessions in the first 6 months, with at least monthly contact for weight loss maintenance) is appropriate for this patient. It is the responsibility of the HCP to help their patients access such care if desired. Health insurance plans are increasingly paying for such interventions, but reimbursement remains inconsistent. If the HCP is not able to provide a program like this in their office, then they should recommend participation in such a program and to be aware of high-quality, low-cost options in their practice setting and/or local community that provide evidence-based intensive treatment of obesity. The intervention may be provided in the health system where the provider practices, or through an outside referral to a commercial or nonprofit group behavioral intervention. In this case, the patient is resistant to participating in such interventions and has attempted lifestyle change on his own, but without success. The HCP's responsibility is to explain the benefit of high-intensity lifestyle intervention and the importance of self-monitoring and of specific targets for reduced calorie intake and increased physical activity. If the patient continues to be resistant to group intervention, then the HCP should attempt to further engage the patient in lifestyle intervention with more aggressive self-monitoring and employing a 1:1 approach with an RDN. The HCP also should advise his/her patient that (1) pharmacotherapy for obesity does not cause weight loss on its own; rather, it is used as a tool to help the patient make lifestyle changes; and (2) the combination of high-intensity behavioral intervention and pharmacotherapy is expected to nearly double the weight loss achieved, compared with either therapy alone.

The second issue in this case relates to the choice of agent for pharmacotherapy, in the context of lack of insurance coverage. Medicare Part D excludes medications for weight management, and many employers and private health insurers also do not cover medications. Newer agents (naltrexone HCL/bupropion HCL, phentermine-topiramate extended release, and liraglutide 3.0 mg) can range in price from $100 to $1,200 per month, putting them out of reach for many patients. Some clinicians may have concerns about the effect of a cardiac stimulant in an elderly patient, such as the one described in the case (e.g., the risk of inducing a cardiac arrhythmia). One appropriate response in this case would be to explain the insurance coverage issue to the patient. If the patient still wants to pursue pharmacotherapy, medications with lower risk can be used, such as low-dose phentermine (8 mg, 15 mg, or ½ of a 37.5 mg). The HCP should also explain that if the medication is beneficial, the patient will need to take it long term and have regular monitoring done to ensure efficacy and safety. *It is important to note that at the time of the writing of this book, some states have laws restricting or limiting long-term prescribing of phentermine, so it is important for the HCP to know the laws in the state in which they practice.*

QUIZ QUESTIONS

1. You are seeing a patient with body mass index (BMI) 38.3 for a weight management consultation. The patient also has prediabetes and hypertension.

   Which of the following are the most appropriate billing codes?

   A. Primary diagnosis I10 (hypertension); secondary diagnosis E66.01 (severe obesity)
   B. Primary diagnosis E66.9 (obesity); secondary diagnosis Z68.38 (BMI 38 to 38.9)
   C. Primary diagnosis E66.01 (severe obesity); secondary diagnosis Z68.38 (BMI 38 to 38.9)
   D. Primary diagnosis Z68.38 (BMI 38 to 38.9); secondary diagnosis E66.01 (severe obesity)

   Answer: C. *A is not correct because you are seeing the patient for weight management; thus, the weight should be billed as the primary diagnosis. B is not correct because the patient's BMI is in the range of "**severe obesity equivalent**" (BMI 35 to 39.9 with a comorbid condition). D is not correct because the medical diagnosis of obesity is billed first, followed by the BMI code.*

2. With regard to culturally tailored communication around weight and health, which of these racial-ethnic subgroups has the *lowest* risk of medical complications at a given body mass index (BMI)?

   A. Caucasians
   B. Mexican Americans
   C. East Asians
   D. African Americans
   E. South Asians

   Answer: D. *At a given BMI, east and south Asian patients have a higher degree of visceral adiposity, compared with whites, and African American patients have slightly lower visceral adiposity compared with whites.*

PRACTICAL RESOURCES

Clinical Guidelines and Practice Management Resources

- The Obesity Society (www.obesity.org)
- The Obesity Medicine Association (www.obesitymedicine.org)
- The American Board of Obesity Medicine (www.abom.org)

- American Academy of Clinical Endocrinologists (obesity.aace.com)

Patient Education Materials and Treatment Protocols (others listed in Chapter 5 and Chapter 13)

- Academy of Nutrition and Dietetics (www.eatright.org)
- The Model-IBT Program (Intensive Behavioral Therapy) for Obesity (https://onlinelibrary.wiley.com/doi/full/10.1002/oby.22594)

- Free or Low-Cost Patient Resources
  - Spark People (www.sparkpeople.com)
  - Calorie King (www.calorieking.com)
  - MyFitnessPal (www.myfitnesspal.com)
  - Take Off Pounds Sensibly (www.tops.org)

Advocacy

- Obesity Action Coalition (www.obesityaction.org)
- Rudd Center (www.uconnruddcenter.org)

REFERENCES

1. Wadden TA, Berkowitz RI, Sarwer DB, Prus-Wisniewski R, Steinberg C. Benefits of lifestyle modification in the pharmacologic treatment of obesity: a randomized trial. *Arch Intern Med*. 2001;161(2):218-227.

2. Wadden TA; Look AHEAD Research Group. Eight-year weight losses with an intensive lifestyle intervention: the look AHEAD study. *Obesity*. 2014;22(1):5-13.

3. Turner M, Jannah N, Kahan S, Gallagher C, Dietz W. Current knowledge of obesity treatment guidelines by health care professionals. *Obesity*. 2018;26(4):665-671.

4. American Medical Association. *CME Report 3*. AMA Annual Meeting; 2017.

5. Kushner RF, Butsch WS, Kahan S, Machineni S, Cook S, Aronne LJ. Obesity coverage on medical licensing examinations in the United States. What is being tested? *Teach Learn Med*. 2017;29:(2):123-128. doi:10.1080/10401334.2016.1250641

6. American Society for Metabolic, Bariatric Surgery. Find a Provider. Accessed May 26, 2020. https://www.asmbs.org/find-a-provider

7. Obesity Action Coalition. Action Through Advocacy: Weight Bias. Accessed October 28, 2019. https://www.obesityaction.org/action-through-advocacy/weight-bias

8. Puhl R, Brownell KD. Confronting and coping with weight stigma: an investigation of overweight and individuals with obesity. *Obesity*. 2006;14(10):1802-1815.

9. American Academy of Family Physicians. 2019 Congress of Delegates. Accessed October 28, 2019. https://www.aafp.org/news/2019-congress-fmx/20191002cod-hops.html

10. Center for Medicare and Medicaid Services. Decision memo for intensive behavioral therapy for obesity (CAG-00423N). Published November 29, 2011. Accessed April 2, 2019. https://www.cms.gov/medicare-coverage-database/details/nca-decision-memo.aspx?NCAId=253

11. Ogden CL, Fakhouri TH, Carroll MD, et al. Prevalence of obesity among adults, by household income and education — United States, 2011-2014. *MMWR Morb Mortal Wkly Rep*. 2017;66:1369-1373. doi:10.15585/mmwr.mm6650a1

12. Dorsey RR, Eberhardt MS, Ogden CL. Racial/ethnic differences in weight perception. *Obesity*. 2009;17(4):790-795.

13. Foster GD, Wadden TA, Vogt RA. Resting energy expenditure in obese African American and Caucasian women. *Obes Res*. 1997;5(1):1-8.

14. Zhu S, Heymsfield SB, Toyoshima H, Wang Z, Pietrobelli A, Heshka S. Race-ethnicity-specific waist circumference cutoffs for identifying cardiovascular disease risk factors. *Am J Clin Nutr*. 2005;81(2):409-415.

15. IDF Consensus Statement on Metabolic Syndrome. 2006. Accessed May 26, 2020. https://www.idf.org/e-library/consensus-statements/60-idfconsensus-worldwide-definitionof-the-metabolic-syndrome.html

16. Bleich SN, Bennett WL, Gudzune KA, Cooper LA. Impact of physician BMI on obesity care and beliefs. *Obesity*. 2012;20:999-1005.

17. Forhan M, Risdon C, Solomon P. Contributors to patient engagement in primary health care: perceptions of patients with obesity. *Prim Health Care Res Dev*. 2013;14:367-372.

18. Leske S, Strodl E, Hou XY. Patient-practitioner relationships desired by overweight/obese adults. *Patient Educ Couns*. 2012;89(2):309-315. doi:10.1016/j.pec.2012.07.002

19. Stewart-Higgins S. *Perspective of Obese Minority Women on Weight Issues within a Primary Care Setting: A Qualitative Study*. PhD Defense. University of Missouri-Kansas City; 2008.

20. Lewis KH, Fischer H, Ard J, et al. Safety and effectiveness of longer-term phentermine use: clinical outcomes from an electronic health record cohort. *Obesity*. 2019;27(4):591-602. doi:10.1002/oby.22430

21. Apovian CM, Aronne LJ, Bessesen DH, et al. Pharmacological management of obesity: an endocrine Society clinical practice guideline. *J Clin Endocrinol Metab*. 2015;100(2):342-362. doi:10.1210/jc.2014-3415

22. American Medical Association. Code of Medical Ethics: Sale of Health-Related Products. Accessed May 19, 2020. https://www.ama-assn.org/delivering-care/ethics/sale-health-related-products

23. American Medical Association Policy H440.842. Recognition of Obesity as a Disease. Accessed May 19, 2020. https://policysearch.ama-assn.org/policyfinder/detail/H-440.842?uri=%2FAMADoc%2FHOD.xml-0-3858.xml

24. Thomas CE, Mauer EA, Shukla AP, Rathi S, Aronne LJ. Low adoption of weight loss medications: a comparison of prescribing patterns of antiobesity pharmacotherapies and SGLT2s. *Obesity*. 2016;24(9):1955-1961. doi:10.1002/oby.21533

25. Center for Disease Control and Prevention. International Classification of Diseases, 10th revision, clinical modification (ICD-10-CM). Accessed October 28, 2019. www.cdc.gov/nchs/icd/icd10cm.htm

26. Current Procedural Technology. Accessed October 28, 2019. https://www.ama-assn.org/amaone/cpt-current-procedural-terminology

27. Costa SA, Ferris E, Huang TT. What the obesity prevention field can learn from the gay marriage movement. *Obesity*. 2015;23(10):1939-1940. doi:10.1002/oby.21225

TEAM CARE, REFERRALS, AND PRACTICE RESOURCES

Deborah Bade Horn

CASE STUDY

Grace is 50-year-old woman with hypertension, uncontrolled type 2 diabetes, and arthritis in both knees. Three months ago, you broached the topic of her weight during a diabetes follow-up visit and its effect on her other health problems. At that time, she chose to implement self-directed dietary changes and to try to be more physically active. However, she found that walking for exercise hurts her knees too much and she returns today frustrated that she has not lost any weight.

Medications include ramipril 5 mg, metformin 1,000 mg BID, and diclofenac sodium 50 mg/day. On examination, blood pressure (BP) is 136/88, heart rate (HR) 92, and body mass index (BMI) 34 kg/m². Laboratory testing shows HgbA1c is 8.1%. You ask her to consider additional tools for weight management and the use of an antiobesity medication (AOM).

CLINICAL SIGNIFICANCE

Providing obesity care within a primary care practice can be challenging, but it is essential for successful disease treatment. Just as there will never be enough endocrinologists to treat the 30 million individuals living with diabetes in the United States, there will also not be enough obesity medicine specialists to treat the 93 million individuals living with obesity.[1,2] Patients believe it is the "responsibility of the primary care provider" to initiate the conversation about weight management and to do so in a nonjudgmental, knowledgeable and respectful manner.[3] Furthermore, delivering obesity care is dependent upon disease recognition and utilization of the essential and varied resources for chronic disease management.

Patient outcomes will vary depending upon how the practice functions. For example, failure to diagnose obesity is associated with a decrease in the likelihood of successfully sustaining meaningful weight loss.[4] A healthcare professional's (HCP's) recognition of a patient's previous attempts at weight loss increases the odds of success. Identifying the disease, acknowledging effort, and providing resources that improve motivation can improve patient outcomes.[4] These brief examples highlight the importance of the three key topics covered in this chapter: Team Care, Referrals, and Practice Resources.

In reviewing each of the three key areas, it is important to acknowledge that primary care practice models vary widely. Some practices exist as part of a larger healthcare system or network, while others operate as private practices in single or multiple sites. There are also a wide range of collaborative business models that fall in between. This variation in practice models can result in just as many variations in team member structure, including team members that are practice employed, outsourced, multisite shared, or system/network shared. Regardless of structure, the resources available to patients with obesity should be consistent across all practice models, from team access to referrals to treatment options.

TEAM-BASED CARE

Team-based healthcare is defined by the National Academy of Medicine as "...the provision of health services to individuals, families and/or their communities by at least 2 health providers who work collaboratively with patients and their caregivers—to the extent preferred by each patient—to accomplish shared goals within and across settings to achieve coordinated, high quality care."[5] The advantages of team-based care in primary care include improvements in effectiveness and efficiency in delivering patient education, behavioral health, and care coordination.[6] The practical advantages of team-based care include increased job satisfaction and provision of high-quality care. Team-based care can be implemented across different practices and for a variety of chronic diseases. For example, an HCP can treat low back pain with basic advice and pain medications, but the implementation of a treatment plan is best provided by a physical therapist.

Obesity is complex, and successful treatment requires frequent patient visits and additional resources beyond the typical brief patient/HCP encounter. This alone drives the need for team-based care. As mentioned above, a team care approach can improve both quality and efficiency of patient care.[7] For example, team care is essential in making a diagnosis of obesity which requires an accurate documentation of height and weight, typically performed by a medical assistant, so that a meaningful discussion can be initiated between the patient and HCP.[8] Additional team members (registered dietitian nutritionist [RDN], psychologist) can implement treatment and provide individualized resources beyond the brief medical encounter. Additionally, it is recognized that high-intensity behavioral counseling is effective in promoting weight loss and can be delivered by many different types of healthcare team members in primary care.[9,10] Obesity care requires a multidisciplinary team to successfully deliver care and take advantage of the strengths of each team member.

The Team Lead

The first step in building an obesity care team is identifying the team lead or champion. Most often this will be a physician, but it can also be delegated to an advanced practice provider (APP: nurse practitioner [NP] or physician assistant [PA]) with physician oversight. In some states, nurse practitioners can practice independently. In a single-provider private practice, the team lead will be the solo HCP. From a team perspective, in a multi-HCP single-site practice, one HCP most commonly is identified to serve as the champion lead. Similarly, in a multisite healthcare system or multisite private practice, an overarching team lead is necessary for consistent obesity care initiatives across multiple sites. In this scenario, each site would identify a champion HCP who works together with the overarching team lead to ensure consistent implementation of practice protocols and improvements.

Ideally the team lead will either have or pursue additional expertise in obesity treatment. This can take the form of continuing medical education (CME), certificates of completion of dedicated obesity-focused CME, or attaining American Board of Obesity Medicine Diplomate status. See *Team Education* below for more information. The team lead should plan the practice's approach to patient care and action steps for practice improvement activities for increasing and maintaining quality of obesity care. Examples of practice improvements include engaging all team members in obesity stigma and bias training, adding a question to patient satisfaction surveys already in use, and documenting the diagnosis of obesity in the electronic health record to help encourage providers and teams to treat obesity as a disease. The Healthy Teams Model is one approach to building an effective healthcare team. It is based on six key characteristics of a productive team: purpose, goals, communication, leadership, cohesion, and mutual respect.[7] The team lead can build on these key characteristics to help team members engage and adopt new practice procedures regarding obesity care. Examples of these team-focused procedures may include documenting discussions around weight for purposes of quality improvement, or training team members on the principles and techniques of using motivational interviewing to solicit patient change talk. Creating a unified "team" work environment is critical to successful obesity patient care.

Team Members and Team Structure

The obesity care team involves many key players that may have overlapping roles. It is essential to identify and plan for which team members should be employed internally (within the practice) versus referred to externally (remain outside of the practice but still consistently utilized). Many of the team members necessary for delivering obesity treatment are already part of an existing primary care practice. These team members are covered in detail in Chapter 12. For example, these include the front and back office staff, e.g., receptionists, schedulers, patient advocates, and medical assistants. Other important key team members may or may not already be part of an existing practice. These include RDNs, APPs, exercise physiologists/trainers or physical therapists, behavioral specialists (including coaches, social workers, counselors, and psychologists), and clinical pharmacists. There are many options to providing access to this broader network of team members. In a university system or an integrated healthcare system, these team members might exist elsewhere in the practice system and available for referral. In a private group practice, they might be hired by the practice and shared between multiple practice sites. For single private practices, they might be outsourced to the community via building a referral network of providers with whom the practice collaborates on patient care.

For example, currently it is uncommon for a primary care practice to have an exercise physiologist or a certified personal trainer on staff, and yet physical activity is an essential component of obesity treatment. (The training and skill set of an exercise physiologist are described in Chapter 12.) Therefore, a patient could be referred to resources outside the practice but inside the larger healthcare system or community to receive this component of care. Alternatively, the practice could hire an exercise physiologist or certified personal trainer as a contracted consultant (not an employee) to deliver interactive lectures or workshops to patients in a group setting. Practices that use this strategy often pay a flat class or hourly rate to the exercise physiologist and charge the patients a class fee for attending. This option can keep the cost down for both the practice and patients, provide essential physical activity guidance for patients, and build revenue for the practice. In this example, a resource that potentially costs the practice money is converted into a resource that increases practice revenue.

As the obesity care team becomes defined, it is important to remember that not every patient needs to see every type of clinician in the team; the care plan should be individualized. For example, some patients may need the accountability and additional behavioral support provided by a behavioral coach to build a skill set for long-term success, while others may need guidance from a physical therapist or certified personal trainer to develop a physical activity program that meets their treatment needs and physical abilities. This individualization of care must be considered as a practice determines its patients' needs and plans for provision of resources.

When a specialty member of the obesity care team is not accessible or available, a practice may be able to train other team members to deliver those aspects of obesity treatment. For example, in some practices, medical assistants receive additional training in nutrition, sleep hygiene, stress reduction, and physical activity guidance. This additional training allows them to teach group classes to patients using a slide deck, leader guide, and handouts. The content delivered has been preapproved by the entire team and provides a consistent message to patients. This consistency is important since it ensures that patients receive the same education regardless of who is available to teach the class on any given clinic day. Practices will need to have some flexibility in staffing, as classes may start or end outside of the normal clinic workday to accommodate patient work schedules.

When considering whether to hire, refer to a resource inside a system, or outsource team members,

it is important to confirm that they have a thorough understanding of the practice's overall treatment goals and philosophy, thus ensuring that patients receive consistent messaging about their disease treatment. If a patient receives one set of instructions from the HCP at a clinic visit but a different set of recommendations in a class or from another provider, it can create confusion, frustration, and inconsistent implementation.

Team Treatment Flow

Treatment flow refers to the frequency and sequence of patient visits within the practice. Questions to consider include whether treatment flow changes based on the intervention chosen by a patient and their HCP, when does a patient see each member of the team, and what health data points need to be collected and when. Each of these decisions will affect treatment flow. High-intensity treatment is the most effective approach to successful obesity treatment, regardless of the nutritional intervention selected. Low- to moderate-intensity treatments often produce minimal results and often fail to meet patient and provider expectations.[10-12] This evidence can guide decisions around frequency of visits as well as which and when providers are utilized.

What does treatment flow look like in an effective high-intensity treatment plan? High-intensity treatment is defined as ≥14 visits in 6 months that can be individual or group visits[13] and including at least monthly contact for maintenance of weight loss. Emerging data support that the HCP does not always have to be the team member delivering this care. Studies demonstrate effective use of medical assistants, RDNs, and psychologists for successful treatment of obesity between HCP visits.[14,15] Obesity is a chronic metabolic disease, and the initial assessment and evaluation of the patient should be done by a medical professional (physician, NP, or PA). The ability to delegate care between HCPs and other professionals highlights the need for an effective team.

The treatment flow also depends on the team members available and the structure of the clinic. When considering treatment flow pathways, consider all the possible types of visits: individual visits, shared medical appointments (group visits), intensive behavioral programs (both inside and outside of the practice or healthcare system), peer support groups, or any visit in which the patient's support network of family/friends might be involved. Some patients may be resistant to group meetings, but clinicians should be aware that group interventions are at least as effective as 1:1 treatment, even among patients who express a preference for individual treatment.[16]

Being flexible in considering different types of visit structures can alleviate some barriers that a practice may initially perceive in delivering care. For example, the patient may see the HCP at the start of treatment, and then see an RDN, nurse, or medical assistant for frequent check-ins over a 3- to 6-month period of intensive treatment. The patient then returns to the HCP after a set period of treatment or after achieving a weight loss of 5% to 10% of initial body weight.

While there are multiple pathways to arrange the treatment flow, in general it may be useful for the practice to strive to match high-intensity treatment models (≥14 visits in the first 6 months) that studies have demonstrated to be the most effective. At this frequency, visits could be weekly in the beginning and then less frequent in later months, or visits could be every other week for 6 months. The goal is to provide patients with the opportunity for frequent follow-up to allow for individualized adjustments in their treatment plan as needed over time and supportive accountability as they focus on lifestyle changes.

As a practice evaluates treatment flow for delivering a high-intensity intervention, it is important to consider that patients can also be referred to an obesity medicine specialist or an intensive treatment program that is already in the practice's healthcare system or community. However, as the patient's primary care provider, the HCP should remain involved. For example, the HCP may continue to comanage comorbidities as the patient loses weight, reducing the need for diabetes, hypertension, lipid, or pain medications.

Team Communication

Most primary care practices already have a method in place for communicating between providers, allied health professionals, and each of the key front and back office staff members. Obesity care is likely to test the robustness of that communication structure. Unlike a patient coming in for an acute care visit or well patient examination, obesity is like diabetes in that it requires chronic care management. In this sense, obesity has similarities with major depression or chronic low back pain, in that the condition requires frequent contact to produce clinically significant improvement. In the beginning weeks of treatment when frequency of visits and the number of involved providers are higher, team communication is essential. Good team communication involves communication about new or updated processes of care, as well as information specific to an individual patient's treatment plan.

A simple example of the need for process communication is the delegation of tasks for a practice that has decided to take a small step toward improved obesity care by improving identification of the disease and then referring, known as Assess-Advise-Refer. In this sequence of care, the HCP documents the BMI as normal, overweight, or one of the obesity classifications; reviews the diagnosis with the patient; and refers to a high-intensity intervention. The medical assistant can then follow up with patient education handouts and provide the patient with contact information if they are being referred to an outside treatment program. Finally, the front desk can be trained to recognize when a patient is referred for obesity treatment and scheduled for follow-up with the HCP (e.g., 3 months into treatment). In this well-planned treatment flow, the HCP can maintain a vital connection with the patient and monitor progress. All three team members in this scenario are well prepared for the next step, and the patient has a positive and productive healthcare experience.

Communication between providers is essential in each patient's plan of care. There are many examples of this collaborative, multidisciplinary care in other areas of medicine. One of the best examples is spinal cord injury care teams and their weekly team meeting to review progress and plan of care. These meetings often involve the physical medicine and rehab physician as the team lead, respiratory therapist, wound care specialist, nurses, social workers, clinical pharmacists, and, at some meetings, the patient and family of the patient. The analogous members in an obesity team meeting could include the HCP, nurse, medical assistant or front desk staff, RDN, and possibly additional allied health team members like the behaviorist or exercise physiologist/physical therapist.

The structure of patient treatment communication can vary widely. At a minimum, team members can communicate through the electronic medical record (EMR) by both reviewing each other's notes and by messaging within the EMR. However, this can be time consuming. A second option is to schedule team meetings to review patients' treatment plans, such as a morning huddle, which provides a daily opportunity to quickly review patients coming to clinic for the day and what resources the team needs to deliver effective and efficient care. It helps identify patients that have outstanding diagnostic tests, laboratory test results, medication prior authorizations, or other provider referrals and ensures that the clinician seeing the patient that day has the results and resources ready to review with the patient. Morning huddle for an average clinic day can usually be accomplished in 10 minutes. This affords the team, specifically the medical assistant, time to locate any missing data before the visits begin, as opposed to trying to locate the data in the middle of clinic when many other tasks are going on simultaneously. It also provides efficient exchange between providers. For example, if the team RDN has seen the patient for the previous one to three visits and can be present for huddle, they can offer insights into nutritional changes and goals for which the patient may need encouragement during the upcoming provider visit. This reinforces unified messaging to the patient and can help promote success.

Finally, the practice team might consider a monthly team meeting to review complicated obesity cases or patients that need a referral outside of the practice to a more intensive medical or surgical treatment program. A successful example of this has been seen in bariatric surgery practices. At some surgical practices, the bariatric surgery team and the obesity medicine specialists convene monthly for what is called "Revision Team Meeting." This meeting focuses on the team review of obesity surgery cases that have had a primary bariatric surgical procedure but are regaining weight. Together as a team of physicians, surgeons, RDNs, psychologists, advanced practice providers, and patient advocates, they discuss which treatment options should be considered to improve the patient's long-term outcome. This example does not need to be limited to bariatric surgical care. Any practice could consider a monthly or quarterly meeting to discuss patients struggling with initial or long-term successful obesity treatment.

Team Education

Once a practice has dedicated itself to treating obesity, identified the treatment team, and assembled care resources, it is time to plan for obesity education for the team. Up-to-date medical treatment of obesity in the primary care setting is still a novel offering for most primary care practices. Every staff member should have a basic understanding of obesity and the fund of knowledge appropriate for their role on the team.

At the most fundamental level, care needs to be empathetic and free from the bias and stigma that many patients with obesity experience in all areas of medicine. Obesity is different from most other chronic diseases that are treated in primary care settings, in that patients often feel a sense of shame and self-blame about their excess body weight. Even today, many patients and HCPs often do not understand that obesity is a disease and continue to feel that it is a "choice" that a patient needs to correct on their own. Thus, the first step in effective team education is providing resources on how to identify and correct explicit and implicit obesity bias and stigma. See Chapter 12 for additional discussion on weight bias.

HCPs (and the public) need better education on the nature of obesity as a chronic condition. Both patients and HCPs often believe that obesity is a lifestyle choice, rather than a chronic metabolic disease. In the ACTION (Awareness, Care, and Treatment In Obesity MaNagement) study, 82% of patients with obesity felt that losing weight was completely their responsibility.[8] Similarly, 72% of HCPs in the ACTION study stated they have a responsibility to "actively contribute to my patient's successful weight loss effort," but only 30% of them felt that prescribing antiobesity medication (AOM) was an effective treatment.[8] In another study,

51% of HCPs "rarely" or "never" prescribed AOM and only 9% (14 of 160) indicated they prescribe medication in the management of obesity.[17] Thus, the HCP belief that obesity is a lifestyle choice translates into a reluctance to use pharmacotherapy as a treatment modality. Unfortunately, the view of HCPs regarding obesity are not consistent with the underlying science. Obesity, once established, is not a lifestyle choice. Rather, it is a chronic, often progressive metabolic disease, with alterations in hormones and neuropeptides that affect appetite control.[18] Similarly, metabolism drops disproportionately in response to successful weight loss, thus working against patients' efforts.[19] Research has demonstrated that HCPs do not feel adequately trained to treat obesity and therefore do not feel they have the skills to deliver effective care.[20-22] Thus, practices can consider additional obesity education that may include fundamental concepts of obesity as a disease for some team members and more advanced training for the HCPs that will be directly delivering care.

REFERRALS

Outgoing Referrals and Referrals Beyond the In-House Practice Team

As discussed earlier in this chapter, a practice is likely to refer some components of care to clinicians/providers outside of the practice. Depending on the practice treatment flow and resources, patients may need to be referred out to see RDNs, exercise physiologists, physical therapists, behaviorists, obesity medicine specialists, or bariatric surgeons. In this situation, as discussed previously, the most important variable is consistent messaging for patient. The HCP should expect and receive reports/feedback from these other HCPs to help manage treatment cohesively.

Like other areas of chronic disease, there will also be referrals for necessary testing that may be outside the scope of the practice, such as sleep studies, stress tests/cardiac evaluations, and imaging/orthopedic evaluations. Many of these referrals are already in the flow of treatment that is provided in a primary care office and thus just needed to be applied to the treatment of obesity. A curated list of specialists that can be used for referrals and shared readily with patients improves efficiency of care. For example, the practice should know which gastroenterologist has expertise in nonalcoholic fatty liver disease, or which reproductive endocrinologist has expertise in obesity and infertility.

Among the referrals that are specific to weight management, there are three that HCPs would be expected to make most commonly. The first is referral to an intensive behavioral program (when the practice cannot provide that service). The second is referral to an obesity medicine specialist for advanced medical treatment. The third is referral to a bariatric surgeon. How does a provider know when to refer a patient on for these types of specialty care?

The first step is knowing when to consider a referral. Like every other chronic disease, medical providers must make decisions regarding whether they will begin treatment with the patient or refer the patient out for care. Consider diabetes as an analogy. The HCP may feel comfortable with oral antidiabetes agents and once- or twice-daily insulin, but then refer to an endocrinologist to start insulin pump therapy if the patient requests that form of treatment. The same model should be applied to obesity. Perhaps a provider feels comfortable starting a patient on lifestyle intervention and a single AOM (i.e., phentermine or diethylpropion), but might refer to an obesity medicine specialist if a more complex medical regimen is needed. Each HCP must decide their level of provision of care and, if it is insufficient to control the disease, provide the patient with a referral for advanced intervention. Stated another way, the HCP should either treat obesity themselves, or refer to a provider who can treat it.

Referral to an Intensive Lifestyle Program

When is it appropriate to refer for an intensive lifestyle treatment program? Depending on what resources the practice has decided to provide within the office, it is important to remember that high-intensity treatment (≥14 visits in the first 6 months, followed by monthly contact for maintenance of weight loss) provides the best opportunity for successful lifestyle management of obesity.[9,10] Thus, following diagnosis, a referral to an RDN for one counseling session is unlikely to help the patient succeed at lasting change. If the current practice resources do not provide for high-intensity treatment, then the HCP should begin the care and education that is available and refer the patient to a treatment program in the system or community that can deliver a high-intensity intervention. For example, the HCP can get the patient started on AOM and refer the patient for more intensive intervention outside of the practice. Similarly, there may be data or assessments that a patient may benefit from during obesity care that can be obtained by sending the patient to a specialized obesity clinic. These might include body composition analysis, resting metabolic rate, or genetic testing.

Referrals to an Obesity Medicine Specialist Clinic

Obesity medicine specialists typically provide consultative, comprehensive, and team-based care. As with a consultation for any other medical specialty, the referring HCP should expect communication from the obesity medicine specialist with practical recommendations for treatment. Follow-up communication also should occur when there is a change in medications, new test results are available, or the patient succeeds in reaching a weight loss milestone.

Some obesity medicine specialists will adjust or discontinue medications that need to be changed as a result of weight loss, such as those for diabetes, hypertension, hyperlipidemia, or pain control. Conversely, some obesity medicine specialists do not adjust any medications other than AOMs and leave management of comorbidities to the HCP. The obesity medicine specialist may also review the patient's concurrent medication therapy and recommend changes (e.g., changing paroxetine [weight gaining] for treatment of depression to bupropion [associated with weight loss]). It is important that the HCP and obesity medicine specialist establish a working relationship regarding comanagement of the patient. At some point in time, long-term management of the patient's obesity will fall back to the HCP.

Referral for Consideration of Bariatric Surgery

For patients in whom a high-intensity lifestyle intervention with or without adjunctive use of AOMs is not successful (i.e., a clinically significant weight loss that reduces the burden of comorbid disease) and meet the BMI criteria for bariatric surgery, the patient should be offered a referral to a bariatric surgeon to discuss the surgical options. Patients have the right to know all the evidence-based treatment options available to treat their disease and rely on their HCP and specialists to help them determine the best treatment approach. To qualify for bariatric surgery, a patient must have a BMI ≥40 kg/m² or a BMI ≥35 kg/m² with at least one comorbidity. The comorbidities that can be used for the second of these qualifications have been narrowed over time by insurers and can vary from plan to plan.[23] Despite the variability, HCPs should have at least some understanding of the comorbidities that generally qualify a patient for surgery. HCPs also play an important role in managing comorbidities preoperatively to reduce operative risk. See Chapter 9 for a detailed discussion on bariatric surgery.

Many surgeons handle the preoperative and immediate postoperative care for their bariatric surgery patients. Updates on shared patients should be similar to those described above for medical referrals. Like medical obesity treatment, at some point postsurgically, the patient will return to the care of their HCP. To be prepared for these changes in care and potential complications that come with bariatric surgery, HCPs should become knowledgeable about the most common aspects of perioperative care. Understanding the nutritional deficiencies to monitor and manage is an essential area of care for the postsurgery patient.

(See Chapter 10 for additional detail on this topic.) The guidelines for perioperative care of the bariatric patient arc an excellent resource.[23]

Barriers to Referrals and Appropriate Care

Each of the three major referrals and their treatment interventions discussed above are woefully underutilized in the US healthcare system. A recent Government Accountability Office (GAO) report in August 2019 found that, among the US adults with obesity who also reported trying to lose weight, only 3% reported taking a prescription medication as part of their effort.[24] It is predicted that of all individuals that could qualify for AOMs, less than 2% receive a medication. Similarly, even though 62% of HCPs surveyed indicated that obesity surgery is an effective option, less than 1% of the patients that qualify for bariatric surgery will receive it.[8,25] With the projection that 50% of the United States will be living with obesity by 2030, this pattern of underutilization of effective treatments must change.[26]

There are many potential barriers for a referral to an obesity medicine specialist that include:

- HCP bias toward recognizing obesity as a disease and lack of familiarity regarding effective care,
- patient misinformation about effectiveness of care,[8]
- patient willingness to complete the referral and lack of patient perceived need for care,
- the stigma of receiving the diagnosis of obesity and receiving care,
- cost of care if the specialist is not in the patient's healthcare system or does not accept insurance,
- overall poor insurance coverage for obesity care including provider visits, RDN visits, and physical activity education
- lack of insurance coverage for AOMs.

Perhaps one of the most concerning of these barriers to care is the HCP and patient potential bias and lack of information regarding effectiveness of care. When surveyed, only 36% of patients with obesity and 53% of HCPs perceived referral to an obesity medicine specialist as an effective treatment option. Even fewer in both groups thought that AOM was an effective option.[8] In fact, "general improvement in eating habits/reducing calories" was thought to be the most effective therapy by both patients and HCPs. This view will likely hinder a referral to a specialist. In summary, the barriers to referral to an obesity medicine specialist are related to weight bias, stigma, and unfamiliarity of treatment options, as well as economic factors (cost, lack of insurance coverage).

How can the HCP help to mitigate these barriers? The HCP can explain that obesity medicine specialists have expertise in the medical management of obesity and access to a broad range of resources. However, insurance coverage remains an issue. As of 2020, most Medicare plans still do not cover any AOMs for any patients.[27] Private insurance coverage is improving, but the GAO reported that only 42% of payments for obesity drugs were through insurance.[24] RDN visits under medical nutritional therapy are often limited to patients with diabetes or chronic kidney disease. Some patients have insurance that provides a limited number of RDN visits per year for obesity. Other providers have used "incident to" billing combined with preventive medicine visit codes to allow for RDN reimbursement.

It becomes clear even after a brief discussion about the complex nature of billing and lack of reimbursement that obesity medicine specialists often forgo trying to solve the billing problems and instead develop a fee for service practice. There are two major problems with this practice solution: (1) it creates a disparity in care, as only select patients will be able to afford cash-based care; and (2) the practice will never fully integrate into the traditional referral process, because many patients will not seek care that their insurance does not cover. (See Chapter 12 for additional discussion of billing.) When referring to an obesity medicine specialist, it is important that the HCP can direct patients to programs that meet their expectations with regard to both medical need and cost.

Regarding the barriers to bariatric surgery referrals, affordability and coverage of care are again a major issue. Ironically, most patients now have insurance coverage for bariatric surgery, despite inconsistent reimbursement for RDN visits, intensive behavioral programs, obesity medicine specialist visits, and medications. Patients with insurance coverage for surgery often have a large coinsurance payment (often 30% to 50% of the total cost of the surgery). Under the Affordable Care Act, slightly more than half of the states in the United States have coverage for obesity surgery in their state health insurance exchange. In comparison, only five states have coverage of medical treatment for obesity. Furthermore, HCP beliefs about obesity affect access to bariatric surgery.[28] As described above, some HCPs recognize obesity as a disease,[8] but other studies report that 50% of primary care physicians, cardiologists, and endocrinologists think that the cause of obesity is a lack of patient self-control.[29]

How can the HCP mitigate the barriers to surgical treatment of obesity? The HCP can explain to the patient that obesity is a chronic disease and that bariatric surgery is currently the most effective and durable treatment to help patients that have been unsuccessful with nonsurgical approaches.

Incoming Referrals to the Practice

The effort that a practice puts into team building and improved obesity care can result in benefits to the practice as well. As colleagues in the practice, healthcare system, and community become aware of the focus on comprehensive obesity care, referrals to the practice are likely. Initially these may come from partners within the practice of the HCP who has developed expertise in obesity management. Patients themselves will also seek a primary care physician that is willing to assist them with weight management. Finally, it gives the practice an opportunity to help other practices transition to better care for obesity as they see their own patients succeed.

In summary, it is clear there is still more work to be done to reduce the barriers for all patients in need of obesity treatment. Using an analogy to primary care practice, an HCP that decided not to treat diabetes would very likely not be able to survive in practice. The same should be true for treating obesity, although in 2020 this is not yet the case. The decision to treat or to refer may change in scope and detail over time, but as stated above, the HCP should be able assess and treat patients with obesity or to refer them for treatment.

RESOURCES

Obesity-Specific Onsite Resources

The continuum of resources to treat obesity is broad. From simple educational handouts to high tech measurements, the resources (both onsite and offsite) chosen by a practice directly affect treatment flow and level of care provided (see Table 13.1). A practice might choose to offer some resources in order to deliver most of the patient care, but also refer the patient to an obesity medicine specialty clinic for advanced testing.

The results can then be used by the HCP in the overall treatment plan. For example, an HCP might choose to have a bioelectrical impedance analysis (BIA) machine for body composition analysis but refer a patient out for resting metabolic rate testing. Similarly, patients with implantable cardiac devices cannot use a BIA machine, and so that patient group might be referred out for air displacement plethysmography, and then the results can be used by the HCP to manage care.

mHealth Resources

Smart technology can be a tremendous resource for HCPs and patients in the treatment of obesity. It can help streamline the information that patients provide so that the team can work on individualized, patient-targeted goals. Fifty percent of individuals worldwide use one to two health apps to manage their health conditions.[30] There are more than 2.7 million apps for Android users and 1.8 million apps available in the Apple store.[31] Only 15% of individuals use no health app, and the remaining 35% of individuals are extremely high users of mHealth. Individuals who are successful at long-term maintenance of weight loss share several behaviors; one of those essential behaviors is self-monitoring. Successful weight loss maintainers self-monitor their health habits, i.e., diet, stress, sleep, and physical activity, in addition to their body weight.[32] There are hundreds of free and subscription nutrition and physical activity apps available. Some are combined with wearable devices, while some

TABLE 13.1 Within-Practice Resources for Obesity Treatment

RESOURCE	OPTIONS	EXAMPLES
Educational handouts	Practice developed Downloadable	AACE (www.aace.com), OMA (obesitymedicine.org), OAC (www.obesityaction.org), TOS (www.obesity.org).
Image banks for positive patient images to be used in handouts/marketing	Practice developed Image banks	Obesity Canada (www.obesitycanada.ca) World Obesity Federation (www.worldobesity.org) Rudd Center (www.uconnruddcenter.org)
Peer support groups	Practice-led Practice supported but patient-led	Hospital and private bariatric surgery programs often have support groups already staffed
BIA (bioelectrical impedance analysis) (to measure body composition)	Single frequency Triple frequency Research level	Inbody (www.inbodyusa.com) Seca (www.seca.com) Tanita (www.tanita.com/en/howbiaworks)
Bod Pod (air displacement plethysmography) (to measure body composition)		Cosmed (https://www.cosmed.com/en/)
Resting metabolic rate, indirect calorimetry (to measure energy expenditure)	Requires single-use disposables	Med Gem (https://metabolicratetest.com/medgem-fda-approved-indirect-calorimeter/) Korr (https://korr.com/)

TABLE 13.2 Physical Activity Apps and Resources		
APP	**CATEGORY**	**SPECIAL FEATURES**
MapMyFitness MapMyWalk MapMyRun	Physical activity tracking and analytics	Tracks time, distance, speed of land-based activities. Can synchronize with wearables like Fitbit, Garmin, or Polar
Fitocracy	Physical activity tracking + motivation	Uses social networks. Virtual coaches are available
Daily Yoga	Discipline specific exercise	
7-Minute Workout	Physical activity routines	Time based for quick use; provides instructional videos
Sworkit	Buildable physical activity routines	Tailors to areas of need; provides demonstration videos for correct form
Fitbit	Tracks physical activity and sleep. Used with a wearable	Weekly summaries of distance, calories, weight, sleep

are data entry only. Table 13.2 displays physical activity smartphone apps (food tracking apps are listed in Chapter 5). In addition to apps where the patient interacts or manually enters data, one in six US consumers uses wearable technology to quantify adherence to goals and/or to improve behavior and habit change through "self-hacking."[33] The top reasons for using a wearable like pedometers, accelerometers, or other wearable technology like smart watches included physical activity tracking (54%); weight loss (40%); improved sleep (24%); and stress management (18%). Data are inconsistent on whether wearable technology improves weight loss. Initial smaller studies demonstrated greater weight loss with wearable technology.[34] However, a larger more recent study of 471 subjects found that those who used wearable technology lost slightly less than the standard intervention group.[35] Perhaps most interesting is the idea that an app or wearable technology may need to be able to evolve and tailor its messaging to an individual user over time to be successful at supporting long-term behavior change. For example, when a smartphone application surveyed the subjects and changed the cycle of messaging based on their individual responses to these intermittent surveys, overall walking increased by 1 mile per day and baseline steps increased by 4,000 steps per day.[36]

Helping a patient choose an app or wearable device can be individualized, just like other areas of obesity treatment. Table 13.3 lists unique features that should be considered when choosing a product. Specific features will be more or less important to certain patients and can affect successful adoption of use.

Home Resources

Developing a treatment plan includes assessing what resources the patient already has at home or is willing to consider purchasing. Examples that support dietary counseling include food scales and measuring cups or utensils. A body weight scale is important to self-monitor weight between visits. From a practice and treatment flow plan, having a Wi-Fi scale that transmits data back to the practice allows the HCP to utilize evaluation and management codes for reimbursement for monitoring weight between visits and adjusting care if needed. This monitoring can often be done by an RDN or nurse. Treatment of obesity using objectively measured home weights is similar to home blood pressure monitoring or cardiac monitoring. For example, a Health Insurance Portability and Accountability Act (HIPAA)–compliant remote monitoring scale may cost the practice $50 but can be recouped in the first month of remote monitoring data acquisition billable to the patient's insurance.

TABLE 13.3 Features of Weight Loss Smartphone Applications	
APP FEATURES TO CONSIDER	
Syncs with other apps/ devices	Real-time personalized feedback
Social media networking/ peer support	Customizable to skill or fitness level
Periodic summaries	Coaching/live chat Consultation available
Evidence-based information	Adaptive to user feedback
User friendly	Uses science-based behavioral models
Allows for goal setting	Free trial vs. free vs. cost

Probably the most important home resources to assess revolve around physical activity. Many patients enjoy exercise and prefer to be active at a health club or office gym. However, some individuals do not like or feel comfortable in the gym environment. This may be related to many variables including preference, low confidence in their physical ability, or stigma related to physical appearance. Patients may also need special consideration around orthopedic and other physical issues that limit their physical activity choices. For example, some patients need to be in an aquatic or gravity-mediated environment to manage osteoarthritis pain. Developing practice resources and recommendations to be active at home is essential. Consider having a handout with a list of recommended resources, exercises, and equipment. Some practices teach patients physical activity as part of their treatment. For examples, the practice can develop a physical activity kit that includes low-cost, low-risk physical activity equipment like exercise bands, physiology balls, and stretching straps. Handouts with a preplanned workout using the equipment can be given to patients. Some practices hold classes to teach patients how to use home equipment. The use of mHealth and apps can help facilitate home exercise, as discussed above. Like nutrition, physical activity goals and plans need to be individualized to each patient. Physical activity is discussed in greater detail in Chapter 6.

Finally, many patients need behavioral health support at home. This may include sleep health, stress reduction, contingency management plans, time management, anxiety management, and motivation. Home resources can include apps for deep breathing exercises, calendar reminders, and motivational encouragement. Behavioral coaching by phone from the HCP office or utilizing a coaching service can also allow for behavioral support at home.

Work Resources

The workspace itself can provide support for a patient's weight management efforts but may require resourcefulness and assertiveness. Work is where individuals spend most of their waking hours and often contributes to the obesogenic environment. However, some common pitfalls can be overcome. For example, patients can request a standing desk or a treadmill desk to transition from a sedentary workday to a light-activity workday by adding many hours of standing. Physiology balls can be used as chairs to encourage active sitting. Some work environments allow time in the day for employees to be more active, some provide discounts to gym memberships, while others provide flexible work schedules which may allow for more consistent health-targeted physical activity. Employee wellness programs also often offer programs around stress management.

Employers may also provide financial incentives for employees to meet health improvement benchmarks. So-called nongrandfathered health plans offered via state health insurance exchanges are required to cover high-intensity behavioral treatment of obesity by mandate of the Affordable Care Act (ACA). The ACA mandates coverage of services that have received a positive recommendation from the US Preventive Services Task Force.

Many of the home resources described previously could also be kept at work. For example, patients that struggle with getting physical activity due to time barriers might consider doing 5- to 10-minute bouts of exercise at work. They can do quick strength exercises using resistance bands while on conference calls, at the lunch hour, or while waiting for rush hour traffic to die down. An office gym or wellness program can also be helpful in reducing time-based barriers.

Similarly, keeping healthy snacks and protein-rich foods and supplements at work can help patients make better decisions when otherwise they might skip lunch or delay eating. If the work environment includes personal office space, patients can stock a small refrigerator with healthy food choices. Otherwise, a drawer of healthy snacks (e.g., protein bars) or even a cooler are all simple resources to consider. Whether it relates to food, stress, or physical activity, consider having a handout that shares all these ideas with patients to foster a more efficient counseling session during their medical visit.

Community Resources

Commercial weight loss programs (covered in Chapter 5 and briefly in Chapter 12) are a useful resource to consider when obesity treatment goals cannot be met within the practice. Evidence-based commercial programs are recommended in obesity treatment guidelines as an alternative for providing high-intensity behavioral treatment. Hospitals with bariatric surgery practices often have peer support groups that are open to individuals regardless of what dietary regimen they are employing.

Nutritionally, patients may want to utilize services that help make choosing healthier food easier. Many meal-delivery plans that provide entire meals proportioned and ready to cook are now available. Preproportioned and precooked meals are also available for pick up at commercial nutrition businesses. These nutritional services will provide the nutritional data that can be easily inputted into a food tracking app.

Regarding physical activity resources in the community, there are many different types of gyms, health clubs, and specialized exercise studios from which to choose. If cost is an issue, community resources such as city recreation centers, YMCAs, city parks, and schools are a good option. These physical activity facilities often have reduced rates based on geographic residence, sliding scales based on financial need, and free programs like Silver Sneakers and aqua arthritis programs. Many have free or minimal-fee day cares to support parents who have childcare responsibilities. The HCP should also consider virtual community resources such as Sparkpeople. com, which combines technology and resources to link individuals together to provide support.

TRAINING THE CURRENT AND NEXT GENERATION IN PRIMARY CARE

Competency in Obesity Knowledge

In the current medical training system, comprehensive obesity education from fundamental physiology to clinical treatment is minimal at best.[37] Improving fund of knowledge in the treatment of obesity can be achieved through three basic pathways: (1) continuing medical education (CME), (2) undergraduate, graduate, and postgraduate training pathways, (3) mentorship. In 2019, the Obesity Medicine Education Collaborative (OMEC) published the first obesity-focused competencies for HCPs and outlined in six major areas the knowledge and skills that HCPs should have to treat obesity.[38] The OMEC competencies can be downloaded and used as a guide to building education for students, residents, fellows, practicing providers, and healthcare systems. For example, all HCPs should be able to "Apply knowledge of obesity treatment guidelines to the development of a comprehensive personalized obesity management care plan" for a patient. HCPs should also be able to "Elicit a comprehensive obesity-focused medical history.... and physical exam for the assessment of obesity." At a more individual level, the competencies can be used to guide an HCP's continuing education. The competencies and a guide for use can be found at www.obesitymedicine. org/omec. HCPs are at the frontline of treatment and must have the knowledge, skills, and confidence to treat obesity as they treat other chronic diseases.

Fellowship

While obesity medicine is still in the process of obtaining American Board of Medical Specialties (ABMS) formal recognition, clinical fellowships to train obesity medicine specialists have existed for over a decade. Both graduating residents and practicing physicians can be accepted for fellowship training. Typically, the background of applicants for an obesity medicine fellowship is family medicine, internal medicine, endocrinology, or pediatrics. Most obesity medicine fellowships are 1 year in duration with a focus on clinical care. Fellowship completion also fulfills the requirements necessary to take the American Board of Obesity Medicine board examination. Detailed information on applying for fellowship or for starting a new fellowship is available at www.omfellowship.org.

Continuing Medical Education

For HCPs already in practice, education on obesity care is available at CME conferences, live or recorded online webinars and lectures, online enduring content, and obesity-focused journals. Most of the training offered is valuable to both physicians and APPs and may offer certificates of completion and/or certification. Table 13.4 shows some of the common obesity resources that provide obesity-focused continuing education.

Education as a Team

While there are many opportunities for discipline-specific education and training, several of the obesity-focused societies have diverse training options at in-person yearly conferences. These can provide the option for team members to attend sessions of their choice and then regroup as a team to strategize about improved patient care at the practice. For example, the Obesity Medicine Association, The Obesity Society, and the American Society of Metabolic and Bariatric Surgeons all have annual national educational meetings. These annual meetings provide an opportunity to learn from colleagues in the field about advances in science and clinical care. At the American Society for Metabolic and Bariatric Surgery (ASMBS), there is a track of sessions that are specific for allied health practitioners that run simultaneously to a track of sessions for physicians. At Obesity Week (The Obesity Society), there are several tracks that cover a wide diversity of topics, including basic science, clinical care, behavior, and population health. There are also section meetings that allow providers with specific interests in obesity like pediatrics, surgery, gastroenterology, clinical care, and research to come together. At the Obesity Medicine Association (OMA), there are some meeting days where a practice team can learn together, and some days where team members might select different tracks to attend based on different areas of focus in patient care. Many of these sessions at OMA provide case-based learning which can be valuable for a clinical team. Each of the meetings provide session breaks where the team can come back together and discuss changes to make in the practice to increase effectiveness and efficiency. In addition to the formal education which typically provides CME credits, the networking opportunities allow team members to talk to other practices and share successes, challenges, and clinical pearls.

In addition to yearly national meetings, there are also local education programs that can be a first step toward these larger, more time-intensive conferences. Many of the organizations have 1 day or weekend regional educational events that can be easier and more cost effective. For example, the OMA provides

TABLE 13.4 Societies, Certifications, and Academic Resources Supporting Obesity Education and Treatment		
ORGANIZATIONS		
AACE	American Academy of Clinical Endocrinologists	www.aace.org
ASMBS	American Society of Metabolic and Bariatric Surgery	www.asmbs.org
OMA	Obesity Medicine Association	www.obesitymedicine.org
TOS	The Obesity Society	www.obesity.org
Obesity Canada	Obesity Canada	www.obesitycanada.ca
WOF	World Obesity Federation	www.worldobesity.org
Certifications	**Providing Organization**	**Website and Candidates**
ABOM Certification	American Board of Obesity Medicine	www.abom.org Examination-based certification for physicians only
CDR's Interdisciplinary Obesity and Weight Management Certification	Commission on Dietetic Registration	www.cdrnet.org/interdisciplinary Examination-based certification for advanced practitioners, exercise physiologists, clinical psychologists, social workers, pharmacists, physical therapists, or dietitians
Certified Bariatric Nurse	American Society of Metabolic and Bariatric Surgery	https://asmbs.org/integrated-health/cbn-certification
Certificates of Learning	**Providing Organization**	**Requirements**
NP/PA Certificate of Advanced Education in Obesity Medicine	Obesity Medicine Association	Completion of 60 CE hours (no examination) www.obesitymedicine.org
Certificate in Primary Care Obesity Management	Obesity Medicine Association	For nurse practitioners and physicians' assistants
Strategic Center for Obesity Professional Education (SCOPE)	World Obesity Federation	Offers a series of online learning modules and a certification. Available to any healthcare professional
Obesity Journals		
Obesity	*Obesity Reviews*	*Obesity Science and Practice*
Surgery for Obesity and Related Diseases	*Obesity Surgery*	*Pediatric Obesity*
Clinical Obesity	*Diabetes, Obesity and Metabolism*	*International Journal of Obesity*
Journal of the Academy of Nutrition and Dietetics	*American Journal of Clinical Nutrition*	

a 1-day Fundamentals in Obesity Treatment course in four to six major US cities each year. Additionally, there are now local obesity organizations that offer opportunities to meet and learn about obesity care with colleagues in the practice's own community. These are typically quarterly dinner meetings and are likely to grow in number and size in the next few years. For example, there is the Illinois Obesity Society which meets in Chicago, the HOPE (Houston Obesity Partnership in Excellence) which meets quarterly in Texas, and similar organizations in many other US cities.

SUMMARY

Primary care providers are essential in the treatment of obesity. HCP practices will always have varying levels of resources to offer patients based on the clinic structure, provider knowledge, and resource availability. Deciding the level of obesity care a practice can offer and then ensuring that the practice team is prepared includes developing and evaluating the following elements: team structure, treatment flow, provider education, access to additional obesity testing, lifestyle intervention resources, referrals, medication and surgical treatments, web-based/mobile health resources, and community resources. Provision of these resources is essential to successful obesity treatment. Given the prevalence of obesity, all HCPs need at least a basic fund of knowledge in the evaluation and treatment of obesity. Collaborating with specialists in obesity treatment is essential to understanding and implementing excellent care and will ultimately improve patient experience and outcomes. Obesity is a serious chronic progressive disease that all HCP's should be prepared to treat.

WHEN TO REFER?

- Need for high-intensity treatment intervention program.
- Need for advanced medical evaluation and consideration for pharmacotherapy with an obesity medicine specialist.
- Need for advanced testing resources like metabolic or body composition testing.
- Continued weight gain or inability to lose weight using the tools available.
- Comorbidity history that complicates AOM decision-making.
- Need for bariatric surgery consultation.

CASE STUDY

Discussion

Grace would currently be documented as having Class I obesity (BMI between 30 and 34.9). At her last primary care visit, you helped her begin to link her weight and the disease of obesity to her other health issues. She had the opportunity to start to make healthy changes, but she has run up against a few barriers: her physiology and her pain. By opening the door to changing behaviors at the first visit, she is ready to consider other options and is more likely to take action. From a team standpoint, you are already succeeding. You and your team documented her BMI, recognized the relationship to other chronic conditions, and started the conversation with your patient.

The next steps in Grace's obesity treatment is to consider your resources and ability to deliver a high-intensity treatment intervention to give her the best opportunity to succeed. Your patient would benefit from a more thorough assessment of her disease which includes a detailed history of diet, physical activity, sleep, concurrent medications, and barriers for change. Consider asking Grace to begin to more formally track her food intake and physical activity, based on targets that you set together. Nutritional targets will include a reduction in calorie intake as well as change in type and quantity of foods or number of meals/snacks throughout the day. This level of detail and patient learning requires time. Grace can begin by using an app to facilitate food logging. Consider a referral to a previously defined RDN to expand on the details of the goals that you set together.

This visit is also an appropriate time to discuss starting an AOM with Grace. If you feel comfortable prescribing, consider starting an AOM at this visit. If you are not familiar enough to prescribe an AOM at this time, then it is time to consider taking advantage of multiple educational opportunities. An option for this visit would be to refer her to an obesity medicine specialist to get an AOM started to support her behavior change efforts by changing her physiology (controlling hunger). Finally, based on Grace's needs, consider the other resources you might want to include in her care plan. Does she need a physical therapy evaluation to guide her physical activity given the knee pain? Does Grace have access to gravity-mediated exercise choices to put in place of walking? Aqua aerobics, swimming, seated stationary bikes, or elliptical machines are all possibilities that would partially unweight the knee forces caused by gravity but still let her begin to recruit large muscle groups and raise her heart rate. Lastly, schedule follow-up so that together you can track her progress and offer changes in her treatment plan as needed.

CLINICAL HIGHLIGHTS

- All primary care providers can and need to manage obesity in their patients.
- Team care is essential to delivering effective obesity care.
- Successful treatment requires a bias- and stigma-free environment, including staff training and appropriate equipment.
- Referrals should be used to extend care needed when it goes beyond the practice resources.
- Patient resources range from handouts, apps, advanced testing, to intensive behavioral treatment programs.
- Successful obesity treatment depends on engaged patients and engaged providers.
- mHealth tools can extend care and provide for meaningful monitoring.
- Competency-based provider training and education is the key to improving provider knowledge, confidence, and delivery of effective care.

QUIZ QUESTIONS

1. A primary care team is considering how to improve its treatment of obesity. The electronic medical record automatically calculates BMI. However, the HCPs in the practice (two physicians, one nurse practitioner) do not routinely discuss weight with all patients. The next most appropriate step is:

   A. The medical assistant flags the charts of patients with BMI ≥30 kg/m²
   B. The HCPs undertake a chart audit to evaluate frequency of weight management counseling
   C. The HCPs refer all patients with BMI ≥30 kg/m² to an RDN
   D. The practice employs a registered nurse (RN) to conduct weight management counseling

   Answer: B. *A is not correct because the electronic record already calculates BMI and the HCPs are aware of it. B is the most correct answer to obtain a baseline for quality improvement. C is not correct, since it is the job of the HCP to make the initial diagnosis and select a treatment strategy. D is not correct since an RN does not have the practice scope of an HCP to assess a patient's weight-related health risk.*

2. An HCP is considering how to decide which patients are referred for a bariatric surgery evaluation. The most appropriate criterion for the HCP to use is:

   A. The patient has tried and failed pharmacotherapy for obesity
   B. The patient meets BMI criteria
   C. The patient has the nutrition knowledge needed to succeed with surgery
   D. The patient has tried and failed repeated courses of lifestyle modification

   Answer: D. *A is not correct because there is no requirement to have tried medication before being referred for a surgical evaluation. B is a necessary prerequisite for a surgical referral but is not an appropriate indication on its own. C is not correct because knowledge or perceived motivation are not reliable predictors of outcome after bariatric surgery. D is the most correct, as repeated courses of lifestyle modification with inability to maintain weight loss is an appropriate referral criterion.*

PRACTICAL RESOURCES

- Obesity Action Coalition (www.obesityaction.org); this resource provides patient handouts, patient first language, and how to become an advocate for patients.
- The Obesity Society (www.obesity.org); this resource offers further online education, all levels of scientific input from bench to bedside, and *Obesity* the journal.
- American Association of Clinical Endocrinologists (www.aace.com); AACE offers a complication centric treatment algorithm.
- Obesity Medicine Association (www.obesitymedicine.org); this organization provides physician/advanced practitioner online education and an ongoing clinical educational home.
- American Society of Metabolic and Bariatric Surgery (www.asmbs.org); this resource offers bariatric surgery guidelines and description of center of excellence qualifications.
- Positive Patient-Focused Image Banks
  - Rudd Center Image Gallery (www.uconnruddcenter.org/image-library)
  - Obesity Canada Image bank (https://obesitycanada.ca/resources/image-bank/)
  - World Obesity federation Image bank (www.worldobesity.org/resources/image-bank)
- Project Implicit (www.implicit.harvard.edu/implicit/); this resource includes testing for obesity bias.
- Sparkpeople (www.sparkpeople.com); this is a healthy living online community.
- TOPS—Take Off Pounds Sensibly (www.TOPS.org); TOPS is a nonprofit weight-loss support and wellness education organization.

REFERENCES

1. Diabetes policy brief. Centers for Disease Control and Prevention website. Accessed January 2020. https://www.cdc.gov/ruralhealth/diabetes/policybrief.html

2. Hales CM, Carroll MD, Fryar CD, Ogden CL. *Prevalence of Obesity Among Adults and Youth: United States, 2015-2016. NCHS Data Brief No. 288.* National Centre for Health Statistics; 2017. Accessed January 2020. https://www.cdc.gov/nchs/data/databriefs/db288.pdf

3. Torti J, Luig T, Borowitz M, Johnson JA, Sharma AM, Campbell-Sherer DL. The 5A's team patient study: patient perspectives on the role of primary care in obesity management. *BMC Fam Pract.* 2017; 18:19.

4. Dhurandhar NV, Kyle T, Stevenin B, Tomasceqski K; The ACTION Steering Group. Predictors of weight loss outcomes in obesity care: results of the National ACTION Study. *BMC Public Health.* 2019; 19:1422.

5. Mitchell P, Wynia M, Golder R, McNellis B, Okun S, Webb CE. *Core Principles and Values of Effective Team-Based Health Care*. Discussion Paper. 2012. Accessed April 2020. https://nam.edu/wp-content/uploads/2015/06/VSRT-Team-Based-Care-Principles-Values.pdf

6. Schottenfeld L, Petersen D, Peikes D, Ricciardi R, Burack H, McNellis R, Genervro J. *Creating Patient-Centered Team-Based Primary Care*. White Paper for Agency for Healthcare Research and Quality. Accessed April 2020. https://pcmh.ahrq.gov/sites/default/files/attachments/creating-patient-centered-team-based-primary-care-white-paper.pdf

7. Mickan SM, Rodger SA. Effective health care teams: a model of six characteristics developed from shared perceptions. *J Interprof Care*. 2005;19(4):358-370.

8. Kaplan LM, Golden A, Jinnett KJ, et al. Perceptions of barriers to effective obesity care: results from the national ACTION study. *Obesity*. 2018;26:61-69.

9. Wadden TA, Butryn ML, Hong BA, Tsai AG. Behavioral treatment of obesity in patients encountered in primary care settings: a systematic review. *J Am Med Assoc*. 2014;213(17):1779-1791.

10. Tsai AG, Remmert JE, Butryn ML, Wadden TA. Treatment of obesity in primary care. *Med Clin North Am*. 2018;102:35-47.

11. Martin PD, Dutton GR, Rhode PC, Horswell RL, Ryan DH, Brantley PJ. Weight loss maintenance following a primary care intervention for low income minority women. *Obesity*. 2008;16(11):2462-2467.

12. Christian JG, Bessesen DH, Byers TE, Christian KK, Goldstein MG, Bock BC. Clinic-based support to help overweight patients with type 2 diabetes increase physical activity and lose weight. *Arch Intern Med*. 2008;168(1):141-146.

13. Jensen MD, Ryan DH, Apovian CM, et al. 2013 AHA/ACC/TOS guidelines for the management of overweight and obesity in adults: a report of the American College of Cardiology/American Heart Association task force on practice guidelines and the Obesity Society. *J Am Coll Cardiol*. 2014;63(25 pt B):2985-3023.

14. ter Bogt NCW, Bemelmans WJE, Beltman FW, Broer J, Smit AJ, van der Meer K. Preventing weight gain by lifestyle intervention in a general practice setting: three-year results of a randomized controlled trial. *Arch Intern Med*. 2011;171(4):306-313.

15. Kumanyika SK, Fassbender JE, Sarwer DB, et al. One-year results of the Think Health! study of weight management in primary care practices. *Obesity*. 2012;20(6):1249-1257.

16. Renjilian DA, Perri MG, Nezu AM, McKelvey WF, Shermer RL, Anton SD. Individual versus group therapy for obesity: effects of matching participants to their treatment preferences. *J Consult Clin Psychol*. 2001;69(4):717-721.

17. Falvo AM, Philp FH, Eid GM. Primary care provider management of patients with obesity at an integrated health network: a survey of practices, views, and knowledge. *Surg Obes Relat Dis*. 2018;14(8):1149-1154.

18. Sumithran P, Prendergast LA, Delbridge E, et al. Long-term persistence of hormonal adaptations to weight loss. *N Engl J Med*. 2011;365(17):1597-1604.

19. Lam YY, Ravussin E. Analysis of energy metabolism in humans: a review of methodologies. *Mol Metab*. 2016;5(11):1057-1071.

20. Rueda-Clausen CF, Benterud E, Bond T, Olszowka R, Vallis MT, Sharma AM. Effect of implementing the 5As of Obesity Management framework on provider-patient interactions in primary care: 5As of obesity management in primary care. *Clin Obes*. 2014;4(1):39-44.

21. Jay M, Kalet A, Ark T, et al. Physicians' attitudes about obesity and their associations with competency and specialty: a cross-sectional study. *BMC Health Serv Res*. 2009;9(1):106.

22. Fitzpatrick SL, Wischenka D, Appelhans BM, et al; on behalf of the Society of Behavioral Medicine. An evidence-based guide for obesity treatment in primary care. *Am J Med*. 2016;129(1):115.e1-115.e7.

23. Mechanick JI, Apovian C, Brethauer S, et al. Clinical practice guidelines for the perioperative nutrition, metabolic, and nonsurgical support of patients undergoing baritric procedures – 2019 update: Cosponsored by American Association of Clinical Endocrinologists/American College of Endocrinology, The Obesity Society, American Society for Metabolic & Bariatric Surgery, Obesity Medicine Association, and American Society of Anesthesiologists. *Endocr Pract*. 2019;25(12):1346-1359.

24. US Government Accountability Office. *Report to Congressional Committees. Obesity Drugs: Few Adults Used Prescription Drugs for Weight Loss and Insurance Coverage Varied*. 2019. Accessed January 2020. https://www.gao.gov/assets/710/700815.pdf

25. Ponce J, Nguyen NT, Hutter M, Sudan R, Morton JM. American Society for Metabolic and Bariatric Surgery estimation of bariatric surgery procedures in the United States, 2011-2014. *Surg Obes Relat Dis*. 2015;11(6):1199-1200.

26. Ward ZJ, Bleich SN, Cradock AL et al. Projected U.S. State-level prevalence of adult obesity and severe obesity. *N Engl J Med*. 2019;381(25):2440-2450.

27. Centers for Medicare and Medicaid Services. *Decision Memo for Intensive Behavioral Therapy for Obesity*. 2011. Accessed January 2011. https://www.cms.gov/medicare-coverage-database/details/nca-decision-memo.aspx?NCAId=253

28. Imbus JR, Voils CI, Fund LM. Bariatric surgery barriers: a review using Andersen's Model of Health Services Use. *Surg Obes Relat Dis*. 2018;14:404-412.

29. Glauser TS, Roepke N, Stevenin B, Dubois AM. Physician knowledge about and perceptions of obesity management. *Obes Res Clin Pract* 2015;9(6):573-583.

30. The Statistics Portal. Number of health apps being used by patients worldwide to manage their conditions as of 2017. Accessed July 2018. https://www.statista.com/statistics809394/health-apps-number-usage-share-by-known-patients

31. The Statistics Portal. Number of apps available in leading app stores as of 2nd quarter of 2020. Accessed November. https://www.statista.com/statistics/276623/number-of-apps-in-leading-app-stores/

32. Thomas JG, Bond DS, Phelan S, Hill JO, Wing RR. Weight-loss maintenance for 10 years in the national weight control registry. *Am J Prev Med*. 2014;46(1):17-23.

33. Piwek L, Ellis DA, Andrews S,Joinson A. The rise of consumer health wearables: Promises and Barriers. *PLoS Med*. 2016;13(2):e1001953.

34. Pellegrini CA, Verba SD, Otto AD, Helsel DL, Davis KK, Jakicic JM. The comparison of a technology-based system and an in-person behavioral weight loss intervention. *Obesity (Silver Spring)*. 2012;20(2):356-363.

35. Jakicic JM, Davis KK, Rogers RJ, et al. Effect of wearable technology combined with a lifestyle intervention on long-term weight loss: the IDEA randomized clinical trial. *J Am Med Assoc*. 2016;316(11):1161-1171.

36. Korinek EV, Phatak SS, Martin CA, et al. Adaptive step goals and rewards: a longitudinal growth model of daily steps for smartphone-based walking intervention. *J Behav Med*. 2018;41(1):74-86.

37. Butsch WS, Kushner RF, Alford S, Smolarz BG. Low priority of obesity education leads to lack of physician' preparedness to effectively treat patients with obesity: results from the U.S. medical school obesity education curriculum benchmark study. Presentation at WGEA/WGSA/WOSR Collaborative Spring Conference. 2019.

38. Kushner RF, Horn DB, Butsch WS, et al. Development of obesity competencies for medical education: a report from the obesity medicine education collaborative. *Obesity*. 2019;27(7):1063-1067.

Appendices

APPENDIX

RESOURCES FOR THE HEALTHCARE PROFESSIONAL

TABLE 2.3 Using the Mnemonic "OPQRST" to Take the Weight History	
	SAMPLE QUESTIONS
Onset	"When did you first begin to gain weight?" "Have you struggled with your weight since childhood?" "Do you remember how much you weighed in high school, college, early 20s, 30s, 40s?" "Did the weight gain begin when you started taking a new medication?"
Precipitating	"What life events led to your weight gain, e.g., college, long commute, marriage, divorce, financial loss, depression, illness, etc.?" "How much weight did you gain with pregnancy?" "How much weight did you gain when you stopped smoking?" "How much additional weight did you gain when you started insulin?"
Quality of life	"At what weight did you feel your best?" "What is hard to do at your current weight?" "How does your weight affect how you feel and function?"
Remedy	"What have you done or tried in the past to control your weight?" "Have you made any changes to your diet?" Have you made any changes to your physical activity?" "Have you taken any medications to help control your weight?" "What is the most successful approach you tried to lose weight?" "What do you attribute the weight loss to?" "What caused you to regain your weight?" "What are the biggest challenges in maintaining your weight?"
Setting	"What was going on in your life when you last felt in control of your weight?" "What was going on when you gained your weight?" "What role has stress played in your weight gain?" "How important is social support or having a buddy to help you?" "Do you currently have social support from your family and friends to help you manage your weight?"
Temporal pattern	"What is the pattern of your weight gain?" "Did you gradually gain your weight over time, or is it more cyclic (yo-yo)?" "Are there large swings in your weight, and if so, what is the weight change?" "What was your lightest weight and heaviest weight as an adult?"

Reprinted from Kushner RF, Batsis JA, Butsch WS, et al. Weight history in clinical practice: The state of the science and future directions. Obesity. 2020;28:9-17.

1. What is the least you have weighed as an adult (21 years and older)? _____

2. What is the most you have weighed as an adult, not including pregnancy (21 years and older)? _____

3. At what ages have you been overweight? *(Check all that apply)*

☐ Childhood (under 12 years old)   ☐ Middle adulthood (40 to 65 years old)

☐ Adolescence (12 to 18 years old)   ☐ Late adulthood (65 years and older)

☐ Early adulthood (18 to 40 years old)

4. What was the cause of your weight gain? *(Check all that apply)*

☐ Genetics   ☐ Menopause

☐ Unhealthy diet   ☐ Quitting smoking

☐ Not enough physical activity   ☐ Medications

☐ Pregnancy   ☐ Depression/grief/stress

☐ Medical problem   ☐ I don't know

5. What are your concerns about excess weight?

_____

_____

6. What methods have you tried to lose weight in the past? *(Check all that apply)*

☐ Nothing   ☐ Commercial diet programs

☐ Keeping track of the food I eat   ☐ Working with a registered dietitian

☐ Counting calories   ☐ Weight-loss medication

☐ Exercise   ☐ Weight-loss surgery (bariatric)

☐ Specific eating plans (Atkins/keto,
   South Beach, Zone, etc.)

7. What was your greatest amount of weight loss, and what strategies did you use to lose weight at that time?

_____

_____

8. What are your barriers to losing weight and/or keeping it off?

_____

_____

9. Please list what you typically eat and drink for meals and snacks. Please provide as much detail as you can (portion size, method of preparation, etc.)

Meal	Foods and beverages that I usually eat
Breakfast	
Snack	
Lunch	
Snack	
Dinner	
Snack	

FIGURE 2.2 (Continued)

10. Do you normally plan your meals and snacks? *Circle* **YES** *or* **NO**

11. Please check a box to tell us how often you eat or drink the following.

	Never	Once a week	Several times per week	Every day
Fast food				
Fruits and vegetables				
Any sugared drink (soda, juice, sweet tea, sports drinks)				

12. How may we help you manage your weight and eating habits? *(Check all that apply)*

☐ Diet and nutrition education   ☐ Stress-induced eating education

☐ Portion control education   ☐ Binge-eating education

☐ Meal planning education   ☐ Food preparation education

How many hours per day are you sitting? _____

13. Do you track your activity or your total calories burned on a device? *Circle* **YES** *or* **NO**

If **YES**, what is your usual daily activity level (steps, minutes, distance)?

_____

14. How many minutes per week do you do physical activity (such as brisk walking)?

_____

15. Do you exercise (swim, bike, run, or use a cardio machine)? *Circle* **YES** *or* **NO**

If **YES**, what do you do and how often?

_____

_____

16. Do you do strength training? *Circle* **YES** *or* **NO**

If **YES**, how many times per week? _____

17. What barriers stand in your way of increasing your physical activity? *(Check all that apply)*

☐ Time limitations   ☐ Access to equipment or safe environment

☐ Lack of enjoyment   ☐ Lack of peer or family support

☐ Physical limitations   ☐ I don't know

18. Are you interested in any of the following assistance options? *(Check all that apply)*

☐ Weight-loss handouts/books   ☐ Health psychologist consultation

☐ Weight-loss websites   ☐ Weight-loss medication

☐ Commercial weight-loss program   ☐ Bariatric surgery

☐ Registered dietitian consultation   ☐ I am not ready for assistance at this time

19. If you are interested in assistance, what is your preferred method of support? *(Check all that apply)*

☐ In-person consultation   ☐ In-person classes

☐ Phone call consultation   ☐ Online seminars

FIGURE 2.2 Weight management previsit questionnaire.

TABLE 2.5 DSM-5 criteria for diagnosis of Binge Eating Disorder (DSM-5)

A. Recurrent episodes of binge eating. An episode of binge eating is characterized by both of the following:

1. Eating, in a discrete period of time (e.g., within any 2-hour period), an amount of food that is definitely larger than most people would eat during a similar period of time and under similar circumstances.
2. A sense of lack of control over eating during the episode (e.g., a feeling that one cannot stop eating or control what or how much one is eating).

B. The binge-eating episodes are associated with three (or more) of the following:

1. Eating much more rapidly than normal.
2. Eating until feeling uncomfortably full.
3. Eating large amounts of food when not feeling physically hungry.
4. Eating alone because of feeling embarrassed by how much one is eating.
5. Feeling disgusted with oneself, depressed, or very guilty afterward.

C. Marked distress regarding binge eating is present.

D. Binge eating occurs, on average, at least once a week for three months.

E. The binge eating is not associated with the recurrent use of inappropriate compensatory behavior as in bulimia nervosa and does not occur exclusively during the course of bulimia nervosa or anorexia nervosa.

Specify if:

In partial remission: After full criteria for binge-eating disorder were previously met, binge eating occurs at an average frequency of less than one episode per week for a sustained period of time.

In full remission: After full criteria for binge-eating disorder were previously met, none of the criteria have been met for a sustained period of time.

Specify current severity:

The minimum level of severity is based on the frequency of episodes of binge eating (see below). The level of severity may be increased to reflect other symptoms and the degree of functional disability.

Mild: 1-3 binge-eating episodes per week.

Moderate: 4-7 binge-eating episodes per week.

Severe: 8-13 binge-eating episodes per week.

Extreme: 14 or more binge-eating episodes per week.

TABLE 2.6 Practical Assessment of Physical Activity

- What is the most physically active thing you do in the course of the day? (examples may include walking as needed, walking the dog, stair climbing, house or yard work, exercising)
- How do you spend your working day and leisure time?
- What types of physical activity do you enjoy? How often do you do them?
- How many hours of TV do you watch every day? How many hours are you at a computer or desk every day?
- Are you *currently exercising regularly?*
- If answer yes (ask the following questions):
  - How many days per week do you exercise?
  - How many minutes per exercise session?
  - What type of activity do you engage in?
  - What is the intensity of your exercise? Low, moderate, or vigorous
- If answer no (ask the following questions):
  - How do you feel about/what are your thoughts on initiating/are you ready to initiate physical activity?
  - What are the barriers to initiating physical activity for you (i.e., access to gym, access to safe environment, injuries, or physical limitations)?
  - What are the benefits of physical activity for you?
  - Describe your previous experiences with exercise?
- Do you have any negative feelings about exercise or had any bad experiences with exercise?
- Do you have a support system to encourage you to exercise or exercise with you?
- How much time are you able to commit to exercise?

TABLE 2.7 Practical Assessment of Sleep

- What time do you usually go to bed?
- What time do you usually wake up in the morning?
- Do you fall asleep within 30 minutes of lying on the bed?
- How many times do you wake up at night?
- What is the reason you wake up at night?
- Do you feel well rested in the morning?
- How many times have you used sleep aids in the past month?

TABLE 2.8 Practical Assessment of Stress

PERCEIVED STRESS SCALE 4

For each of the four questions, a range of scores is assigned based from 0 = never to 4 = very often. Reverse scores for questions 2 and 3 like this: 0 = 4, 1 = 3, 2 = 2, 3 = 1, 4 = 0.
Now add up scores for each item to get a total score which varies between 0 and 16.
Higher scores indicative of higher perceived stress.

(Continued)

TABLE 2.8 Practical Assessment of Stress   (Continued)

PERCEIVED STRESS SCALE 4

_____ 1. In the last month, how often have you felt that you were unable to control the important things in your life?

_____ 2. In the last month, how often have you felt confident about your ability to handle your personal problems?

_____ 3. In the last month, how often have you felt that things were going your way?

_____ 4. In the last month, how often have you felt difficulties were piling up so high that you could not overcome them?

Modified from Cohen S, Kamarck T, Mermelstein R. A global measure of perceived stress. J Health Soc Behav. *1983;24:385-396.*

TABLE 2.9 Obesity-Related Organ Systems Review

Cardiovascular	Respiratory
Hypertension	Dyspnea/deconditioning
Congestive heart failure	Obstructive sleep apnea
Cor pulmonale	
Varicose veins	Obesity hypoventilation syndrome, also known as Pickwickian syndrome
Pulmonary embolism	Asthma
Coronary artery disease Atrial fibrillation	**Gastrointestinal**
Endocrine	Gastroesophageal reflux disease
Metabolic syndrome	Nonalcoholic fatty liver disease
Type 2 diabetes	Cholelithiasis
Dyslipidemia	Hernias
Polycystic ovarian syndrome	Colon cancer
Cushing syndrome	
Hypogonadism/erectile dysfunction	
Musculoskeletal	**Genitourinary**
Hyperuricemia and gout	Urinary stress incontinence
Immobility	Obesity-related glomerulopathy

TABLE 2.9 Obesity-Related Organ Systems Review   (Continued)

Osteoarthritis (knees and hips)	Breast and uterine cancer
Low back pain	Pregnancy complications
Carpal tunnel syndrome	
Psychological	**Neurologic**
Depression/low self-esteem	Stroke
Body image disturbance	Idiopathic intracranial hypertension
Internal stigmatization	Meralgia paresthetica
Integument	Dementia
Striae distensae	
Stasis pigmentation of legs	
Lymphedema	
Cellulitis	
Intertrigo, carbuncles	
Acanthosis nigricans	
Acrochordons (skin tags)	
Hidradenitis suppurativa	

TABLE 2.10 Physical Examination of the Patient With Obesity: Domains of Special Interest

DOMAIN	WHAT TO EXPECT	WHAT TO DO
Vital signs	Body mass index (BMI) requires accurate measurement of weight and height Miscuffing wide arm circumferences leads to spurious blood pressure readings	Have scales with wide base and weight limit >350 lb; use wall-mounted stadiometer if possible Have large blood pressure cuffs available
Head and neck	Crowded oropharynx may suggest obstructive sleep apnea Patients may have insulin resistance	Use Mallampati score I to IV (Figure 2.4) to describe the pharynx Examine the neck and axillae for acanthosis nigricans (Figure 2.5)

TABLE 2.10 Physical Examination of the Patient With Obesity: Domains of Special Interest (Continued)

DOMAIN	WHAT TO EXPECT	WHAT TO DO
Abdomen	Upper body fat distribution signifies increased risk for metabolic syndrome	Have paper or plastic tape measure available to measure waist circumference (if BMI 25 – <35 kg/m^2) Examination of the abdominal skin
Cardio-vascular	Patients may have peripheral edema and venous status of the lower extremities	Check for pitting edema and examine the lower extremities with socks removed
Skin	Patients with excessive skinfolds are prone to develop carbuncles, furuncles, and fungal infections Bruising and purplish striae >1 cm may signify Cushing syndrome	Examine all skinfolds, particularly under the breasts and abdominal panniculus

Adapted from Silk AW, McTigue KM. Reexamining the physical examination for obese patients. J Am Med Assoc. *2011;305:193-194.*

TABLE 2.11 Ethnic Specific Values for Waist Circumference (cm)

COUNTRY/ ETHNIC GROUP	MALE	FEMALE
North American	≥102 cm	≥88 cm
European	≥94 cm	≥80 cm
South Asian/ Chinese	≥90 cm	≥80 cm
Japanese	≥85 cm	≥90 cm
Ethnic South and Central Americans	Use South Asian recommendations	Use South Asian recommendations
Sub-Saharan Africans	Use European data	Use European data

TABLE 2.11 Ethnic Specific Values for Waist Circumference (cm) (Continued)

COUNTRY/ ETHNIC GROUP	MALE	FEMALE
Eastern Mediterranean and Middle East (Arab) populations	Use European data	Use European data

Modified from Alberti KG, Zimmet P, Shaw J. Metabolic syndrome – A new world-wide definition. A Consensus Statement from the International Diabetes Federation. Diabet Med. *2006;23:469-480.*

TABLE 3.1 Aggravating Factors and Social and Environmental Determinants

	FACTORS AFFECTING INDIVIDUALIZED CARE PLAN	POSSIBLE INTERVENTIONS
Medications	Examples: insulin, TZDs, sulfonylureas; β-adrenergic receptor blockers; antipsychotics; certain antidepressants; antiepileptics; glucocorticoids	• Assess the need for offending medication • Substitute with weight neutral alternative

Psycho-logical/ psychiatric factors	• Depression
	• Anxiety disorder
	• Psychosis
	• Binge eating disorder
	• Night eating syndrome
	• Stigmatization
	• Stress
		• Psychological screening
		• Counseling
		• Referral
		• Medications
		  • Antide-pressants
		  • Anxiolytics
		  • Antiobesity medications to address cravings

Social and environ-mental deter-minants	• Behaviors • Cultural factors • Time management • Access to unprocessed foods • Physical activity resources • Work related • Health literacy • Access to clinics/hospitals • Economic status • Health insurance	• Motivational interviewing • Counseling (personal and family) • Dietitian referral • Education • Social work referral • Information regarding community resources

TZDs, thiazolidinediones.

TABLE 3.2 Underlying Causes of or Aggravating Factors Causing Obesity

CAUSE OF OBESITY	SPECIFIC DISORDER	SIGNS AND SYMPTOMS
Monogenic or syndromic	Prader-Willi syndrome	• Onset in childhood • Strong family history • Infertility/hypogonadism • Delayed or absent puberty • Short stature or macrosomia • Intellectual disability • Behavior problems • Unexplained organ system defects (e.g., heart, kidney) • Visual or olfactory impairment • Dysmorphic features (e.g., face, digits)
	MC4R deficiency	
	Leptin deficiency	
	Leptin receptor deficiency	
	POMC deficiency	
	Alström syndrome	
	Bardet-Biedl syndrome	
	Beckwith-Wiedemann syndrome	
	WAGR-O syndrome (BDNF deficiency)	
	Wilson-Turner syndrome	
Aggravating endocrine disorders	Hypothyroidism	• Cold intolerance, lethargy, weakness • Constipation • Delayed reflexes • Bradycardia
	Hypercortisolism	• Weakness, poor concentration • Bruising and purple striae • Acne, moon facies • Thin skin and central fat redistribution
	Hypothalamic/CNS injury	• Lethargy • Decreased libido • Polyuria
Aggravated by disability	Immobilization	• Muscle weakness • Gait abnormality • Disability evident on presentation
	Neuromuscular disease or injury	
	Movement disorder	
Idiopathic/common type		• Most common • Diagnosis of exclusion • No identifiable causal influence

BDNF, brain-derived neurotrophic factor; CNS, central nervous system POMC, pro-opiomelanocortin, WAGR-O, Wilms tumor, aniridia, genitourinary anomalies, and mental retardation and obesity.

TABLE 3.3 Examination, Review of Systems (ROS), and Laboratory Findings for the Identification of Weight-Related Complications

ORGAN SYSTEM	ROS	EXAMINATION	LABORATORY FINDING	COMPLICATION	FURTHER TESTING
Anthropometric Component of the Diagnosis of Obesity					
Adipose tissue		BMI, waist circumference Exclude: muscularity, edema, sarcopenia, solid tumor mass, lipodystrophy		• **Increased adipose tissue mass**	Impedance plethysmography, DEXA scan
Clinical Component of the Diagnosis of Obesity					
Diabetes	Symptoms of hyperglycemia	Foot examination	Fasting glucose, HbA1c	• **Prediabetes** • **Diabetes**	HbA1c 5.7%-6.4% or fasting glucose 100-125 mg/dL HbA1c ≥ 6.5% or fasting glucose ≥126 mg/dL
Insulin resistance		Waist circumference, blood pressure, acanthosis nigricans	Fasting glucose, lipid panel	• **Metabolic syndrome** • **Dyslipidemia** • **Hypertension**	Non-HDL-c or apoB-100 may further define risk; ambulatory BP monitoring
Liver		Enlarged liver, firm liver edge	LFTs, NASH biomarker scoring	• **NAFLD** • **NASH**	Ultrasound, consider referral, biopsy
Cardiovascular	Chest pain, syncope, orthopnea, SOB, claudication, stroke/TIAs	Heart examination, ABI, carotid auscultation, edema	ECG	• **CAD** • **CVD** • **PVD** • **CHF**	Stress test, imaging, arteriography, or ultrasound, consider referral
Pulmonary	Fatigue, snoring, poor sleep, SOB, poor exercise tolerance	Neck circumference, lung examination (wheezing, rales)		• **Obstructive sleep apnea** • **Asthma**	Polysomnography (clinical laboratory or home testing), spirometry, consider referral
Endocrine	Lethargy, weakness, skin changes, hair loss, trouble concentrating, acne, decreased libido, cold intolerance	Skin and hair abnormalities, pigmented striae, fat distribution, proximal muscle weakness, abnormal muscle reflexes, abnormal thyroid		• **Hypothyroidism** • **Hypercortisolism** • **Hypopituitarism** • **Hypothalamic/ CNS injury**	Hormone testing, endocrine gland imaging, consider referral
Sex steroids	Oligomenorrhea, infertility	Hirsutism	Testosterone, estradiol LH/ FSH	• **PCOS** • **Infertility**	Imaging of ovaries, consider referral

(Continued)

TABLE 3.3 Examination, Review of Systems (ROS), and Laboratory Findings for the Identification of Weight-Related Complications   (Continued)

ORGAN SYSTEM	ROS	EXAMINATION	LABORATORY FINDING	COMPLICATION	FURTHER TESTING
Musculoskeletal	Joint pain, limited motion	Swelling, crepitus		• **Osteoarthritis**	Radiographic imaging
Gastrointestinal	Heartburn, abdominal pain	Abdominal tenderness	LFTs	• **GERD** • **Cholelithiasis/cystitis**	Endoscopy, esophageal motility study, abdominal imaging, consider referral
Urinary tract	Stress incontinence			• **Urinary stress incontinence**	Urine culture, consider referral, urodynamic testing
Psychological	Depressed, suicidal ideation, anxiety, stigmatization, binge eating, drugs, and alcohol			• **Depression** • **Anxiety disorder** • **Psychosis** • **Binge eating syndrome** • **Night eating syndrome** • **Stigmatization** • **Stress**	Validated questionnaires, psychological testing and evaluation, consider referral
Impaired functional capacity	Impaired activities of daily living, immobility	Weakness, paralysis, limited motion		• **Immobilization** • **Neurological disease/injury**	Functional testing may be helpful

ABI, ankle-brachial index; BMI, body mass index; BP, blood pressure; CAD, coronary artery disease; CHF, congestive heart failure; CNS, central nervous system; CVD, cardiovascular disease; DEXA, dual-energy X-ray absorptiometry; ECG, electrocardiograph; GERD, gastroesophageal reflux disease; HDL-c, high-density lipoprotein cholesterol; LFT, liver function tests; LH/TSH, luteinizing hormone/follicle-stimulating hormone; NAFLD, nonalcoholic fatty liver disease; NASH, nonalcoholic steatohepatitis; PCOS, polycystic ovary syndrome; PVD, peripheral vascular disease; SOB, shortness of breath; TIA, transient ischemic attack.

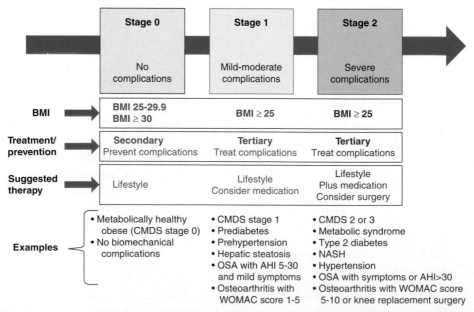

FIGURE 3.4 Staging the severity of obesity using the AACE clinical practice guidelines. AHI, apnea-hypopnea index; BMI, body mass index; CMDS, cardiometabolic disease staging; NASH, nonalcoholic steatohepatitis; OSA, obstructive sleep apnea; WOMAC, Western Ontario and McMaster Universities Osteoarthritis Index and is a patient-reported outcome measure for osteoarthritis registering pain, stiffness, and function.[12]

TABLE 3.5 ATP III Criteria for Metabolic Syndrome (Must Have at Least Three of These Five Risk Factors)

RISK FACTOR	DEFINING LEVEL
1. Waist	≥40 in (102 cm) men ≥35 in (88 cm) women
2. Triglycerides	≥150 mg/dL (1.7 mmol/L)
3. HDL-c	<40 mg/dL (1.03 mmol/L) men <50 mg/dL (1.29 mmol/L) women
4. Blood pressure	≥130/≥85 mm Hg
5. Fasting glucose	≥100 mg/dL (5.6 mmol/L)

ATP III, Adult Treatment Panel III; HDL-c, high-density lipoprotein cholesterol.

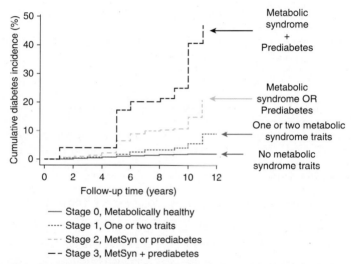

FIGURE 3.6 Cumulative risk of developing diabetes among patients with overweight or obesity. Validation of the prediction of incident diabetes in the CARDIA study cohort. (Modified from Guo F, Moellering DR, Garvey WT. The progression of cardiometabolic disease: validation of a new cardiometabolic disease staging system applicable to obesity. *Obesity*. 2014;22:110-118.)

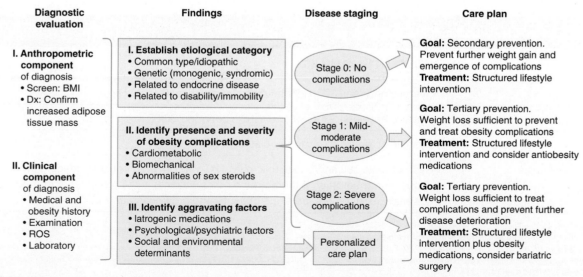

FIGURE 3.7 Diagnostic evaluation and disease staging: implications regarding therapy. Staging provides a guide for selecting the modality and intensity of therapy as well as treatment goals. BMI, body mass index; ROS, review of systems.

TABLE 3.6 Disease Staging for the High-Risk Case Study Patient

COMPLICATION		AACE STAGE	RATIONALE
Cardiometabolic	Metabolic syndrome	AACE Stage 2	Meets criteria for both prediabetes and metabolic syndrome placing the patient in the highest CMDS risk stratum for future diabetes
	Prediabetes		
	Hypertension	AACE Stage 2	Blood pressure not at target despite two hypertension medications
Biomechanical	Obstructive sleep apnea	AACE Stage 2	The AHI at polysomnography consistent with moderate severity but symptom of marked daytime lethargy indicates that this complication should be treated at a higher level of severity

Aggravating Factors to Be Considered in Developing an Effective Treatment Plan

Category	Factor	Solution
Iatrogenic	Atenolol and paroxetine could contribute to obesity	Switch to calcium channel blocker for hypertension and bupropion or venlafaxine for depression
Psychological	Depression	Consider referral to psychologist; continue medication
	Nighttime food cravings	Antiobesity medication to blunt cravings; dietitian referral
	Stigmatization (guarded in social settings)	Consider referral to psychologist; counseling; education about obesity as a disease; motivational interviewing
	Feelings of ineffectiveness	
Social and environmental	Sedentary job (paralegal)	Engage in progressively longer walks with dog in the evening
	Reliance on fast food	Encouraged to have "dinner nights" with coworker taking turns several times per week to prepare dinner with leftovers for lunch on the next day. Dietitian referral

AACE, American Association of Clinical Endocrinologists; CMDS, Cardiometabolic Disease Staging.

TABLE 4.1 Criteria for the Diagnosis of HTN[a]

NORMAL	LESS THAN 120/80 MM HG
Elevated	Systolic between 120-129 and diastolic less than 80 mm Hg
Stage 1	Systolic between 130-139 or diastolic between 80-89 mm Hg
Stage 2	Systolic at least 140 or diastolic at least 90 mm Hg
Hypertensive crisis	Systolic over 180 and/or diastolic over 120 mm Hg, with patients needing prompt changes in medication if there are no other indications of problems, or immediate hospitalization if there are signs of acute end organ damage

HTN, hypertension.
[a]Based on accurate measurements and average of at least 2 readings on at least 2 occasions.
Adapted from Whelton PK, Carey RM, Aronow WS, et al. 2017 ACC/AHA/AAPA/ABC/ACPM/AGS/APhA/ASH/ASPC/NMA/PCNA guideline for the prevention, detection, evaluation, and management of high blood pressure in adults: a report of the American College of Cardiology/American Heart Association Task Force on Clinical Practice Guidelines. J Am Coll Cardiol. 2018;71(19):e127-e248.

TABLE 4.2 Lifestyle Modification and Its Effect on Blood Pressure and Treatment of Hypertension

	NONPHARMACOLOGIC INTERVENTION	DOSE	APPROXIMATE IMPACT ON SBP	
			HYPERTENSIVE	NORMOTENSIVE
Weight loss	Weight/body fat	Ideal body weight is best goal but at least 1 kg reduction in body weight for most adults who are overweight. Expect about 1 mm Hg for every 1 kg reduction in body weight	−5 mm Hg	−2/3 mm Hg
Healthy diet	DASH dietary pattern	Diet rich in fruits, vegetables, whole grains, and low-fat dairy products with reduced content of saturated and trans fat	−11 mm Hg	−3 mm Hg
Reduced intake of dietary sodium	Dietary sodium	<1,500 mg/d is optimal goal but at least 1,000 mg/d reduction in most adults	−5/6 mm Hg	−2/3 mm Hg
Enhanced intake of dietary potassium	Dietary potassium	3,500-5,000 mg/d, preferably by consumption of a diet rich in potassium	−4/5 mm Hg	−2 mm Hg
Physical activity	Aerobic	• 90-150 minutes/week • 65%-75% heart rate reserve	−5/8 mm Hg	−2/4 mm Hg
	Dynamic resistance	• 90-150 minutes/week • 50%-80% 1 rep maximum • Six exercises, three sets/exercise, 10 repetitions/set	−4 mm Hg	−2 mm Hg
	Isometric resistance	• 4 × 2 minutes (hand grip), 1 minute rest between exercises, 30%-40% maximum voluntary contraction, three sessions/week • 8-10 weeks	−5 mm Hg	−4 mm Hg
Moderation in alcohol intake	Alcohol consumption	In individuals who drink alcohol, reduce alcohol to • Men: ≤2 drinks daily • Women: ≤1 drink daily	−4 mm Hg	−3 mm Hg

DASH, Dietary Approaches to Stop Hypertension; SBP, systolic blood pressure.
Modified from Whelton PK, Carey RM, Aronowthe WS, et al. 2017 ACC/AHA/AAPA/ABC/ACPM/AGS/APhA/ASH/ASPC/NMA/PCNA guideline for the prevention, detection, evaluation, and management of high blood pressure in adults: a report of the American College of Cardiology/American Heart Association Task Force on Clinical Practice Guidelines. J Am Coll Cardiol. *2018;71(19):e127-e248.*

TABLE 4.3 Risk factors for Testing for Diabetes or Prediabetes in Asymptomatic Adults

1. First-degree relative with diabetes
2. High-risk race/ethnicity (e.g., African American, Latino, Native American, Asian American, and Pacific Islander)
3. History of cardiovascular disease
4. Hypertension
5. Dyslipidemia (HDL cholesterol level < 35 mg/dL and/or a triglyceride level >250 mg/dL)
6. Polycystic ovary syndrome
7. Other clinical conditions associated with insulin resistance

Modified from American Diabetes Association. Standards of Medical Care in Diabetes-2019 Abridged for Primary Care Providers. Clin Diabetes. *2019;37(1):11-34.*

TABLE 4.5 Drug-specific and Patient Factors to Consider When Selecting Antihyperglycemic Treatment in Adults With DM2

	HYPOGLYCEMIA	EFFECT ON WEIGHT	CARDIOVASCULAR EFFECTS		ORAL/SQ	RENAL EFFECTS	OTHER
			ASCVD	CHF		PROGRESSION OF CKD	
Biguanide: Metformin	No	Modest weight loss	Potential benefit	Neutral	Oral	Neutral	Gastrointestinal side effects B12 deficiency
SGLT-2 inhibitors: Canagliflozin Empagliflozin Dapagliflozin Ertugliflozin	No	Loss	Benefit	Benefit	Oral	Benefit	FDA black box: Risk of amputation (canagliflozin)
GLP-1 agonists: Liraglutide Semaglutide Exenatide ER Dulaglutide	No	Loss	based on agent	Neutral	SQ	Benefit	FDA black box: thyroid C-cell tumors. GI side effects
DPP-4 inhibitors: Saxagliptin Alogliptin Sitagliptin Linagliptin	No	Neutral	Neutral	Risk	Oral	Neutral	Risk of acute pancreatitis
Thiazolidinediones: Pioglitazone	No	Gain	Benefit	Risk	Oral	Neutral	FDA black box: CHF
Sulfonylureas: Glyburide Glipizide Glimepiride	Yes	Gain	Neutral	Neutral	SQ	Neutral	Injection site reactions
Insulin	Yes	Gain	Neutral	Neutral	SQ	Neutral	Higher risk of hypoglycemia with human insulin vs. analogs

ASCVD, atherosclerotic cardiovascular disease; CHF, congestive heart failure; CKD, chronic kidney disease; DM2, diabetes mellitus type 2; ER, extended release; FDA, U.S. Food and Drug Administration; GI, gastrointestinal; SQ, subcutaneous.
Modified from American Diabetes Association. 9. Pharmacologic approaches to glycemic treatment: standards of medical care in diabetes-2019. Diabetes Care. 2019;42(suppl 1):S90-S102.

TABLE 4.6 OSA Screening Questionnaires and Prediction Tools

BERLIN QUESTIONNAIRE[49]	EPWORTH SLEEPINESS SCALE[50]	STOP-BANG[51]
Are there changes in weight? **Category 1:** Do you snore? Snoring loudness Snoring frequency Has snoring bothered others? Frequency of witnessed apnea? **Category 2:** Morning fatigue? Frequency of morning fatigue Have you fallen asleep at the wheel? **Category 3:** History of hypertension BMI ≥30 mg/m²	How likely are you to doze off or fall asleep in the following situations, in contrast to feeling tired (0-3)? 1. Sitting and reading 2. Watching TV 3. Sitting, inactive in public place 4. As a passenger in a car for an hour without break 5. Lying down to rest in the afternoon when circumstances permit 6. Sitting and talking to someone 7. Sitting quietly after a lunch without alcohol 8. In a car, while stopped for a few minutes in the traffic	Do you **snore** loudly? Do you feel **tired**, fatigued, or sleepy during the daytime? Has anyone **observed** you stop breathing or choking/gasping during sleep? Do you have high blood **pressure**? **BMI** ≥ 35 mg/m² **Age** ≥ 50 years old **Neck** size (male ≥ 17 inches, females ≥ 16 inches) **Gender** = Male
High risk: If there are two or more categories where the score is positive	**High risk:** A score of ≥10	**High risk:** Yes to five to eight questions Yes to more than two STOP questions + male gender or BMI ≥ 35 kg/m² or neck circumference

BMI, body mass index; OSA, obstructive sleep apnea.

TABLE 4.8 Society Cancer Screening Recommendations

United States Preventive Services Task Force (USPSTF) A and B Recommendations

Breast cancer screening	Screening mammography for women, with or without clinical breast examination, every 1-2 years for women aged 50 years or older. The decision to start screening mammography in women prior to age 50 years should be an individual one.
Cervical cancer screening	The USPSTF recommends screening for cervical cancer every 3 years with cervical cytology alone in women aged 21-29 years. For women aged 30-65 years, the USPSTF recommends screening every 3 years with cervical cytology alone, every 5 years with high-risk human papillomavirus (hrHPV) testing alone, or every 5 years with hrHPV testing in combination with cytology.
Colorectal cancer screening	The USPSTF recommends screening for colorectal cancer starting at the age of 50 years and continuing until the age of 75 years.

American Association for the Study of Liver Disease recommendations

Liver cancer screening*	The AASLD recommends abdominal ultrasound and/or AFP every 6 months for patients with cirrhosis from NAFLD based on laboratory test, imaging, or biopsy. No screening is recommended for noncirrhosis NAFLD.

AASLD, American Association for the Study of Liver Diseases; AFP, alpha-fetoprotein; NAFLD, nonalcoholic fatty liver disease.
*No screening is recommended for gastric cardia cancer, pancreatic cancer, or gallbladder cancer in the asymptomatic population.
Adapted from Heimbach JK, Kulik LM, Finn RS, et al. AASLD guidelines for the treatment of hepatocellular carcinoma. Hepatology. 2018;67(1):358-380.

TABLE 4.9 Comparison of PHQ9 to PHQ2 Depression Screening Tests

PATIENT HEALTH QUESTIONNAIRE-9 (PHQ-9[b])	PATIENT HEALTH QUESTIONNAIRE-2 (PHQ-2[a])
Over the past 2 weeks, how often have you been bothered by any of the following problems? (0-Not at all, 1-Several days, 2-More than half the days, 3-Nearly every day)	
Little interest in doing things	Little interest in doing things
Feeling down, hopeless or depressed	Feeling down, hopeless or depressed
Trouble falling asleep or staying asleep, or sleeping too much	
Feeling tired or having little energy	
Poor appetite or overeating	
Feeling bad about yourself, feeling like a failure	
Trouble concentrating on things	
Moving or speaking slowly, or the opposite, restless and fidgety	
Thoughts that you would be better off dead, or thoughts of hurting yourself	

[a]PHQ-2: Score of >3 is positive, proceed with PHQ-9.
[b]PHQ-9: Scoring 1 to 4 = minimal depression; 5 to 9 = mild depression; 10 to 14 = moderate depression; 15 to 19 = moderately severe depression; 20 to 27 = severe depression.
Adapted from Maurer DM, Raymond TJ, Davis BN. Depression: screening and diagnosis. Am Fam Physician. 2018;98(8):508-515.

TABLE 4.10 Antidepressant Medications Effect on Weight

WEIGHT GAIN	WEIGHT NEUTRAL/ LESS WEIGHT GAIN	WEIGHT LOSS
Tricyclics MAOIs SSRIs (Paroxetine) Mirtazapine	SSRIs (Fluoxetine, Sertraline) SNRIs (Duloxetine, Venlafaxine)	Bupropion

MAOIs, monoamine oxidase inhibitors; SNRIs, serotonin norepinephrine reuptake inhibitors; SSRIs, selective serotonin reuptake inhibitors.
Adapted from Igel LI, Kumar RB, Saunders KH, Aronne LJ. Practical use of pharmacotherapy for obesity. Gastroenterology. 2017;152(7):1765-1779.

TABLE 5.1 Weight Management Resources and Tracking Tools for Internet and Smartphone Apps[a]

WEIGHT MANAGEMENT RESOURCES AND TRACKING TOOLS FOR INTERNET AND SMARTPHONE APPS	SPECIAL FEATURES
Calorie King www.calorieking.com	Food nutrition database
Bitesnap www.bitesnap.com	Photo food tracker
Cooking Light www.cookinglight.com	*Cooking Light* magazine recipes
EatingWell www.eatingwell.com	Healthy recipes and meal plans
Fitday www.fitday.com	Food tracker
Fooducate www.fooducate.com	Scans barcodes of items and gives it a nutritional grade with information
Hungry Girl www.hungrygirl.com	Low-calorie recipes
Livestrong www.livestrong.com	Food tracker
Lose It! www.loseit.com	Food tracker
MyFitnessPal www.myfitnesspal.com	Food tracker
My-Food-Diary www.myfooddiary.com	Food tracker
Noom www.noom.com	Digital weight management program using cognitive behavioral therapy
Skinny Taste www.skinnytaste.com	Healthy recipes
Spark People www.sparkpeople.com	Online weight management program
USDA Foodkeeper www.choosemyplate.gov	US Department of Agriculture food tracker that uses the MyPlatefood groups and meal plans
WW (formally Weight Watchers) www.weightwatchers.com	Digital and in-person comprehensive weight management program

[a]Selected items as of May 2020.

TABLE 5.2 Dietary Counseling in the Office Setting

DIETARY PATTERNS	CLINICAL CONSIDERATIONS	KEY NUTRITIONAL FEATURES	RESOURCES (ACCESSED MAY 2020)
DASH (dietary approaches to stop hypertension)	Hypertension	High intake of fruits (4-5 servings/day); vegetables (4-5 servings/day); legumes; low-fat dairy	https://www.nhlbi.nih.gov/files/docs/public/heart/dash_brief.pdf https://www.nhlbi.nih.gov/files/docs/public/heart/new_dash.pdf http://www.healthyinfo.com/consumers/ho/nut.dash.diet.pdf
Mediterranean	Type 2 diabetes mellitus Prediabetes Metabolic syndrome CVD	Vegetables (3-9 servings/day); fresh fruit (up to 2 servings/day); cereals: mostly whole grain (from 1 to 13 servings/day); oil (up to 8 servings of olive oil/day); fat—mostly unsaturated—up to 37% of the total calories; nuts, legumes, fish, and poultry	https://health.usnews.com/best-diet/mediterranean-diet https://oldwayspt.org/traditional-diets/mediterranean-diet https://www.medicalnewstoday.com/articles/149090
Low-fat diet	Hyperlipidemia CVD	<30% of total calories from fat <10% saturated fats	https://health.usnews.com/wellness/food/articles/what-is-a-low-fat-diet https://www.healthline.com/nutrition/healthy-low-fat-foods

CVD, cardiovascular disease.

TABLE 5.3 Three Evidence-based National Commercial Programs

	WW (FORMALLY WEIGHT WATCHERS)	JENNY CRAIG	NUTRISYSTEM
Meal plan	Based on point system, subscribers choose one of three food-based programs	Provides preprepared low-calorie foods that are shelf-stable for three meals and two snacks per day; patients supplement with fruits, vegetables, and dairy	Provides preprepared low-calorie foods that are shelf-stable, with patients supplementing fruits and vegetables. Eat six times per day. Foods are delivered every 4 weeks
Counseling services	Begins with personal assessment, followed by options of digital, in-person, and virtual workshops and personal coaching; social community support	Weekly 1:1 meeting with a coach for weight loss guidance (in-person or telephonic), personalized feedback, and meal planning	No counseling services are offered

TABLE 5.4 Intermittent Fasting Strategies

Intermittent Fasting Strategies	Fast Day	Nonfasting Day
ADF (alternate-day fasting)	Complete fasting	Ad libitum eating
mADF (modified alternate-day fasting)	Modified fasting = 25% of daily calories	125% of daily calories
1:6	Fasting 1 day/week	6 days ad libitum eating
2:5	75% of daily requirements 2 days/week	Isocaloric diet 5 days/week
Time-Restricted Eating Strategies	**Fasting Period**	**Eating Period**
18:6[a]	18 hours fasting	6 hours eating
16:8	16 hours fasting	8 hours eating

[a]Early time-restricted eating 8 AM-3 PM (dinner meal before 3:00 PM) has been associated with greater metabolic benefit.

TABLE 6.1 Summary of Key Recommendations From the 2018 Physical Activity Guidelines for Americans

KEY RECOMMENDATIONS

1. Adults should move more and sit less throughout the day. Some physical activity is better than none. Adults who sit less and do any amount of moderate-to-vigorous physical activity gain some health benefits.

2. For substantial health benefits, adults should do at least 150 minutes (2 hours and 30 minutes) to 300 minutes (5 hours) a week of moderate-intensity aerobic physical activity, or 75 minutes (1 hour and 15 minutes) to 150 minutes (2 hours and 30 minutes) a week of vigorous-intensity aerobic physical activity, or an equivalent combination of moderate-intensity and vigorous-intensity aerobic activity. Preferably, aerobic activity should be spread throughout the week.

3. Additional health benefits are gained by engaging in physical activity beyond the equivalent of 300 minutes (5 hours) of moderate-intensity physical activity a week.

4. Adults should also do muscle strengthening activities of moderate or greater intensity and that involve all major muscle groups on 2 or more days a week, as these activities provide additional health benefits.

TABLE 6.2 Physical Activity and Exercise Terminology	
TERMS	**DEFINITION**
Metabolic equivalents (METs)	A method of standardizing the intensity of an activity. This method is based on the energy cost of an activity. 1 MET is equivalent to the resting energy expenditure. 3 METs, which is considered moderate-intensity physical activity, means that the activity elicits an energy cost that is threefold resting energy expenditure.
Aerobic activity	Activities where the energy demand is met via aerobic pathways; also known as cardiovascular activities; typically associated with increases in breathing and heart rate.
Strength/resistance activity	A form of physical activity that focuses on muscular contraction and seeks to improve muscular strength and endurance. Typically done for shorter periods of time compared with aerobic activity.
Rating of perceived exertion (RPE)	The perceived intensity of an activity. Usually rated on a 0-10 scale. Moderate intensity is typically associated with an RPE of 3-5.
Sedentary behavior	Time spent awake with a low energy expenditure (<1.5 METs) in a sitting/reclining posture. Examples: watching TV, desk work, driving
Light physical activity	Activities where heart rate is not elevated much above resting (≥1.5-<3.0 METs). Examples: normal daily activity, intermittent periods of normal walking, some forms of yoga
Moderate physical activity	Activities where heart rate is moderately elevated (50%-70% of maximum heart rate); ≥3.0-<6.0 METs. Examples: brisk walking, cycling <10 miles/hour, water aerobics
Vigorous physical activity	Activities where heart is elevated (70%-85% of maximum heart rate); ≥6.0 METs. Examples: running, swimming, cycling >10 miles/hour
Moderate-to-vigorous physical activity	Any activity ≥3.0 METs. Commonly used in public health recommendations. This is a summary measure that includes both moderate and vigorous physical activity
Dose/volume	The total dose or volume of activity is usually a summary of weekly activity. For overall health benefits, the dose of physical activity should progress up to 300 minutes/week. For weight loss and weight loss maintenance, even higher amounts of physical activity may be necessary. Energy expenditure per week: Physical activity and exercise can be prescribed based on the energy expenditure of activity. This type of prescription is difficult and requires careful measurements. It is typically done in controlled research studies. MET-minutes per week: This prescription takes into account the intensity and duration of physical activity. The MET value of each activity is multiplied by the duration of the activity. Measuring physical activity as MET-min is typically done in research studies only.

TABLE 6.3 Strategies to Overcome Common Barriers to Physical Activity

COMMON BARRIERS TO PHYSICAL ACTIVITY	SUGGESTED STRATEGIES TO OVERCOME BARRIERS
Time	Is it true that you do not have time for one more step? Or, is it that you do not have a full 30 minutes to spare, so you think it's not worth doing anything at all? Most people find it's the latter. You can almost always choose to modify your plans and just move—even if it's only a few more steps.
Family commitments	1. Communicate with your family about your self-care needs. Bring your partner and children on board with your plans and let them know things that you may need help with in order to be more active. Examples include asking your partner to make dinner two nights a week, telling your child that during their soccer practice, you will be walking at an area nearby but that you will be back in time to pick them up, etc. 2. Incorporate your family into your physical activities. You can go for a family walk, bike ride, or hike. You can play with the kids at the playground, instead of sitting and watching them play.
Work commitments	Physical activity and your work commitments do not have to conflict. In fact, physical activity can help you be more productive at work, reduce anxiety/stress, and improve your memory and cognition. 1. Communicate with your boss and/or coworkers about your self-care needs. Some language you could use include, "I know that you are used to me working at the office past 5:00 PM, but I wanted to communicate with you that I am trying to take better care of myself. I'd like to plan to be out of the office by 5:00 PM on Mondays and Wednesdays so that I can get to a Zumba class. On these days, I'll be sure to be in by 8:00 AM." 2. Working walk/walking meeting: Many people find that they have better ideas and feel freed up for creativity when they walk and work outside of the office environment. 3. Standing work station: Instead of sitting at your desk, try standing up and working.
Weather	Think creatively about things you can do when the weather is poor. 1. Walk around an indoor mall. 2. Wear proper gear so you can be active outside. For the winter, activities like snow shoeing or cross-country skiing can be quite enjoyable. 3. Try out your local gym. Most gyms offer a complimentary day pass. 4. Search YouTube for exercise videos to do at home.
Illness/injury	1. For any serious illness/injury, seek a healthcare professional. 2. Ease back into being physically active and take it slow. 3. Modify the activity. For lower body injuries, try the arm ergometer. For overuse injuries, try swimming or water aerobics—these can help take pressure off your joints.
Boring	1. Focus on enjoyment. What are movements that you actually enjoy doing? Try those instead! 2. Try moving while spending time with a friend or family member. Go for a hike, call someone just to catch up while walking around a park. 3. Try a sport. For example, pickleball is easy to learn and easy on your body.

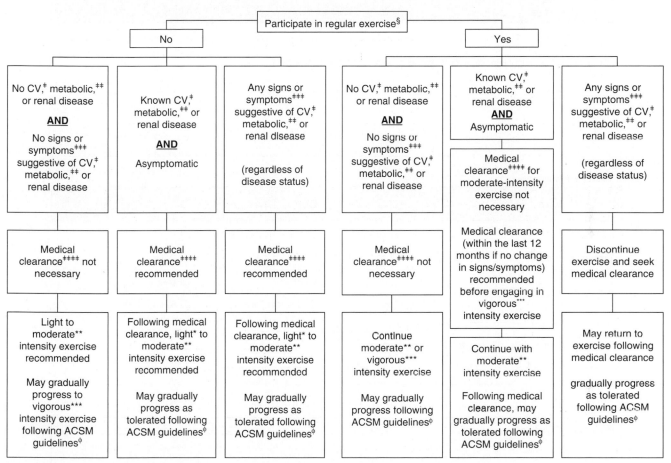

§Exercise participation, performing planned, structured physical activity at least 30 min at moderate intensity on at least 3 d.wk⁻¹ for at least the last 3 months.

*Light-intensity exercise, 30% to < 40% HRR or VO₂R, 2 to <3 METs, 9-11 RPE, an intensity that causes slight increases in HR and breathing.

**Moderate-intensity exercise,40% to, <60% HRR or VO₂R, 3 to <6 METs, 12-13 RPE, an intensity that causes noticeable increases in HR and breathing.

***Vigorous-intensity exercise ≥60% HRR or VO2R, ≥6 METs, ≥14 RPE, an intensity that causes substantial increases in HR and breathing.

‡CVD, cardiac, peripheral vascular, or cerebrovascular disease.

‡‡Metabolic disease, type1 and 2 diabetes mellitus.

‡‡‡Signs and symptoms, at rest or during activity, include pain, discomfort in the chest, neck, jaw, arms, or other areas that may result from ischemia; shortness of breath at rest or with mild exertion; dizziness or syncope; orthopnea or paroxysmal nocturnal dyspnea; ankle edema; palpitations or tachycardia; intermittent claudication; known heart murmur; or unusual fatigue or shortness of breath with usual activities.

‡‡‡‡Medical clearance, approval from a health care professional to engage in exercise.

ᶲACSM Guidelines, see *ACSM's Guidelines for Exercise Testing and Prescription, 9th edition, 2014.*

FIGURE 6.2 American College of Sports Medicine preparticipation screening algorithm. (Reprinted from Riebe D, Franklin BA, Thompson PD, et al. Updating ACSM's recommendations for exercise preparticipation health screening. *Med Sci Sports Exerc.* 2015;47(11):2473-2479.)

Name: _____ Date: _____

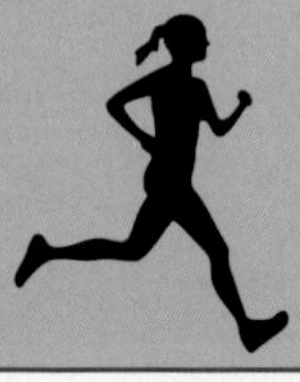

Physical Activity Prescription Pad

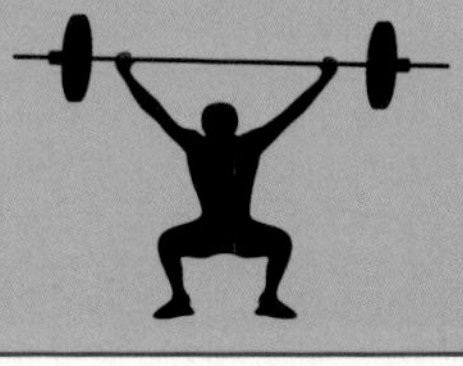

Current Physical Activity Level: _____

Patient Goals (i.e. weight loss, increase fitness level, walk up a flight of stairs, etc.):

   a. _____

   b. _____

   c. _____

Exercise Prescription:

Frequency (days/week):	☐ 1	☐ 2	☐ 3	☐ 4	☐ 5	☐ 6	☐ 7

Intensity: ☐ Light (casual walk)   ☐ Moderate (brisk walk)   ☐ Vigorous (jogging)

Time (minutes/day):   ☐ 10 ☐ 20 ☐ 30 ☐ 40 ☐ 50 ☐ 60 ☐ Other_____

Type: ☐ walk   ☐ Run   ☐ Bike

      ☐ Group Class   ☐ Strength Training   ☐ Swim

      ☐ Other _____

Details (i.e. Progressions, HR goal, follow-up in a month, etc.): _____

_____

_____

_____

Prescriber's Signature: _____

FIGURE 6.3 Physical activity prescription pad.

TABLE 7.1 Problem-Solving Steps

STEP	DESCRIPTION
1. Problem identification	• Establish that the patient agrees that there is a problem • Agree on the definition of the problem/target for intervention
2. Brainstorming	• Develop a list of potential solutions to the target problem • Use behavioral analysis to facilitate the development of a wide variety of potential solutions
3. Pro/con analysis	• Help patient select a strategy that will be acceptable and also likely to effectively resolve the problem • Discuss the patients' perceived benefits and costs associated with each possible solution
4. Selection of a plan	• Select and write down a plan of action including a target behavior/problem, well-defined goal, detailed plan of action tailored to the individual, specified period during which the effectiveness will be evaluated, and specified target goal defined in objective terms
5. Evaluation of effectiveness	• After a specified period of time, evaluate strategy to determine if it achieved predetermined goal • If successful, continue solution • If unsuccessful, discuss process of behavior change, problems with implementation, examine new intervention options, and repeat steps

TABLE 7.2 The 5 *A*'s for Obesity Treatment in Primary Care

CMS'S 5 *A*'S	DEFINITION	EXAMPLES
Assess	Ask whether the patient feels comfortable having a discussion regarding their weight. Assess patient readiness to manage weight through behavioral changes. Assess BMI, waist circumference, "root causes" of obesity, and effects of weight on psychosocial factors.	"Would it be alright if we talked about your weight?" "Can you tell me about your diet and exercise habits?" "How confident are you that you will be able to change your eating and exercise habits?"
Advise	Encourage patient that there are benefits to healthier lifestyles regardless of their weight. Provide specific and personalized behavior change recommendations.	"You might want to try self-monitoring with a food journal and activity log." "Since it sounds like you travel a lot for work, let's brainstorm some on-the-go meals that would fit your calorie goals."
Agree	Collaborate with patient to come up with realistic behavioral changes and goals with the patient's personal interests in mind. Place emphasis on changing behavior rather than pounds lost.	"How many days a week do you think you could realistically go to the gym after work?" "How would you feel about trying to food log on just the weekdays to start?"
Assist	Help patient to identify and address any barriers or obstacles that might challenge their goals. Recommend weight-management resources or refer patient to IBT programs that could provide more specialized care.	"How do you think your friends and family could support you in your diet changes?" "Would you be interested in making an appointment with a dietitian?
Arrange	Schedule follow-up contacts with patient to check in with patient and adjust the treatment plan as needed.	"I will give you a call in 2 weeks to see how our plan is going."

BMI, *body mass index; CMS, Centers for Medicare and Medicaid Services; IBT, intensive behavioral treatment.*

TABLE 8.3 Medications Approved in the United States: Common Side Effects and Safety Issues[a]

DRUG, GENERIC NAME	COMMON SIDE EFFECTS	CONTRAINDICATIONS AND SAFETY ISSUES
Phentermine	• Headache, elevated BP, elevated HR • Insomnia, dry mouth, constipation, anxiety • Cardiovascular: palpitation, tachycardia, elevated BP, ischemic events • Central nervous system: overstimulation, restlessness, dizziness, insomnia, euphoria, dysphoria, tremor, headache, psychosis • Gastrointestinal: dryness of the mouth, unpleasant taste, diarrhea, constipation, other gastrointestinal disturbances • Allergic: urticaria • Endocrine: impotence, changes in libido	• Anxiety disorders (agitated states), history of heart disease, uncontrolled hypertension, • Seizure • MAO inhibitors • Pregnancy and breastfeeding, • Hyperthyroidism • Glaucoma • History of drug abuse • Sympathomimetic amines
Orlistat	• Steatorrhea • Oily spotting • Flatulence with discharge • Fecal urgency • Oily evacuation • Increased defecation • Fecal incontinence	• Contraindicated in pregnancy • Warning: ↑cyclosporine exposure • Liver failure (rare) • Requires coadministration of multi-vitamin • Increased risk of gall bladder disease • Increased urine oxalate; monitor renal function

(Continued)

TABLE 8.3 Medications Approved in the United States: Common Side Effects and Safety Issues[a]   (Continued)

DRUG, GENERIC NAME	COMMON SIDE EFFECTS	CONTRAINDICATIONS AND SAFETY ISSUES
Phentermine/ Topiramate ER	• Insomnia • Dry mouth • Constipation • Paresthesias • Dizziness • Dysgeusia (altered taste)	• Contraindicated in pregnancy • Fetal toxicity; monthly pregnancy test suggested • Contraindicated with hyperthyroidism, glaucoma • Do not use with MAOIs or sympathomimetic amines • Metabolic acidosis and kidney stones • Acute myopia—angle closure glaucoma (rare)
Naltrexone SR/ Bupropion SR	• Nausea • Constipation • Headache • Vomiting • Dizziness	• Boxed warning: suicide risk in depression • Contraindicated in pregnancy • Contraindicated in seizure disorders, uncontrolled hypertension • Do not use with opioids, MAOIs • Hepatotoxicity (rare) • Warning: angle closure glaucoma
Liraglutide 3.0 mg	• Nausea • Vomiting • Diarrhea • Constipation • Headache • Dyspepsia • Fatigue • Dizziness • Abdominal pain	• Boxed warning: thyroid C-cell tumors in rodents • Contraindicated with personal or family history of medullary thyroid cancer or multiple endocrine neoplasia • Pancreatitis • Hypoglycemia in diabetes • Increased risk of gall bladder disease

BP, blood pressure; HR, heart rate; MAOI, monoamine oxidase inhibitor.
[a]*Information from product labels of prescribing information, except where noted.*

TABLE 8.4 Dual Benefits to Guide Obesity Medication Selection

IF PATIENT HAS OBESITY AND	CONSIDER THIS MEDICATION (BUT NOT EXPLICITLY APPROVED)
Smoking	Naltrexone/Bupropion
Depression	Naltrexone/Bupropion
Migraines	Phentermine/topiramate
Diabetes	Liraglutide 3.0 mg
Chronic constipation	Orlistat
Elevated LDL	Orlistat

LDL, low-density lipoprotein.

TABLE 8.5 Medications Which Promote Weight Gain and Alternative Approaches

WEIGHT GAIN ASSOCIATED WITH USE	ALTERNATIVES (WEIGHT REDUCING IN PARENTHESES)
Medications for diabetes • Insulin • Sulfonylureas • Thiazolidinediones • Meglitinide	• (Metformin) • Alpha-glucosidase inhibitors • DPP-4 inhibitors • (Pramlintide) • (GLP-1 receptor agonists) • (SGLT 2 inhibitors)
Antidepressants/mood stabilizers: **Tricyclic antidepressants** • Amitriptyline • Doxepin • Imipramine • Nortriptyline • Trimipramine • Mirtazapine	• (Bupropion) • Nefazodone • Fluoxetine, short term • Sertraline, given <1 year
Antidepressants/mood stabilizers: **Selective Serotonin Reuptake Inhibitors** • Paroxetine • Fluvoxamine	
Antidepressants/mood stabilizers: **Monoamine Oxidase Inhibitors** • Phenelzine • Tranylcypromine	
Mood stabilizers • Lithium	
Antipsychotic medications • Clozapine • Risperidone • Olanzapine • Quetiapine • Haloperidol • Perphenazine	• Ziprasidone • Aripiprazole
Anticonvulsants • Carbamazepine • Gabapentin • Valproate	• Lamotrigine • (Topiramate) • (Zonisamide)

TABLE 8.5 Medications Which Promote Weight Gain and Alternative Approaches   (Continued)

WEIGHT GAIN ASSOCIATED WITH USE	ALTERNATIVES (WEIGHT REDUCING IN PARENTHESES)
Hypertension medications • α-blocker • β-blocker, i.e., atenolol, metoprolol, nadolol, propranolol	• ACE inhibitors • Calcium channel blockers • Angiotensin-2 receptor antagonists
Contraceptives • Injectable progesterone • Oral progesterone	• Barrier methods • IUDs • Oral contraceptives preferable to injectable
Endometriosis treatment • Depot leuprolide acetate	• Surgical treatment
Chronic inflammatory diseases • Glucocorticoids	• Nonsteroidal anti-inflammatory drugs • Disease-modifying antirheumatic drugs
AIDS treatment • Antiretroviral therapies may adversely affect body fat distribution	• No therapeutic alternatives but monitoring and counseling are appropriate

ACE, angiotensin-converting enzyme; AIDS, acquired immunodeficiency syndrome; IUD, intrauterine device.
Adapted from Apovian CM, Aronne LJ, Bessesen DH, et al. Pharmacological management of obesity: An Endocrine Society clinical practice guideline. J Clin Endocrinol Metab. 2015;100(2):342-362. Erratum in: J Clin Endocrinol Metab. 2015;100(5):2135-2136.

TABLE 9.1 Preoperative Checklist

PREOPERATIVE CHECKLIST FOR METABOLIC AND BARIATRIC SURGERY

• Comprehensive history and physical	• Identify treatable causes of obesity and treat, if present • Look for inclusion criteria meeting the National Institutes of Health and insurance criteria • Note contraindications for surgery, if present • Document medical necessity for surgery including obesity-related comorbidities, weight, body mass index • Assess patient level of commitment • Identify history of cancer, if present • Assess for nicotine use (smoking, vaping, patch, chewing, etc.) and require nicotine cessation; refer for counseling if needed

(Continued)

TABLE 9.1 Preoperative Checklist   (Continued)

PREOPERATIVE CHECKLIST FOR METABOLIC AND BARIATRIC SURGERY

• Routine labs	• Complete blood count and comprehensive metabolic profile, including fasting blood glucose and liver function tests, are routine during initial consultation • Other recommended labs, if indicated, include thyroid function, lipid profile and glycated hemoglobin, urinalysis, prothrombin time, and partial thromboplastin time • Type and screen just prior to surgery
• Additional nutrition labs, if indicated	• Iron, TIBC, ferritin, vitamin B12, folic acid, 25-OH vitamin D, parathyroid hormone levels
• Dietary evaluation	• Educate about dietary behavior required postsurgery • Educate about potential for vitamin and mineral deficiencies in the postoperative period • Review body composition and energy balance • Set weight loss goals and manage discrepancies
• Psychological evaluation (includes lifestyle assessment)	• Assess healthy eating index and identify binge eating and night eating disorder, and treat if present • Assess overall mood and identify untreated depression, and treat if present • Assess for substance and alcohol abuse, and treat if present • Identify medications that may contribute to suboptimal weight loss • Assess overall support structure • Identify need for further behavioral support and counseling
• Cardiology evaluation, if indicated	• Electrocardiogram • Echocardiogram • Stress testing • Cardiac catheterization • Optimization of hypertension

• Pulmonary evaluation, if indicated	• Sleep apnea screening
	  • STOP-BANG questionnaire
	  • Epworth Sleepiness Scale
	• Optimization of COPD, asthma

• Gastrointestinal (GI) evaluation, if indicated	• Esophagogastroduodenoscopy • Upper GI contrast study • *Helicobacter pylori* testing • Gallbladder ultrasound • Colonoscopy

TABLE 9.1 Preoperative Checklist   (Continued)

PREOPERATIVE CHECKLIST FOR METABOLIC AND BARIATRIC SURGERY

• Endocrine evaluation, if indicated	• Optimization of diabetes mellitus • Glycated hemoglobin • Dexamethasone test • 24-Hour urinary cortisol • Thyroid-stimulating hormone • Testosterone • Dehydroepiandrosterone
• Insurance prerequisites, if applicable	• Confirm patient has benefits covering metabolic and bariatric surgery • Preoperative weight management documentation • Documented weight loss prior to surgery

TABLE 9.2 Epworth Sleepiness Scale and STOP-BANG Questionnaire Used for Obstructive Sleep Apnea Screening

Epworth Sleepiness Scale	Use the following point tabulation for each question
0-10: Normal range 10-12: Borderline 12-24: Abnormal	0: No chance of dozing 1: Minimal chance of dozing 2: Moderate chance of dozing 3: High chance of dozing How likely are you to doze off or sleep during the following? 1. Sitting or reading? 2. Watching television? 3. Sitting inactive in a public space? 4. As a passenger in a car for an hour without a break? 5. Lying down to rest when circumstances permit? 6. Sitting and talking to someone? 7. Sitting quietly after lunch without alcohol? 8. In a car, while stopped for a few minutes in traffic?

TABLE 9.2 Epworth Sleepiness Scale and STOP-BANG Questionnaire Used for Obstructive Sleep Apnea Screening (Continued)

STOP-BANG Questionnaire	Use the following point tabulation for each question
0-2: Low risk 3-4: Intermediate risk 5-8: High risk	0: No 1: Yes S: Snore loudly? T: Feel tired during the day? O: Observe apnea while sleeping? P: Treated for high blood pressure? B: Body mass index ≥35 kg/m^2 A: Age ≥50 years N: Neck circumference • Male ≥17 inches • Female ≥16 inches G: Gender—male

TABLE 10.2 Laboratory Screening and Monitoring for Bone Health After Surgery

GUIDELINES FOR MONITORING BONE HEALTH AFTER METABOLIC SURGERY

Laboratory tests used in the evaluation of bone health

- Calcium, phosphorous, magnesium
- 25(OH) vitamin D (and 1,25(OH) vitamin D if renal function is impaired)
- Bone-specific alkaline phosphatase or osteocalcin
- Parathyroid hormone (PTH)
- 24-Hour urinary calcium excretion
- Vitamin A and K_1 levels
- Albumin, prealbumin
- DEXA at baseline and 2-year follow-up

DEXA, dual-energy x-ray absorptiometry.

TABLE 9.4 Late Complications After Metabolic and Bariatric Surgery

RYGB	Incidence
Gastrojejunostomy anastomotic stricture	5.4%-7.3%
Gastrojejunostomy anastomotic (marginal) ulceration	2.3%-4%
Internal hernia	0.2%-2.6%
Small bowel obstruction	1.4%-5.2%
Cholelithiasis requiring cholecystectomy	3%-13%
Nephrolithiasis	7.7%-11%
VSG	**Incidence**
Luminal stenosis	0.1%-1.0%
Staple line leak (after 30 days)	1.1%-3.3%
Symptomatic GERD	28%-33%
Refractory GERD (requiring revision to RYGB)	1.4%-2.9%
New-onset Barrett esophagus	4%-17%

GERD, gastroesophageal reflux disease; RYGB, Roux-en-Y gastric bypass; VSG, vertical sleeve gastrectomy.

TABLE 10.3 Routine Monitoring for Metabolic Bone Disease for Bariatric Surgery Patients

SG/RYGB	BPD w/wo DS
Every 3-6 months for the first year and annually thereafter: 25(OH)D Optional: PTH DEXA monitoring may be indicated at baseline and at about 2 years	Every 3 months for the first year, every 3-6 months thereafter: 25(OH)D Albumin/prealbumin Every 6-12 months: Parathyroid hormone (PTH) 24-Hour urine calcium Annually: Urine N-telopeptide As needed: Osteocalcin DEXA monitoring may be indicated at baseline and at about 2 years

BPD w/wo DS, biliopancreatic diversion with or without duodenal switch; DEXA, dual-energy x-ray absorptiometry; RYGB, Roux-en-Y gastric bypass; SG, sleeve gastrectomy.

TABLE 10.4 Approach to Dietary Treatment of Hypoglycemia

Principles of Dietary Treatment of Postprandial Hypoglycemia

- Avoid high-glycemic carbohydrate food and beverages (cereal, sweets, rice, soda, juices)
- Prioritize protein at every meal and snack (chicken, fish, eggs, meat)
- Small portions of low-glycemic carbohydrate foods (quinoa, nonstarchy vegetables, berries)
- Carbohydrate foods should be consumed last and in small portions

Courtesy of Nicole Rubenstein, RD, Kaiser Permanente Colorado.

TABLE 10.5 Recommended Vitamin and Mineral Supplementation After Bariatric Surgery[a]

	AGB	SG	RYGB	BPD/DS
Vitamin B1[b]	• Minimum 12 mg/d • At risk: at least 50-100 mg/d			
Vitamin B12[b]	• 300-500 µg/d oral, disintegrating tablet, SL or nasal or • 1,000 µg/mo IM			
Folate[b]	• 400-800 µg/d oral • 800-1,000 µg/d F childbearing age			
Calcium	1200-1500 mg/d	1200-1500 mg/d	1200-1500 mg/d	1800-2,400 mg/d
Vitamin A	5000 IU/d	5,000-10,000 IU/d	5,000-10,000 IU/d	10,000 IU/d
Vitamin E[b]	15 mg/d			
Vitamin K	90-120 µg/d	90-120 µg/d	90-120 µg/d	300 µg/d
Vitamin D[b]	At least 3000 IU/d to maintain D, 25 (OH) > 30 ng/mL			
Iron	At least 18 mg/d	M and nonmenstruating F 18 mg/d from multivitamins from multivitamins	At least 65-60 mg/d in F with menses after SG,	RYGB, BPD/DS, and patients with history of anemia
Zinc	8-11 mg/d	8-11 mg/d	8-11 mg/d	16-22 mg/d
Copper	1 mg/d	1 mg/d	1-2 mg/d	2 mg/d

AGB, adjustable gastric banding; BPD/DS, biliopancreatic diversion with duodenal switch; d, daily; F, female; IM, intramuscularly; M, male; mo, monthly; RYGB, Roux-en-Y gastric bypass; SG, sleeve gastrectomy; SL, sublingual.
There are several specialized multivitamin preparations available for bariatric surgery patients. These preparations have higher levels of vitamin B12, iron, and vitamin D in comparison to many standard complete multivitamins in order to meet the supplemental guidelines set forth by the ASMBS. Multivitamins specifically for BPD/DS patients also have additional fat-soluble vitamins (A, D, E, and K). Using such products can help ensure the patient is getting the recommended doses, decrease pill burden, and increase compliance.
[a]Adapted from Parrott J, Frank L, Rabena R, Craggs-Dino L, Isom KA, Greiman L. American society for metabolic and bariatric surgery integrated health nutritional guidelines for the surgical weight loss patient 2016 update: micronutrients. Surg Obes Relat Dis. 2017;13(5):727-741.
[b]Recommended vitamin supplementation same in all bariatric procedures.

TABLE 10.6 Recommended Nutritional Monitoring after Metabolic and Bariatric Surgery[a]

	SCREENING (ADDITION TESTING)	PREOPERATIVELY	3 MO. POSTOPERATIVELY	6 MO. POSTOPERATIVELY	ANNUALLY
Vitamin B1	Whole blood thiamine	X	Any time N/V-	–	–
Vitamin B12	Serum B12 (MMA, homocysteine)	X	RYGB SG BPD/DS	RYGB SG BPD/DS	X
Folate	Folate (RBC folate, homocysteine, MMA)	X	X	X	X
Vitamin A	Plasma retinol (RBP-retinol binding protein)	X		BPD/DS	X
Vitamin D	25(OH)D	X	X	X	X
Vitamin E/K	Plasma α-tocopherol/ Plasma phylloquinone (PT-prothrombin time)	X			X
Iron[b]	Ferritin (serum iron, TSAT, TIBC, CBC)	X	X	X	X
Zinc[b]	plasma or serum zinc (RBC zinc, urine zinc)	X			RYGB SG BPD/DS
Copper[b]	Serum copper (ceruloplasmin, Erythrocyte superoxide dismutase)	X			RYGB SG BPD/DS
PTH	Serum PTH, serum calcium	X	X	X	X
Calcium	Combination: vitamin D25(OH), ALP, serum P, 24 hour urinary calcium in comparison to dietary calcium	X	X	X	X
DEXA		X			Every 2 yrs

X = all bariatric procedures.

ALP, alkaline phosphatase; BPD/DS, biliopancreatic diversion with duodenal switch; CBC, complete blood count; DEXA, dual-energy x-ray absorptiometry; MMA, methylmalonic acid; mo, month; N/V, nausea and vomiting; P, phosphorus; PTH, parathyroid hormone; RBC, red blood cell; RYGB, Roux-en-Y gastric bypass; SG, sleeve gastrectomy; TIBC, total iron binding capacity; TSAT, transferrin saturation; yrs, years.

[a]Adapted from Parrott J, Frank L, Rabena R, Craggs-Dino L, Isom KA, Greiman L. American society for metabolic and bariatric surgery integrated health nutritional guidelines for the surgical weight loss patient 2016 update: micronutrients. Surg Obes Relat Dis. 2017;13(5):727-742.

[b]Ferritin, zinc, and copper are acute phase reactant. Levels fluctuation with infection, inflammation, and age.

TABLE 10.7 Clinical Findings of Vitamin/Mineral Deficiencies[a]

	SIGNS AND SYMPTOMS OF DEFICIENCY
Vitamin B1 (thiamine)	Muscle weakness, ataxia, loss of reflexes Oculomotor dysfunction (nystagmus/ophthalmoplegia), paresthesia, confusion, heart failure/edema (wet beriberi) Wernicke encephalopathy triad: mental status change, oculomotor changes, gait ataxia
Vitamin B12 (cobalamin)	Sensory distal neuropathy Loss of proprioception, ataxia Macrocytic anemia Dementia, depression Glossitis
Folate	Macrocytic anemia, neural tube defects Mild pancytopenia
Iron	Microcytic anemia, fatigue, decrease work performance, glossitis, nail spooning or ridges, pica, restless legs
Calcium	Bone disease, secondary hyperparathyroidism
Vitamin D	Osteomalacia, muscle weakness and pain, cramps, tingling sensation, bone pain, hypocalcemia, tetany
Vitamin A	Bitot spots, night blindness Skin hyperkeratosis Blindness
Vitamin E	Neuropathy (sensor and motor) Ataxia Hemolysis
Vitamin K	Impaired coagulation Osteoporosis
Zinc	Decreased taste/smell, impaired healing, Skin rash, hair loss, glossitis, diarrhea
Copper	Hypochromic anemia, neutropenia, ataxia, paresthesia, myeloneuropathy

[a]Adapted from Parrott J, Frank L, Rabena R, Craggs-Dino L, Isom KA, Greiman L. American society for metabolic and bariatric surgery integrated health nutritional guidelines for the surgical weight loss patient 2016 update micronutrients. Surg Obes Relat Dis. 2017;13(5):727-743.

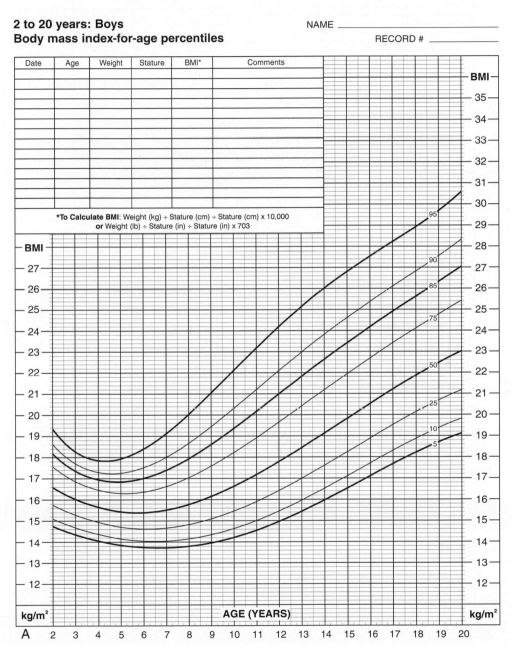

FIGURE 11.1 2002 Centers for Disease Control and Prevention body mass index-for-age growth charts. A, Boys. B, Girls. (Reprinted from Centers for Disease Control and Prevention. *Clinical Growth Charts.* https://www.cdc.gov/growthcharts/clinical_charts.htm#Set1)

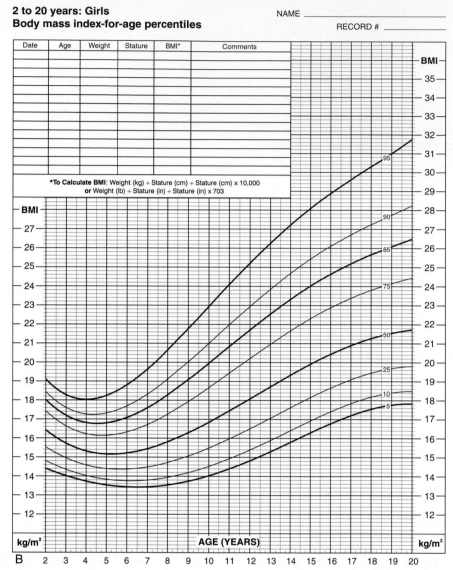

FIGURE 11.1 (Continued)

TABLE 11.1 Classification of Pediatric Body Mass Index Categories

BMI AGE- AND SEX-PERCENTILE	WEIGHT CLASSIFICATION
<5th percentile	Underweight
5th-84th percentile	Healthy weight
85th-94th percentile	Overweight
≥95th percentile *or* absolute BMI ≥30 kg/m²	Obesity
BMI ≥95th percentile *or* an absolute BMI ≥30 kg/m²	Class 1 Obesity
BMI ≥120% of the age- and sex-appropriate 95th percentile *or* an absolute BMI ≥35 kg/m²	Class 2 Obesity[a]
BMI ≥140% of the age- and sex-appropriate 95th percentile *or* an absolute BMI ≥40 kg/m²	Class 3 Obesity[a]

BMI, body mass index.

[a]Class 2 and 3 obesity may both additionally be classified as severe obesity.

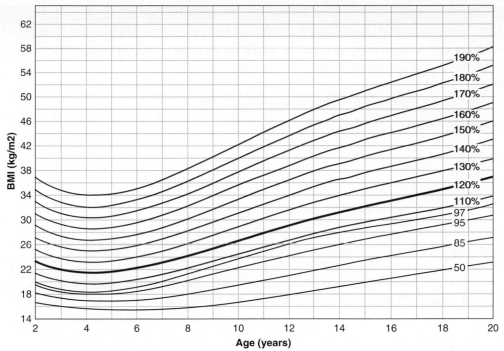

Source: BMI from CDC. BMI calculated as % of 95th percentile.

A

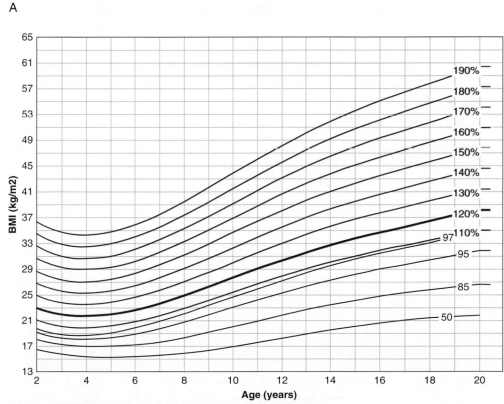

Source: BMI from CDC. BMI calculated as % of 95th percentile.

B

FIGURE 11.2 Modified Centers for Disease Control and Prevention (CDC) body mass index (BMI) growth curves for severe obesity in boys (A) and girls (B). (Reprinted with permission from Kelly AS, Barlow SE, Rao G, et al. Severe obesity in children and adolescents: identification, associated health risks, and treatment approaches. A scientific statement from the American Heart Association. *Circulation*. 2013;128:1689-1712.)

TABLE 11.2 Pediatric Dietary and Physical Activity Questionnaire

Please complete this from as accurately as possible. There are no right or wrong answers. This information will help us get a better picture of your child's current daily patterns.

<u>**Dietary Patterns:**</u>

How many meals does your child eat on a typical day? _____ per day

Does your child regularly eat:

Breakfast	Yes _____ No _____
Lunch	Yes _____ No _____
Dinner	Yes _____ No _____

How many snacks does your child eat on a typical day? _____ per day
What types of snacks does your child typically eat? _____

How many servings of fruits does your child eat on a typical day? (circle one)

None	1	2	3	4	5 or more

How many servings of vegetables does your child eat on a typical day? (circle one)

None	1	2	3	4	5 or more

Select the types of drinks your child normally consumes:

☐ Juice ☐ Lemonade ☐ Sports Drinks ☐ Sweetened Coffee

☐ Regular Soda ☐ Sweetened Tea ☐ Energy Drinks

On a typical day, how many of these types of drinks does your child consume (count them all together & enter the total here)? _____

Who normally prepares the food in the house?

☐ Mom ☐ Dad ☐ Grandparent ☐ This Child ☐ Sibling ☐ Other: _____

Who normally does the grocery shopping in the house?

☐ Mom ☐ Dad ☐ Grandparent ☐ This Child ☐ Sibling ☐ Other: _____

How many times per week do you eat together as a family? (circle one)

Never	1	2	3	4	5 or more

How many times per week does your child eat fast food? (circle one)

Never	1	2	3	4	5 or more

<u>Concerns about your child's eating habits:</u>

Are you satisfied with your child's eating habits?	Yes _____ No _____
Do you have concerns about your child's portion sizes?	Yes _____ No _____
Does your child ever eat in secret or sneak food?	Yes_____ No _____
Does your child ever eat to make himself/herself happy, or to feel better?	Yes _____ No _____
Does your child's weight affect how he/she feels about himself/herself?	Yes_____ No _____

<u>**Physical Activity and Screen Time:**</u>

How many times per week is your child physically active (i.e., His or her breathing gets faster)? (Circle one that best describes a typical week)

Never	1-2 days/week	3-4 days/week	5-6 days/week	Daily

What types of physical activities does your child like to participate in? _____

TABLE 11.2 Pediatric Dietary and Physical Activity Questionnaire (Continued)

How many hours does your child watch TV/movies, sit at the computer, play video games, or spend time on a phone or tablet *on a typical weekday*? _____ hours/day

How many hours does your child watch TV/movies, sit at the computer, play video games, or spend time on a phone or tablet *on a typical weekend day*? _____ hours/day

Sleep Behaviors:

Does your child have a TV or other screen device (e.g., smart phone) in the room where they sleep?

Yes _____ No _____

What time does your child typically go to bed *during the week*? _____

What time does your child typically fall asleep after going to bed *during the week*? _____

What time does your child typically wake up *during the week*? _____

What time does your child typically go to bed *during the weekend*? _____

What time does your child typically fall asleep after going to bed *during the weekend*? _____

What time does your child typically wake up *during the weekend*? _____

Which of the following habits (if any) do you feel ready to help your child and family to change? Check all that apply:

☐ Drink less soda or juice

☐ Choosing healthy snacks

☐ Eating more fruits & vegetables

☐ Eat less fast food

☐ Eat more meals as a family

☐ Plan out meals

☐ Play outside/be more active more often

☐ Spend less time watching TV & playing video games or on the computer

☐ Take the TV/Computer out of the bedroom

TABLE 11.3 Eating Disorder Screener

1. Do you worry you have lost control over how much you eat? YES[a] NO

2. Do you ever eat in secret? YES[a] NO

3. Do you currently have or have you ever had an eating disorder? YES[a] NO

4. Do you make yourself sick when you feel uncomfortably full? YES[a] NO

For use in adolescents aged 12 to 18 years.
[a]*Consider referral to eating disorder specialist for two or more affirmative responses or if YES to Question 3.*
Adapted from Cotton M, Ball C, Robinson P. Four simple questions can help screen for eating disorders. J Gen Int Med. 2003;18:53-56.

TABLE 11.4 Recommended Healthy Sleep Durations for Infants, Children, and Adolescents

CATEGORY	AGE RANGE	RECOMMENDED SLEEP DURATION (HOURS EACH DAY)
Newborns	0-3 months	14-17
Infants	4-11 months	12-15
Toddlers	1-2 years	11-14
Preschoolers	3-5 years	10-13
School-age children	6-13 years	9-11
Teenagers	14-17 years	8-10
Adults	18-64 years	7-9

Adapted from Hirshkowitz M, Whiton K, Albert SM, et al. National Sleep Foundation's sleep time duration recommendations: methodology and results summary. Sleep Health. 2015;1(1):40-43.

TABLE 11.5 Sexual Maturity Rating in Boys and Girls

	BREAST DEVELOPMENT	PUBIC HAIR DEVELOPMENT	TESTICULAR/PENILE DEVELOPMENT
Prepubertal (Stage 1)	No breast buds	Prepubertal (may include some vellus hair)	Prepubertal
Stage 2	Subareolar breast bud	Sparse, fine, straight pubic hairs, typically at the base of penis or along labia	Enlargement of testes and scrotum, no enlargement of the penis
Stage 3	Elevation of the breast contour and enlargement of the areola	Long, dark curly pubic hairs limited to mons pubis	Enlargement of testes and scrotum, penis grows in length
Stage 4	Areola forms a secondary mound above the contour of the breast	Pubic hair is adult in quality, not yet spread to thighs	Further enlargement of testes and scrotum, penis grows in length
Stage 5	Mature female breast with dependent breast contour, recession of areola	Pubic hair has distribution of inverted triangle and spread to thighs	Mature male genitalia

Adapted from Wolf RM, Long D. Pubertal Development. Pediatr Rev. 2016;37(7):292-300.

TABLE 11.6 Recommended Laboratory Screening for Cardiometabolic Risk Factors in Youth With Overweight and Obesity

BMI	RECOMMENDED TESTS
>85th-94th percentile, with no risk factors	Fasting lipid profile
>85th-94th percentile, with risk factors[a]	Fasting lipid profile Screening for glucose intolerance[b] AST and ALT levels
≥95th percentile	Fasting lipid profile Screening for glucose intolerance[b] AST and ALT levels

ALT, alanine aminotransferase; AST, aspartate aminotransferase; BMI, body mass index.
[a]Risk factors include family history of obesity-related diseases such as type 2 diabetes mellitus (T2D); elevated blood pressure; elevated lipid levels; or tobacco use.
[b]Screening for glucose intolerance via one of the following tests: fasting plasma glucose, oral glucose tolerance test, or HgbA₁c.
Adapted from Krebs NF, Himes JH, Jacobson D, Nicklas TA, Guilday P, Styne D. Assessment of Child and Adolescent Overweight and Obesity. Pediatrics. 2007;120(suppl 4): S193-S228 and Styne DM, Arslanian SA, Connor EL, et al. Pediatric obesity-assessment, treatment, and prevention: an endocrine society clinical practice guideline. J Clin Endocrinol Metab. 2017;102(3):709-757.

TABLE 11.7 Pediatric Weight Goals, According to Age and BMI Category

AGE	BMI CATEGORY	WEIGHT GOAL
2-5 years	85th-94th percentile with *no* health risks	Weight velocity maintenance
	85th-94th percentile with health risks	Weight maintenance or slow weight gain
	≥95th percentile	Weight maintenance (weight loss of up to 1 lb/mo may be acceptable if BMI >21 kg/m^2)
6-11 years	85th-94th percentile with *no* health risks	Weight velocity maintenance
	85th-94th percentile with health risks	Weight maintenance
	95th-99th percentile	Gradual weight loss (1 lb/mo or 0.5 kg/mo)
	>99th percentile	Weight loss (maximum is 2 lb/wk)
12-18 years	85th-94th percentile with *no* health risks	Weight velocity maintenance; after linear growth is complete, weight maintenance
	85th-94th percentile with health risks	Weight maintenance or gradual weight loss
	95th-99th percentile	Weight loss (maximum is 2 lb/wk)
	>99th percentile	Weight loss (maximum is 2 lb/wk)[a]

BMI, body mass index; mo, month; wk, week.

[a]More rapid weight loss may be appropriate in adolescents with severe obesity treated with pharmacotherapy or metabolic and bariatric surgery.

Adapted from Barlow SE; Expert Committee. Expert committee recommendations regarding the prevention, assessment, and treatment of child and adolescent overweight and obesity: summary report. Pediatrics. 2007;120(suppl 4):S164-S192.

TABLE 11.8 Key Behavioral Targets for Treatment of Pediatric Overweight and Obesity

- Minimize or eliminate sugar-sweetened beverage intake
- Consume ≥5 serving of fruits and vegetables every day
- Eat a healthy breakfast every day
- Set age-appropriate limits on screen time, including the establishment of screen-free zones (e.g., bedrooms at night) and times (e.g., during meals)
- Be physically active a total of ≥60 minutes each day
- Prepare more meals at home
- Eat family meals at a table five or six times a week
- Establish a regular sleeping schedule according to age-specific recommendations

Adapted from Barlow SE; Expert Committee. Expert committee recommendations regarding the prevention, assessment, and treatment of child and adolescent overweight and obesity: summary report. Pediatrics. 2007;120(suppl 4):S164-S192.

TABLE 11.9 Estimated Pediatric Daily Caloric Needs (Kcal/day) by Age and Sex[a]

AGE (YEARS)	MALES	FEMALES[b]
2	1,000	1,000
3	1,000-1,400	1,000-1,200
4	1,200-1,400	1,200-1,400
5	1,200-1,400	1,200-1,400
6	1,400-1,600	1,200-1,400
7	1,400-1,600	1,200-1,600
8	1,400-1,600	1,400-1,600
9	1,600-1,800	1,400-1,600
10	1,600-1,800	1,400-1,800
11	1,800-2,000	1,600-1,800
12	1,800-2,200	1,600-2,000
13	2,000-2,200	1,600-2,000
14	2,000-2,400	1,800-2,000
15	2,200-2,600	1,800-2,000
16-18	2,400-2,800	1,800-2,000

Adapted from U.S. Department of Health and Human Services and U.S. Department of Agriculture. 2015-2020 Dietary Guidelines for Americans. 8th ed. December 2015. https://health.gov/our-work/food-nutrition/2015-2020-dietary-guidelines/guidelines/appendix-2
[a]Range based on a sedentary to moderate physical activity level; higher caloric needs may be appropriate for more active children. Lower daily caloric targets may be necessary to induce a negative energy balance necessary for weight loss.
[b]Estimates for females do not include women who are pregnant or breastfeeding.

TABLE 12.1 Clinicians Involved in Treatment of Obesity

STAFF	SERVICE
HCP	Prescribe pharmacotherapy Manage comorbidities Refer to other services—RDN, exercise, behavior, psychologist, surgeon Provide perioperative care for patients who undergo bariatric surgery Arrange follow-up
RDN	Within practice or by referral Perform dietary assessment Review food journals Provide individualized structured food planning, intensive lifestyle intervention Provide dietary and nutritional education
Exercise physiologist/ trainer	Typically by referral Assess physical limitations and abilities Develop individualized physical activity program
Psychologist/ therapist	Typically by referral Assess psychological stressors and barriers Perform motivational interviewing Provide cognitive behavioral therapy
Bariatric surgeon	Typically by referral Assess patient appropriateness for bariatric procedures Perform procedures and arrange follow-up

HCP, healthcare professional; RDN, registered dietitian nutritionist

TABLE 12.2 Office Audit for Delivery of Office-based Obesity Care

AUDIT CATEGORIES

Do you routinely assess and evaluate patients for overweight and obesity?

a. measure height, weight, waist circumference, and calculate body mass index (BMI)

b. take a focused obesity history (see Chapter 2)

c. assess readiness for and barriers to weight loss

What kinds of services or programs do you routinely provide to your patients who have obesity?

a. high-intensity dietary and exercise counseling (individual or group)

b. referral to a registered dietitian nutritionist (RDN), exercise specialist, obesity medicine specialist, or bariatric surgeon

c. email correspondence

d. use of antiobesity medications or medically supervised diets

What are the services or programs recorded in the patient's chart?

a. recommended dietary and exercise behavioral changes

b. percent weight loss goal

c. correspondence to an RDN, health psychologist, or exercise specialist

d. uses and risks of antiobesity medication

What policies and procedures do you have in place for providing obesity care?

a. all patients have a height, weight, waist circumference, and BMI measured and recorded in the chart

b. the patient's readiness is assessed before initiating treatment

c. weight loss goals are established and tracked in the progress notes

d. services are in place to provide high-intensity behavioral treatment, individualized physical activity plans, and behavioral treatment

e. patients with a BMI of ≥ 30 kg/m^2 or ≥ 27 kg/m^2 with a comorbidity are assessed for antiobesity medications

f. patients with a BMI of >40 kg/m^2 or ≥ 35 kg/m^2 with a comorbidity are assessed for bariatric surgery

What forms, patient handouts, and educational materials are you using?

a. focused obesity history form

b. diet and exercise history forms

c. guidance on diet (including popular eating plans), physical activity, and behavioral change, as well as emotional and stress eating

d. food and activity logs

e. education sheets on antiobesity medications

f. education sheets on bariatric surgery

How does your office environment support or inhibit delivery of obesity care?

a. sturdy armless chairs

b. large and thigh blood pressure cuffs

c. large gowns

d. measuring of body weight in a private setting

e. a sensitive and informed office staff and including the use of person-first language for obesity

What functions do staff currently serve in the provision of obesity care?

a. office nurse or MA obtains weight, height, and BMI

b. healthcare provider (MD, NP, or PA) reviews food and activity diaries and medication side effects

c. receptionist schedules referral appointments with RDN, exercise specialist, or clinical psychologist

Adapted from Agency for Healthcare Research and Quality. 10 Steps: Implementation Guide. Put Prevention Into Practice. Adapted from The Clinicians' Handbook of Preventive Services. *2nd ed. Publication No. 98-0025. Agency for Healthcare Research and Quality; 1998.*

TABLE 12.3 Models of Obesity Care

Primary care, insurance-based	Obesity is treated as a chronic disease, similar to other diseases. Insurers are billed for the treatments provided.
Specialty care, insurance-based	Comprehensive obesity management practice including medical specialist and other obesity-specific services such as intensive lifestyle modification, exercise training, structured food plans, etc.
Comprehensive care, insurance-based	Similar to above, but offering further services such as exercise therapist, psychologist, individual and group visits, and bariatric surgery.
Cash-based practice	These practices offer obesity care but opt out of insurance assignment. Patients pay practices directly in a fee-for-service model or sometimes pay for bundled services (such as a 12-week weight loss program including medical monitoring, dietitian visits, etc.)

TABLE 12.4A Obesity Codes

ICD-10 CODE	DESCRIPTION
E65	Localized adiposity Fat pad
E66	Overweight and obesity Use additional code to identify body mass index (BMI) Excludes • adiposogenital dystrophy (E23.6) • lipomatosis NOS (E88.2) • lipomatosis dolorosa (Dercum) (E88.2) • Prader-Willi syndrome (Q87.1)
E66.0	Obesity due to excess calories
E66.01	Morbid (severe) obesity due to excess calories Excludes • morbid (severe) obesity with alveolar hypoventilation (E66.2)
E66.09	Other obesity due to excess calories
E66.1	Drug-induced obesity Use additional code for adverse effect, if applicable, to identify drug (T36-T50 with fifth or sixth character 5)
E66.2	Morbid (severe) obesity with alveolar hypoventilation Pickwickian syndrome

TABLE 12.4A Obesity Codes   (Continued)

ICD-10 CODE	DESCRIPTION
E66.8	Other obesity
E66.9	Obesity, unspecified Obesity NOS
R60.9	Lipedema
Z86.39	Personal history of other endocrine, nutritional, and metabolic disease • includes history of obesity, adults • history of obesity BMI 95-100 percentile
Z98.84	Bariatric surgery status Gastric banding status Gastric bypass status for obesity Obesity surgery status Excludes • bariatric surgery status complicating pregnancy, childbirth, or the puerperium (O99.84) Excludes • intestinal bypass and anastomosis status (Z98.0)

TABLE 12.4B Body Mass Index (BMI) Codes

ICD-10 CODE	DESCRIPTION
Z68.3	BMI 30-39, adult
Z68.30	BMI 30.0-30.9, adult
Z68.31	BMI 31.0-31.9, adult
Z68.32	BMI 32.0-32.9, adult
Z68.33	BMI 33.0-33.9, adult
Z68.34	BMI 34.0-34.9, adult
Z68.35	BMI 35.0-35.9, adult
Z68.36	BMI 36.0-36.9, adult
Z68.37	BMI 37.0-37.9, adult
Z68.38	BMI 38.0-38.9, adult
Z68.39	BMI 39.0-39.9, adult
Z68.4	BMI 40 or greater, adult
Z68.41	BMI 40-44.9, adult
Z68.42	BMI 45.0-49.9, adult
Z68.43	BMI 50.0-59.9, adult
Z68.44	BMI 60.0-69.9, adult
Z68.45	BMI 70 or greater, adult

TABLE 12.5 Current Procedural Technology Codes		
HEALTH AND BEHAVIOR ASSESSMENT CODES	**NOTES**	**TIME**
96150	Initial assessment	Billed in 15-minute increments
96151	Follow-up assessment	Billed in 15-minute increments
Health and Behavior Intervention Codes		
96152	Individual	Billed in 15-minute increments
96153	Group	Billed in 15-minute increments
96154	Family (patient present)	Billed in 15-minute increments
96155	Family (patient not present)	Billed in 15-minute increments
Preventive Visit Codes		
99381-99387	New patient	N/A
99391-99397	Established patient	N/A
Counseling/Risk Factor Reduction Codes		
99401	Preventive counseling	15 minutes
99402	Preventive counseling	30 minutes
99403	Preventive counseling	45 minutes
99404	Preventive counseling	60 minutes
Medical Nutrition Therapy Codes		
97802	Initial assessment	Billed in 15-minute increments
97803	Re-assessment	Billed in 15-minute increments
97804	Group	Billed in 15-minute increments
Test Codes		
0358T	BIA whole body composition assessment	

BIA, bioelectrical impedance analysis.

TABLE 13.1 Within-Practice Resources for Obesity Treatment

RESOURCE	OPTIONS	EXAMPLES
Educational handouts	Practice developed Downloadable	AACE (www.aace.com), OMA (obesitymedicine.org), OAC (www.obesityaction.org), TOS (www.obesity.org).
Image banks for positive patient images to be used in handouts/marketing	Practice developed Image banks	Obesity Canada (www.obesitycanada.ca) World Obesity Federation (www.worldobesity.org) Rudd Center (www.uconnruddcenter.org)
Peer support groups	Practice-led Practice supported but patient-led	Hospital and private bariatric surgery programs often have support groups already staffed
BIA (bioelectrical impedance analysis) (to measure body composition)	Single frequency Triple frequency Research level	Inbody (www.inbodyusa.com) Seca (www.seca.com) Tanita (www.tanita.com/en/howbiaworks)
Bod Pod air displacement plethysmography (to measure body composition)		Cosmed (https://www.cosmed.com/en/)
Resting metabolic rate, indirect calorimetry (to measure energy expenditure)	Requires single-use disposables	Med Gem (https://metabolicratetest.com/medgem-fda-approved-indirect-calorimeter/) Korr (https://korr.com/)

TABLE 13.2 Physical Activity Apps and Resources

APP	CATEGORY	SPECIAL FEATURES
MapMyFitness MapMyWalk MapMyRun	Physical activity tracking and analytics	Tracks time, distance, speed of land-based activities. Can synchronize with wearables like Fitbit, Garmin, or Polar
Fitocracy	Physical activity tracking + motivation	Uses social networks. Virtual coaches are available
Daily Yoga	Discipline-specific exercise	
7-Minute Workout	Physical activity routines	Time based for quick use; provides instructional videos
Sworkit	Buildable physical activity routines	Tailors to areas of need; provides demonstration videos for correct form
Fitbit	Tracks physical activity and sleep. Used with a wearable	Weekly summaries of distance, calories, weight, sleep

TABLE 13.4 Societies, Certifications, and Academic Resources Supporting Obesity Education and Treatment

Organizations

AACE	American Academy of Clinical Endocrinologists	www.aace.org
ASMBS	American Society of Metabolic and Bariatric Surgery	www.asmbs.org
OMA	Obesity Medicine Association	www.obesitymedicine.org
TOS	The Obesity Society	www.obesity.org
Obesity Canada	Obesity Canada	www.obesitycanada.ca
WOF	World Obesity Federation	www.worldobesity.org

Certifications	**Providing Organization**	**Website and Candidates**
ABOM Certification	American Board of Obesity Medicine	www.abom.org Examination-based certification for physicians only
CDR's Interdisciplinary Obesity and Weight Management Certification	Commission on Dietetic Registration	www.cdrnet.org/interdisciplinary Examination-based certification for advanced practitioners, exercise physiologists, clinical psychologists, social workers, pharmacists, physical therapists, or dietitians
Certified Bariatric Nurse	American Society of Metabolic and Bariatric Surgery	https://asmbs.org/integrated-health/ cbn-certification

Certificates of Learning	**Providing Organization**	**Requirements**
NP/PA Certificate of Advanced Education in Obesity Medicine	Obesity Medicine Association	Completion of 60 CE hours (no examination) www.obesitymedicine.org
Certificate in Primary Care Obesity Management	Obesity Medicine Association	For nurse practitioners and physicians' assistants
Strategic Center for Obesity Professional Education (SCOPE)	World Obesity Federation	Offers a series of online learning modules and a certification. Available to any healthcare professional

Obesity Journals

Obesity	*Obesity Reviews*	*Obesity Science and Practice*
Surgery for Obesity and Related Diseases	*Obesity Surgery*	*Pediatric Obesity*
Clinical Obesity	*Diabetes, Obesity and Metabolism*	*International Journal of Obesity*
Journal of the Academy of Nutrition and Dietetics	*American Journal of Clinical Nutrition*	

B

QUIZ QUESTIONS

For the correct answers, please see page 292. For detailed explanations, please see the Quiz Questions at the end of each chapter.

Chapter 1: Obesity as a Disease

1. MJ is a 60-year-old man who comes to see you for weight gain. He has had slow, steady progressive weight gain for the last 40 years. He is an engineer and says he is eating exactly the same as he did 40 years ago, and his exercise habits (walking 2 miles 5 days a week) have not changed either over this time period. He says that he must have a metabolic problem underlying his weight gain.

   Which of the following is the most likely cause of his progressive weight gain?

   A. He actually has been eating more and more calories per day over the years, and he is underreporting his food intake

   B. His BMR has gradually declined as he aged which results in a positive energy balance because he is still taking in the same number of calories each day

   C. His exercise habits have actually declined over the years, and he is underreporting his physical activity

   D. He has become more insulin resistant as he has aged, and this is the underlying cause of his weight gain

2. DJ is a 47-year-old woman who is being seen for routine health maintenance. She feels that her health is good and she has no complaints. She reports eating a Mediterranean-style diet and exercises at a moderate intensity for 40 minutes 5 days a week. She also does three bouts of muscle-strengthening activities 3 days a week. She has no family history of diabetes, hypertension, or cardiovascular disease.

On examination, her BMI is 32 kg/m², waist circumference 34 inches, and blood pressure is 122/74 mm Hg. Laboratory tests show a fasting glucose of 85 mg/dL, HbA1c = 5.3%, triglycerides 98 mg/dL, HDL cholesterol 52 mg/dL, LDL cholesterol 93 mg/dL.

Which of the following best describes her future risk for developing metabolic complications of obesity such as type 2 diabetes or cardiovascular disease?

A. Her risk is the same as other people with a BMI of 30 to 35 kg/m² as weight is the primary driver of these comorbidities

B. Her risk is the same as a normal-weight individual with hypertension, hyperlipidemia, and prediabetes

C. Her risk is the same as a normal-weight individual with normal lipids, glucose, and blood pressure as these markers are the drivers of future comorbidities

D. Her risk is higher than a normal-weight individual with normal metabolic markers but lower than a normal-weight individual who has abnormal metabolic markers

Chapter 2: The Obesity Encounter

1. A 36-year-old woman makes an appointment as a new patient. She is concerned about gaining 15 lbs (6.8 kg) over the past 10 years. On history, you learn that she has experienced several major life events over this time that have included marriage, two pregnancies, relocation to the suburbs, and starting paroxetine for depression. She also states that her mother and sister suffer from obesity. On examination, her BMI is 31 kg/m². The remainder of examination is unremarkable.

What is the next best step?

A. Educate her about the health risks of weight gain and obesity

B. Recommend stopping the antidepressant medication since it is the likely cause of the weight gain

C. Inquire about the weight of her two children since obesity has a genetic contribution

D. Ask her what she thinks may have contributed to the weight gain

E. Provide diet and physical activity counseling

2. During the physical examination of a 48-year-old man with class II obesity (BMI 36.5 kg/m²) and upper body fat distribution (waist circumference 42 inches), you obtain a blood pressure measurement of 146/94 mm Hg on the right arm using an adult size cuff. He has been sitting for 5 minutes and both feet are resting on the floor. He does not have a history of hypertension.

What assessment can be made about his blood pressure, and what is the next appropriate step?

A. Accurate but needs to be repeated in the right arm

B. Spuriously high and needs to be retaken using a large adult cuff

C. Spuriously high and needs to be retaken at the level of the wrist

D. Inaccurate and needs to be repeated after another 5 minutes of resting

E. Accurate and a new diagnosis of hypertension should be added to problem list

Chapter 3: Assessment and Staging: Identification and Evaluation of the High-risk Patient

1. SJ is a 49-year-old woman who comes to see you for a variety of symptoms including marked fatigue, knee and back pain, urinary stress incontinence, gastroesophageal reflux unresponsive to H2 blocking therapy, and depression. Because of marked fatigue and joint pain, she feels she is no longer able to work at her job as a cashier at a local grocer. On review of systems, she says that her partner says that she snores and she reports AM headaches and daytime hypersomnolence. Her life situation is making her feel hopeless. On examination, she has a BMI = 38 kg/m², a blood pressure of 155/98 mm Hg, decreased range of

motion at her knees, 2+ edema in her ankles, and a depressed affect. Her HbA1c = 7.5%; her ECG shows q waves inferiorly.

What stage is she using the Edmonton Obesity Staging System?

A. Stage 1

B. Stage 2

C. Stage 3

D. Stage 4

2. JB is a 35-year-old man who comes to see you for help managing his weight. He currently has a BMI of 29 kg/m². His blood pressure is 125/81 mm Hg and his waist circumference is 38 inches. His fasting glucose is 118 mg/dL, his HDL cholesterol is 38 mg/dL and his fasting triglyceride level is 210 mg/dL.

Which stage is he in the Cardiometabolic Disease Staging System for Prediction of Diabetes?

A. Stage 1

B. Stage 2

C. Stage 3

D. Stage 4

Chapter 4: Comanagement of Obesity-related Comorbidities: Assessment, Treatment, and Monitoring

1. AS is a 50-year-old man who is being evaluated for complications from obesity. Known medical problems include prediabetes and hypertension treated with losartan. He takes no other medications and does not smoke or drink alcohol. He has no known family history of liver disease. On physical examination, BMI is 40 kg/m², blood pressure 130/78 mm Hg, and heart rate is 84 bpm. There is no jaundice, ascites, or other signs of end-stage liver disease. On laboratory testing AST is 95, ALT is 88, and platelet count is 100,000. His ferritin is normal and his serological tests for hepatitis are negative. A Fibrosis 4 score is calculated as 5.1, indicating likely advanced fibrosis.

Which of the following is the best next step to address his abnormal liver function tests?

A. Reassure him that his liver will get better with weight loss

B. Refer him to bariatric surgery

C. Refer for an elastography scan

D. Refer him to a gastroenterologist for a liver biopsy

2. DG is a 54-year-old man with prediabetes, dyslipidemia, and nonalcoholic fatty liver disease (NAFLD). His NAFLD was detected incidentally on a CT scan. He takes metformin and atorvastatin. Physical examination is unremarkable except for his BMI of 39 kg/m^2 and abdominal obesity. Laboratory data show HBA1c of 5.9%, HDL 32, fasting triglycerides 178, and normal AST and ALT. The patient has been reading about obesity and elevated cancer risk and wants to know what cancer screenings he should have based on his weight.

Which of the following is the most appropriate response?

A. He should have the same cancer screening regimen as other 54-year-old men who have normal BMI

B. He should have more frequent screening for colon cancer than other 54-year-old men since this occurs at greater frequency in people with obesity

C. He should have more frequent screening for colon cancer than other 54-year-old men, as well as routine screening for esophageal, liver, and kidney cancer

D. He should have more frequent screening for liver cancer than other 54-year-old men because of his diagnosis of NAFLD

Chapter 5: Dietary Treatment

1. Our case study patient decided to pursue a Mediterranean-style diet. She is interested in lowering her risks for diabetes and heart disease. She has visited with an RDN and has a meal plan to create a calorie restriction of 500 calories per day.

Which of the following is true regarding weight loss expectations?

A. She will lose exactly 1 lb per week for the first 6 months

B. She will lose less weight at one year than if she followed a very-low-carbohydrate diet

C. She will lose more weight with a Mediterranean diet if she keeps a food record

D. She will not lose additional weight by joining a behavioral program at this point

2. Our patient returns for follow-up four months into her weight loss effort. Her baseline weight was 106 kg (233 lbs); her current weight is 98.5 kg (217 lbs) (= 7.1% of initial body weight). She has been adhering to the meal plan created by the RDN. She has not been tracking her food intake as regularly as she did at the start. She is not doing planned exercise but is trying to be more active throughout the day and reports that her step count ranges from 5,000 to 7,000 per day. She is frustrated that she has not experienced more weight loss.

What is the most accurate assessment of her current efforts?

A. She is unlikely to continue to lose weight because of metabolic adaptations to weight loss

B. She has reduced her risk for developing type 2 diabetes with the weight loss achieved so far

C. She is currently getting all the benefits of physical activity

D. She would not be a good candidate for weight loss medication because she has already lost more than 5% of initial body weight

E. She likely did not adhere to the meal plan (did not achieve calorie restriction) because her weight loss stopped before she reached a 10% body weight loss

Chapter 6: Physical Activity Treatment

1. Mrs. S is a 47-year-old woman with a BMI of 32 kg/m^2, prediabetes, and mild degenerative joint disease of her knees who comes to see you with concerns about her weight. She is now at her peak lifetime weight and wants to do everything she can to lose weight. Although she was a cheerleader in high school and enjoyed being active, she has engaged in no planned physical activity for the last 10 years due to family responsibilities. She is self-conscious about her appearance, and this has made her avoid exercising.

Which of the following would be the best first suggestion to make to her today?

A. Reduce her time watching television from 2 hour/day to 1 hour/day

B. Begin walking for 10 minutes two times per week

C. Begin walking at a moderate intensity for 30 minutes 5 days a week

D. Over the next month, increase her activity to 60 minutes of walking 6 days/week

2. Mr. J is a 39-year-old man with a BMI of 35 kg/m² who has been seeing you for help managing his weight. He has been on a moderate 1500 kcal/day restricted diet and began a walking program 6 months ago. He has increased his activity from 15 minutes twice a week to his current level of 40 minutes 5 days a week. He is enjoying walking but is finding it hard to make time for these walks. He is interested in increasing his intensity of activity.

   Which of the following could he use during exercise to know he is exercising at a vigorous level?

   A. He is able to say a few words between breaths

   B. His perceived exertion level is 5 out of 10

   C. His heart rate of 118 bpm

   D. His walking pace is >3.5 miles/hour

Chapter 7: Behavioral Treatment

1. A 48-year-old male patient makes an appointment to discuss his body weight. He has gained 10 lbs over the past 6 months and is concerned about his most recent glycohemoglobin blood test of 6.1%. His BMI is 29 kg/m². You begin to counsel him about the benefit of modest weight loss and paying more attention to diet. At that time, the patient responds; "I know what you are going to say. I talked to my wife last night about this. She suggested that I download an app to my phone so that I can track all of the foods that I eat. I happened to look at it this morning. It's pretty cool but not sure I know how to use it."

   The patient is determined to be in which stage of change regarding reducing his dietary calorie consumption?

   A. Precontemplation

   B. Contemplation

   C. Preparation

   D. Action

2. You have been working with a 38-year-old female patient with obesity (BMI 32 kg/m²) and hypertension (BP 138/90 mm Hg) to reduce her caloric and sodium intake over the past 4 months. She is tracking her diet using a smartphone app with the goal of consuming 1300 kcal and 2300 mg sodium per day. During today's visit, she mentions that her husband continues to bring fatty and salty snacks into the house which makes it hard for her to meet her dietary goals, especially when she is stressed. You counsel her to talk to her husband about not bringing these foods into the house, and instead have healthier snacks available.

   This suggestion is an example of which behavioral weight loss technique?

   A. Self-monitoring

   B. Stimulus control

   C. Cognitive restructuring

   D. Stress reduction

   E. Contingency management

Chapter 8: Obesity Pharmacotherapy

1. A 30-year-old man presents to his primary care provider for an annual visit. His BMI has increased from 30 to 32 kg/m² since his last visit one year ago. The patient has a history of major depression and reports a recent worsening of his mood. He was started on a trial of fluoxetine by his psychiatrist and told to address his weight with his primary provider with the hope that weight loss could improve his mood. The patient previously was very active and did yoga regularly. He says he has been trying to address portion size and snacking but finds sweets comforting. He is interested in hearing more about any medication that can help control his weight gain and cravings for sweets. Medically, he uses tramadol on an intermittent basis for low back pain. Upon your evaluation, he denies suicidal ideation and his vital signs, physical examination, and laboratory studies are normal. The patient is on governmental insurance and has limited medication coverage.

   In addition to optimizing his nutrition, sleep, stress, and physical activity, which antiobesity medication would be most appropriate?

   A. Phentermine

   B. Naltrexone/bupropion

   C. Liraglutide

   D. Phentermine/topiramate

   E. Orlistat

2. A 28-year-old woman, BMI of 34 kg/m², comes to you for help with weight loss. She has been following a commercial weight loss program for several months and has lost about 15 lbs but feels as though she is at a plateau and is feeling hungry. Her past medical history is

significant for anxiety and a seizure disorder managed on levetiracetam. She has two children and has had a tubal ligation. The patient is particularly interested in medication that might help control her appetite, especially as she tries to move forward without using the packaged meals her previous weight loss program provided. Her BP is 125/80 mm Hg, HR 70 bpm, and the rest of her physical examination is normal. Her only abnormal laboratory value is a hemoglobin A1c of 6.1%.

In addition to working with you to optimize her lifestyle, which of the following options would be preferred in this patient?

A. Phentermine/topiramate ER

B. Naltrexone ER/bupropion ER

C. Liraglutide

D. Phentermine

E. Orlistat

Chapter 9: Metabolic and Bariatric Surgery

1. Which of the following patients is most likely to experience complete resolution of type 2 diabetes (T2D) within the first year after laparoscopic Roux-en-Y gastric bypass?

   A. A 25-year-old woman (BMI 41 kg/m^2) with a 3-year history of T2D on metformin, and a preoperative glycated hemoglobin level of 6.9%

   B. A 55-year-old man (BMI 44 kg/m^2) with a 11-year history of T2D requiring insulin and two oral hypoglycemic agents (metformin, glyburide), and a preoperative glycated hemoglobin level of 6.5%

   C. A 40-year-old woman (BMI 43 kg/m^2) with a 4-year history of T2D requiring insulin and two oral hypoglycemic agents (metformin, glyburide), and a preoperative glycated hemoglobin level of 8.2%

   D. A 60-year-old woman (BMI 38 kg/m^2) with a 10-year history of type 2 diabetes on two oral hypoglycemic agents (metformin, glyburide) and a preoperative glycated hemoglobin level of 7.8%

2. A 39-year-old woman presents to your office for a routine annual physical. Her medical history includes obesity, gastroesophageal reflux, obstructive sleep apnea, and bipolar disorder. She was admitted to the hospital 6 months earlier with a major depressive episode

and suicide attempt. She has made a marked improvement since being discharged from the hospital and is currently being followed up by a psychiatrist. She has gained 10 lbs in the last 6 months and wants to undergo bariatric surgery to help her lose weight. Her BMI is 37.2 kg/m^2, and her physical examination is unremarkable except for obesity.

Which of the following statements is the best response for this patient?

A. You are a suitable candidate for bariatric surgery, and I will submit a referral for a bariatric surgery consultation

B. You do not meet criteria for bariatric surgery because your BMI is too low, but I am happy to refer you to an obesity medicine specialist for a medical weight loss evaluation

C. You do not meet criteria for bariatric surgery because you have bipolar disorder, but I am happy to refer you to an obesity medicine specialist for a medical weight loss evaluation

D. You do not meet criteria for surgery at this time because of your recent suicide attempt, but we can discuss referring you for a bariatric surgery consultation in 6 months

Chapter 10: Care of the Postbariatric Surgery Patient

1. A 45-year-old woman with class III obesity, type 2 diabetes, and hypertension returns for a follow-up visit 2 months following an uneventful Roux-en-Y-gastric bypass (RYGB) procedure. She has no nausea, vomiting, or abdominal pain. She is consuming three meals and two snacks daily consisting of protein shakes, eggs, cheese sticks, turkey slices, and chicken soup. Over the past week, she has noticed several episodes of lightheadedness and diaphoresis that resolve by eating a yogurt or several crackers. Medications include ramipril 5 mg/day, metformin 500 mg BID, glyburide 5 mg/day, and omeprazole 20 mg/day. Supplements include two chewable multivitamin-mineral tables.

On examination, weight is 220 lbs (she has lost 20 lbs since surgery), BP 100/68 mm Hg, HR 96 bpm. She is comfortable and in no distress. Abdomen reveals well-healing laparoscopic scars, normal active bowel sounds, no tenderness or rebound.

What is the next most appropriate action to take to address the patient's symptoms?

A. Add carbohydrate foods to her diet

B. Discontinue ramipril

C. Discontinue glyburide

D. Increase fluid intake

2. A 52-year-old man presents to the emergency department 3 weeks following an uneventful laparoscopic sleeve gastrectomy (SG) complaining of persistent nausea, vomiting and double vision. He has only been able to tolerate small amounts of water and sugar-free jello. He is feeling lightheaded, and his urine is malodorous and dark colored. He is not taking any medications or nutritional supplements. On examination, he appears lethargic and dehydrated; afebrile; BP 98/68 mm Hg, HR 108 bpm, RR 14; HEENT: notable for nystagmus and unilateral palsy of his extraocular muscles. Cardiac, pulmonary, and abdominal examination is unremarkable. He has weakness of the arms and legs.

In addition to starting an IV line, what is the next most important step in his management?

A. Infuse normal saline with 5% dextrose

B. Inject vitamin B12 1000 μg IM

C. Insert a nasogastric tube

D. Inject thiamine 200 mg IV

Chapter 11: Pediatric and Adolescent Obesity

1. You are evaluating a 13-year-old boy with obesity. The patient's current BMI is 31.8 kg/m². The BMI value that corresponds to the 2000 CDC 95th percentile for 13-year-old males is 25.1 kg/m².

Which of the following would be the most appropriate classification regarding the severity of the child's obesity according to pediatric definitions?

A. Class 1 obesity

B. Class 2 obesity

C. Class 3 obesity

D. Morbid obesity

2. A 10-year-old girl returns for follow-up of obesity. She is accompanied by her mother. At a previous visit, the patient and her mother identified reducing the consumption of energy-dense desserts as one dietary goal in their family-based lifestyle modification plan. When you assess the family's progress, the mother indicates that there has been significant conflict among members of the family regarding the best strategies to achieve the goal. As part of treatment, you have supported the mother in adopting a more-authoritative parenting and feeding style.

Which of the following responses from the mother would be most consistent with this approach?

A. "We need to make some changes, and everyone in the family is going to cut out dessert completely."

B. "Whoever eats all their vegetables at dinner can have dessert."

C. "We have decided to limit dessert to one night per week. What night would we like to enjoy it this week?"

D. "This isn't going to work. We should pick a different goal."

Chapter 12: Practice Management

1. You are seeing a patient with BMI 38.3 kg/m² for a weight management consultation. The patient also has prediabetes and hypertension.

Which of the following are the most appropriate billing codes?

A. Primary diagnosis I10 (hypertension); secondary diagnosis E66.01 (severe obesity)

B. Primary diagnosis E66.9 (obesity); secondary diagnosis Z68.38 (BMI 38-38.9)

C. Primary diagnosis E66.01 (severe obesity); secondary diagnosis Z68.38 (BMI 38-38.9)

D. Primary diagnosis Z68.38 (BMI 38-38.9); secondary diagnosis E66.01 (severe obesity)

2. With regard to culturally tailored communication around weight and health, which of these racial-ethnic subgroups has the *lowest* risk of medical complications at a given body mass index (BMI)?

A. Caucasians

B. Mexican Americans

C. East Asians

D. African Americans

E. South Asians

Chapter 13: Team Care, Referrals, and Practice Resources

1. A primary care team is considering how to improve its treatment of obesity. The electronic medical record automatically calculates body mass index (BMI). However, the HCPs in the practice (two physicians, one nurse practitioner) do not routinely discuss weight with all patients.

   The next most appropriate step is:

   A. The medical assistant flags the charts of patients with BMI ≥30 kg/m²

   B. The HCPs undertake a chart audit to evaluate frequency of weight management counseling

   C. The HCPs refer all patients with BMI ≥30 kg/m² to a registered dietitian nutritionist (RDN)

   D. The practice employs a registered nurse (RN) to conduct weight management counseling

2. An HCP is considering how to decide which patients are referred for a bariatric surgery evaluation.

   The most appropriate criterion for the HCP to use is:

   A. The patient has tried and failed pharmacotherapy for obesity

   B. The patient meets BMI criteria

   C. The patient has the nutrition knowledge needed to succeed with surgery

   D. The patient has tried and failed repeated courses of lifestyle modification

Answers

CHAPTER 1
1. B
2. D

CHAPTER 2
1. D
2. B

CHAPTER 3
1. C
2. C

CHAPTER 4
1. C
2. A

CHAPTER 5
1. C
2. B

CHAPTER 6
1. B
2. A

CHAPTER 7
1. C
2. B

CHAPTER 8
1. A
2. C

CHAPTER 9
1. A
2. D

CHAPTER 10
1. C
2. D

CHAPTER 11
1. B
2. C

CHAPTER 12
1. C
2. D

CHAPTER 13
1. B
2. D

For detailed explanations of all answers, please see the Quiz Questions at the end of each chapter.

INDEX

Note: Page numbers followed by "*f*" indicate figures and "*t*" indicate tables.